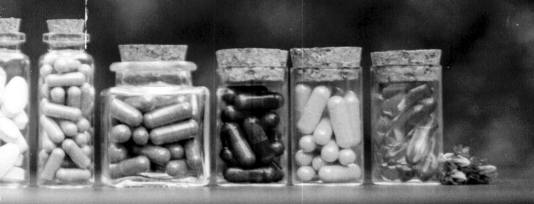

PRAISE FOR THE SUPPLEMENTS DESK REFERENCE

Dr. Olivier Wenker MD, MBA, ABAARM, FAARFM, DEAA
Young Living® Crown Diamond Leader
Bestselling Author and International Speaker www.DoctorOli.com
"Bestselling author Jen O'Sullivan has done what has been overdue for a long time by creating a desk reference guide for Young Living's® supplements. It is not a trivial task as the requirements for supplements vary from person to person, but the way this book is structured makes it easy to find what one searches for. All of Young Living's® supplements can now be found in one single resource. Not only does it provide a way to search for supplements containing certain specific ingredients, it also provides a list of ingredients some people might want to avoid such as dairy, nuts, shellfish, gluten, or listing products that are non-vegan. All in all, this book is a must-have for consumers of Young Living® supplements."

Teri Secrest *Young Living® Royal Crown Diamond Leader*
Bestselling Author and International Speaker www.TeriSecrest.com
"Jen O'Sullivan's *Supplements Desk Reference* book is a gold mine of easy to understand and simple to use information! It is a MUST for all Young Living® distributors! We gift it to each new member we enroll. Finally, we have something compliant that explains what each ingredient does in the human body! As a certified Wellness Coach, I highly endorse this book."

Jessica Laney Petty *Young Living® Royal Crown Diamond Leader*
International Speaker
"My favorite part of this book is the protocols. I think a lot of people come into Young Living® overwhelmed by the number of products. They need help with certain things having to do with their health and don't know which products would best support them and when and how to take them. This book gives people easy to follow protocols for a variety of needs!"

Jordan Schrandt *Young Living® Royal Crown Diamond Leader*
Bestselling Author and International Speaker https://shop.JordanSchrandt.com
"Jen O'Sullivan breaks down Young Living® supplements better than anyone I've heard! It's smart, to the point, and relevant. Supplements are a game changer in our personal health and the health of our teams! I highly recommend this resource to everyone!"

Dr. Doug Corrigan Ph.D. in Biochemistry and Molecular Biology
"Theory Gap" Expert and World-renowned Educator www.StarFishScents.com
"The *Supplements Desk Reference* is a comprehensive repository and reference for the complete supplement product line of Young Living®. It covers everything from A-Z, and provides helpful tips, protocols, and recipes to round out your health wellness program."

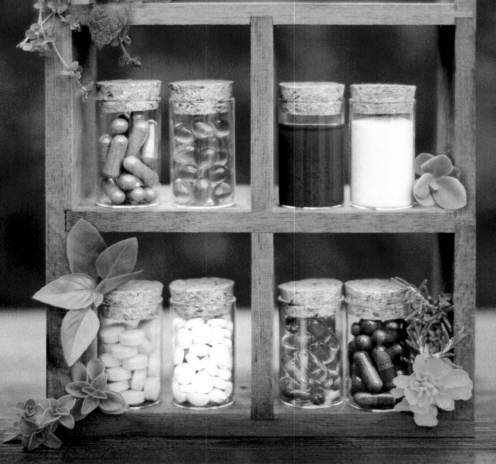

Supplements
DESK REFERENCE
SECOND EDITION

JEN O'SULLIVAN

SUPPLEMENTS DESK REFERENCE: SECOND EDITION

First Edition Copyright © June 2019 by Jen O'Sullivan
Second Edition Copyright © October 2020 by Jen O'Sullivan
www.31oils.com

Cover Design and Photography by Jen O'Sullivan

ISBN: 978-1-7344993-1-5

Updated January 2021
31 Oils, LLC

Printed in the USA.

10 9 8 7 6 5 4 3 2

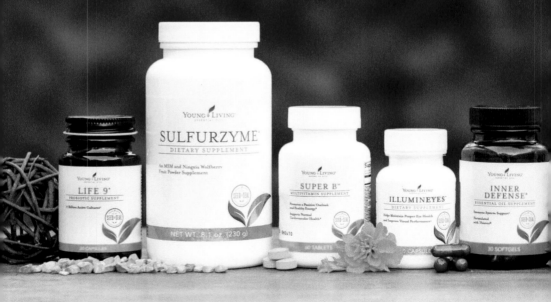

Thank you to Cindy Edens for her hours of new label research for the updated content, and to Tara Adams for the technical editing on this Second Edition. I am forever grateful to my original team of researchers and editors: Caite Bellavia, Cindy Edens, Danah Meyers, Mary White, Michelle Hancock, Stephanie Ward, and Tara Adams. Without their help this book would have never been published. I am blessed to know you all and love doing life with you. A special extra thanks to Caite Bellavia who helped keep us all in line and who is the queen of fact checking, and to Tara Adams who kept me in line with content and formatting. You are all a blessing to me! To my husband, who loves me even when my brain checks out as I am writing, and to my son, who always tells me he loves me as he walks by my office. My two men give me the energy to keep moving forward and Jesus is the reason for everything! Without Jesus, literally I would be lost. Thank you for being my guide, my teacher, my corrector, my warrior, my friend, and the lover of my soul. Thank you, Holy Spirit, for your guidance and words, and thank you, Jesus, for blessing me with breath and life upon life.

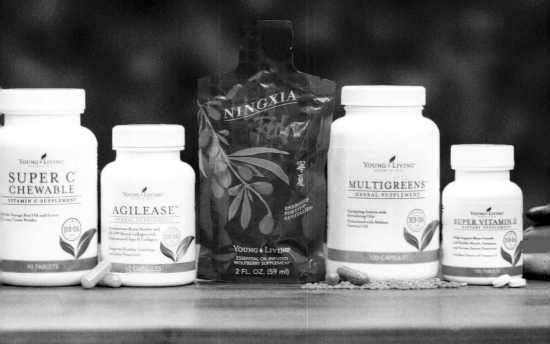

OVERVIEW

The second edition of the "Supplements Desk Reference" by Jen O'Sullivan, covers all of Young Living's® nutrition-based supplements. Each supplement showcases the ingredients and what those ingredients are known to support, so you can be sure if it is the right one for you. It contains specific protocols using Young Living's® recommended directions for areas such as hormone support, liver support, bone health, pregnancy and breastfeeding guidelines, glucose and cholesterol support, weight management, stress and sleep support, along with the basics of child, dog, cat, and horse health. The book contains a comprehensive list of dosage and age requirements, common potential allergens, religious friendly ingredients (halal and kosher), common drug interactions, and cautions, along with a complete list of all the vitamins, minerals, enzymes, amino acids, and herbs found in the Young Living® supplements, so you can easily reference any specific ingredient for which you are searching.

DISCLAIMER

The protocols and supplement descriptions in this book are based on the usage descriptions from the Young Living® website and information readily available online. The amount and timing of each dosage are based on the label on each product. In some instances, lower doses are recommended in this book. When you start a new supplement regimen, it is important to start slowly and pay close attention to your body. Everyone's body is unique and will respond differently. If a product does not work for you, please try another one. Check with your doctor if you are taking prescription medications. Pharmaceutical drugs should not be consumed at the same time as natural supplements. It is best to give a four-hour buffer between them. Always consult your doctor when you start a new regimen.

This book gives suggestions on how to support healthy systems. It is not intended to treat or diagnose existing conditions or illnesses. Each supplement consists of multiple ingredients. Each ingredient listed has a basic description of what it is commonly used for in the medical and holistic practice industries. Herbs and roots have been used for centuries and the traditionally studied uses for each are readily found on sources such as Science Direct, the National Center for Biotechnology Information, U. S. National Library of Medicine, PubMed, and the Food and Drug Administration websites.

The content in this book has not been evaluated by the FDA and the supplements and protocols will not treat or cure any sickness or disease. The author is not a doctor and has published this book as a means to have a compilation of information, in one spot, to make it easier to understand the many supplements Young Living® carries.

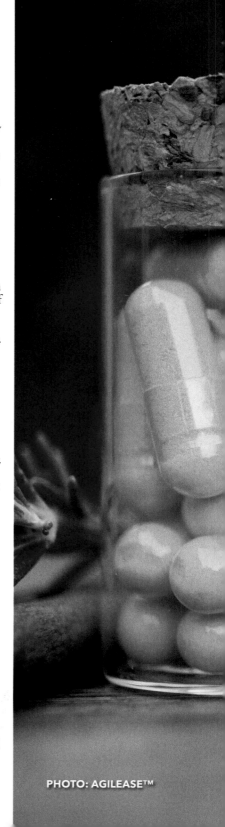

PHOTO: AGILEASE™

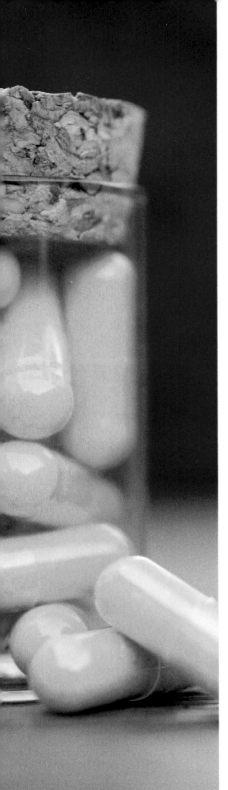

SUPPLEMENTS DESK REFERENCE
BY JEN O'SULLIVAN

CONTENTS

SUPPLEMENTS DESK REFERENCE
BY JEN O'SULLIVAN

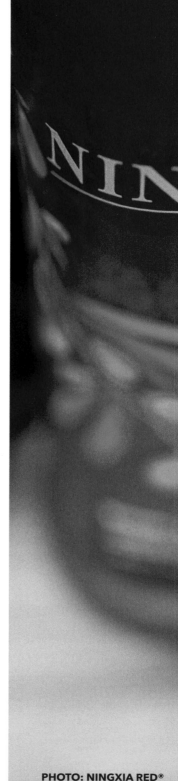

PHOTO: NINGXIA RED®

CHARTS

PROTOCOLS

SUPPLEMENTS

INGREDIENTS

INDEX

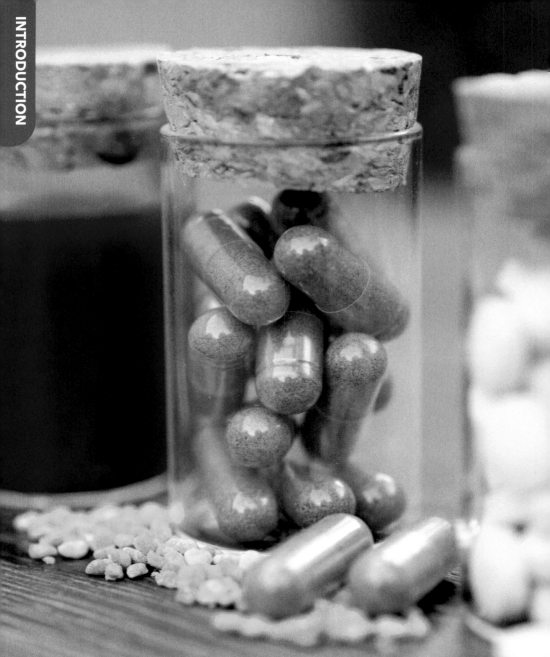

THANK YOU GARY YOUNG FOR DEVELOPING THESE GEMS!

D. Gary Young added essential oils to MultiGreens™ (originally named VitaGreens) and ComforTone® in 1984. Gary was a pioneer. He pushed the natural supplement market forward with great force, yet with incredible ease because he was armed with his powerful and authentic essential oils. Young Living® is the only company on the planet to carry a full line of herbal and whole-food based nutrition infused with true botanical essential oils.

PHOTO: MULTIGREENS™ WITH BEE POLLEN NUGGETS

SECTION ONE
details & charts

INTRODUCTION

We live in a world where supplementation is the norm. We take vitamin C in mass doses, get vitamin B injections, and if you're not on a full-spectrum multivitamin, your mother might just cut you out of her will, if she finds out. Dietary supplements were not a major thing until the U.S. Congress passed the Dietary Supplement and Health Education Act (DSHEA) of 1994.[1] After that, dietary supplement consumption skyrocketed. In the United States alone, the supplement market is a $31 billion dollar industry. Seventy-six percent of all adults in the United States take some form of dietary supplement, as of 2017.[2] It is estimated that there are 80 to 90 thousand dietary supplement products on the market, as of 2016, according to PBS producer, Priyanka Boghani.[3]

The scary reality from the FDA, regarding all of these supplements, can be understood by the following quotes from the FDA.[4]

- "Federal law does not require dietary supplements to be proven safe to FDA's satisfaction before they are marketed."
- "For most claims made in the labeling of dietary supplements, the law does not require the manufacturer or seller to prove to the FDA's satisfaction that the claim is accurate or truthful before it appears on the product."
- "Dietary supplement manufacturers do not have to get the agency's [FDA's] approval before producing or selling these products."

Supplements are exactly what the word means: to add an extra amount of what we are not getting in our nutrition. Whole-food nutrition is the most important aspect to proper health, and the goal is to get as much of that nutrition as possible from what God has created. The reality is, the food sources we currently have access to are very different from those that our grandparents, or even our parents, grew up consuming.

We have massively depleted our soils, but more importantly, even if you are able to get organic, farmer's market type produce and proteins, they are usually picked far before they should be, or the animals are fed from sources that are not ideal. Did you know most produce is picked about two weeks before it is ripe? Did you also know that often the most vital phytonutrients (plant nutrients) are developed during the last few days of ripening?

It is unfortunate, but the reality is, we do not get the right vitamins, minerals, micro minerals, and nutrients in the everyday food sources we eat. Supplementation is a great way to go, but sadly most supplements are synthetic or so isolated that your body does not know what to do with them, so you end up having the supplements you paid good money for go in one end and out the other, without even getting into your system to be used. The act of something going into your body and your body using it is called "bioavailability."

Around 90% of the supplements you can buy today are not fully bioavailable, because they are synthetic.[5] When you consume a synthetic, your body does not know what to do with it. You will simply urinate and defecate your money right down the toilet. Young Living® is different for a couple of reasons. First, they use whole food sources in fruits, vegetables, herbs, and roots for their supplements. Second, they infuse many of their supplements with essential oils. Essential oils are extremely volatile and very small in their molecular structure, making them an excellent vehicle, or pathway, to increase the bioavailability of the supplements.

The essential oils themselves are different than any you can purchase on the market because they are the true unaltered botanical, allowing for a true "entourage effect," which basically means that because the essential oil has not been modified, and the whole of the oil is used, there is much greater action, or synergy, that occurs within the oil, and therefore, within our bodies. Most companies practice what is called "fractional distillation" with their essential oils, simply because the final product smells better and is easier to market to the masses.

With these two important factors in place — whole-plant nutrition infused with unaltered essential oils — you will get dietary supplementation through Young Living® that is second to none. Young Living® offers three types of nutritional supplements: Foundation, Cleansing, and Targeted.

Foundation Nutrition
Noted by the green labeled bottles, the Foundation Nutrition products are the vitamins and minerals that support a healthy lifestyle.

Cleansing Nutrition
Noted by the blue labeled bottles, the Cleansing Nutrition products are specifically designed to support the detox and cleansing of the body.

Targeted Nutrition
Noted by the orange labeled bottles, these are formulated with specific ingredients including powerful essential oils to support specific nutritional needs. These supplements target everything from enzyme support and joint health, heart, brain, and hormone support.

Sources:

1. https://www.ncbi.nlm.nih.gov/books/NBK216048/
2. https://www.crnusa.org/resources/2017-crn-consumer-survey-dietary-supplements
3. https://www.pbs.org/wgbh/frontline/article/can-regulators-keep-up-with-the-supplements-industry/
4. https://www.fda.gov/consumers/consumer-updates/fda-101-dietary-supplements
5. https://myersdetox.com/90-of-vitamins-are-synthetic/

HOW TO GET STARTED

It is important to listen to your body. Start out slowly by taking ¼ to ½ the recommended daily dose. See how you feel. Each week moving forward, increase your dose to the recommended daily dose to figure out what amount is right for you. Once you feel you have the right amount, use that amount for 30 days. After 30 days, stop taking the supplement for 3-7 days to note how you feel, then resume if you determine the supplement is a fit for your needs.

STORE BOUGHT BRANDS

There are many supplements available on the market today. Why should you consider Young Living® supplements over the sea of companies telling you theirs are better? An article on Healthline states, "The majority of supplements available on the market today are made artificially."[6] Artificial or synthetic nutrients are produced in a laboratory to mimic the effects of nature. Synthetic supplements are often less bioavailable than their natural counterpart. While science[7] will tell you that your body will readily "absorb" synthetic versions just as well as it will absorb it in its natural form, they fail to tell you that your body won't readily recognize the synthetic version.

Our ancestral DNA is programed based on thousands of years of genetic code. Your body knows exactly what to do with the thousands of nutrients found in spinach. It gets a little confused when science isolates one vitamin or mineral and decides that is what you need. God created our food source to work synergistically. The entirety of the molecules together are what allow for greater bioavailability. Our bodies know what to do with the 10,000+ phytonutrients found in an apple, but isolating vitamin C and taking it at extremely high doses is something our bodies don't understand how to use, so you end up flushing the majority of your isolated vitamin C right down the toilet.

Isolated nutrients aside, the more frightening reality, when it comes to supplements, is the dangerous ingredients you may not even know you are consuming. Several dangerous ingredients found in supplements[8] are artificial colors such as Blue #1, Red #40, and Yellow #5, hydrogenated oils such as partially hydrogenated soybean oil, lead, mercury, polychlorinated biphenyls (PBCs), talc as a cheap anti-caking substance, and titanium dioxide, all of which cause a myriad of illnesses and disease such as cancer, kidney damage, inflammation, heavy metal poisoning, heart disease and heart attack, autism, autoimmune diseases, and much more! With Young Living® you get naturally derived ingredients that your body knows exactly how to put to good use.

Sources:
6. https://www.healthline.com/nutrition/synthetic-vs-natural-nutrients
7. https://www.scientificamerican.com/article/do-vitamins-in-pills-diff/
8. http://info.achs.edu/blog/dangerous-supplement-ingredients

STORAGE (vertical tab)

EXPIRATION AND STORAGE

Natural supplements have a shorter shelf-life than synthetic medications and supplements. The FDA does not require supplements to have an expiry date on the bottle. That said, some supplements may hold their efficacy for longer than others. Follow these guidelines for optimal freshness. Pharmaceuticals generally never expire because of the synthetic ingredients. Companies must place an expiry for liability reasons. It is always best to keep natural-based supplements in the refrigerator, even if not opened.

EXPIRATION DATE GUIDELINES

- Most natural supplements last for 6-12 months after opened and about three years if not opened.
- Most will not go bad or rancid, they will simply lose their efficacy (effectiveness) over time.
- To tell if a supplement is not good, check the color and smell.
- Do not store supplements where direct sunlight may occur.
- Do not store supplements in the bathroom. The temperature and humidity changes too rapidly and creates an unstable environment.
- Keep all opened supplements in the refrigerator.
- Keep all unopened supplements in a climate controlled dark area in the home or also in the refrigerator.
- Hard tablet supplements usually last longer.
- Powdered supplements (both loose and in a capsule) have a shorter shelf-life.
- Liquid supplements have the shortest shelf-life once opened.

SPECIFIC SUPPLEMENT GUIDELINES

- Life 9® must be refrigerated after opening.
- NingXia Red® bottles must be refrigerated after opening.
- NingXia Red® bottles are clearly marked with instructions to use within 30 days after opening and to store in the refrigerator. The expiration date will be on the bottom of the bottle. If unopened and kept in a cool dark place, it will still be good several years after the expiry has passed. The reason for expiration dates on supplements is for 100% efficacy. If you open a very old bottle of NingXia Red®, smell or taste it to see if it has gone bad.
- Liquid supplements such as Mineral Essence™, K & B™, and Rehemogen™ should all be refrigerated once opened. If you are not planning on using unopened stock for a while, it is best to keep that refrigerated also.

BODY SYSTEM CLEANSING

The human body is a miraculous wonder that is in a constant state of homeostasis. This means your body desires balance. The various systems in the body all contribute to the overall wellbeing of your health and vitality. When one system is out of balance, the others are affected. Flushing various systems and cleansing them through detoxification can have a healthful impact on your mind, body, and spirit. When you begin any cleanse or detox, it is important to support your efforts by getting enough sleep, drinking plenty of water, exercising, limiting or eliminating alcohol, salt, processed sugars and foods, and eating a diet rich in antioxidants such as dark leafy greens and berries.

There are several theories about which body system to cleanse first. It is mostly recommended to start with a colon cleanse and then move on to a liver cleanse, and finish with a kidney cleanse. This book contains a Colon Cleanse Protocol, a Digestive, Gut, and Colon Health Protocol, a Liver Support Protocol, and a Urinary Support Protocol. You are welcome to start with these and then move into other areas. It is advised that you only do one cleanse at a time. Multiple protocols are fine to do at the same time, but you will need to combine schedules. It is advised to not do more than 2-3 at a time. One is a better choice as it will allow you to pay closer attention to your body's response.

THE RED DRINK

An excellent way to start a body system cleansing protocol is with the 30 Day Red Drink Challenge. The Red Drink was developed by Dr. Peter Minke and is one of the most popular recipes with Young Living® members. It supports mobility, the liver, nail and hair growth, as well as a healthy immune system. Dr. Minke states, *"Hydration is essential for life. Drinking water will help flush toxins out of the system. Sulfurzyme® powder has MSM (nutritional sulfur) for detox and hepatoprotective properties, as well as FOS (Fructooligosaccharides) and LPS (Lycium polysaccharides) as prebiotics for gut health. NingXia Red® provides mineral and antioxidant support with an extra boost of LPS for supporting healthy immune function and blood sugar levels. The addition of Lime Vitality™ essential oil adds a refreshing flavor that also supports cleansing the lymphatic system."*

HOW TO MAKE THE RED DRINK
Ingredients:
- 12-16 oz. filtered alkaline water
- 1-2 oz. NingXia Red®
- ½ tsp. Sulfurzyme® powder
  Note: You may substitute two capsules, but do not break them open into the drink. They will not dissolve, nor will they taste good.
- 1-2 drops Lime Vitality™ Essential Oil

Directions: Use a glass or stainless steel drinking container filled with 12-16 oz. of filtered water, preferably alkaline. Add 1-2 oz. NingXia Red®, ½ teaspoon of Sulfurzyme® powder, and 1-2 drops of Lime Vitality™ essential oil. Create two of these drinks per day for 30 days or combine all into one large 25-30 oz. container and drink throughout the day.

For more information and recipes visit www.VitalityEDU.com/reddrink

MEDICAL INTERACTIONS

THE GRAPEFRUIT JUICE EFFECT The cytochrome P450 enzymes are a larger family of almost 60 enzymes that work to metabolize things we consume through the liver. Specific cytochrome P450 enzymes called CYP3A4 and CYP2C19 are metabolized in similar ways to CBD so they might have interactions, but the likelihood is low. Pharmaceutical companies take into consideration the cytochrome P450 enzyme metabolism rate to create their drugs such as anti-depressants, steroids, and beta-blockers.

Certain foods can activate the cytochrome P450 enzyme causing a drug to become useless, voiding out the desired effect. These are items like charcoal-grilled foods and cruciferous vegetables such as broccoli and spinach or even supplements that contain high amounts of phytonutrients from cruciferous vegetables. Other foods or natural supplements can inhibit the cytochrome P450 enzyme causing the drug to not be metabolized, therefore extending its effect in your body with potentially toxic outcomes. We see this in the grapefruit juice effect and possibly with massive dosing of CBD oil.

CBD INTERACTIONS When it comes to understanding CBD and possible drug interactions, many articles that are written on this topic are based on pre-clinical trials, not actual gold-standard clinical studies. These poor pre-clinical trials showed the effects of large doses of CBD that was administered daily over many days to small lab rats. The dosages were in the hundreds of milligrams per day. Normal human dosages are in the tens of milligrams per day. In the pre-clinical trials they found no interaction between a normal dose of CBD and medications. The important thing to note is to always check with your doctor and pay close attention to your body and what supplements and drugs you are using. The internet is full of useful yet sometimes misleading content. Read the full article and do not always trust the title or first few sentences as they are often "click bait" to gain more readers and subscribers.

ADAPTOGENS

Adaptogens are supplements from nature such as herbs and essential oils that have the ability to help your body manage stress responses. While there is not a lot of scientific study on the use of herbs and essential oils as adaptogens, most will agree that the clinical response in your body is evidence enough.
See this study: **https://www.ncbi.nlm.nih.gov/pmc/articles/PMC3991026/**

As it pertains to essential oils, adaptogens can be seen in their ability to regulate or balance the mind and body. For instance, Orange essential oil has the ability to uplift and energize, but also to calm and relax a person. This is a prime example of an adaptogen in essential oils. Other adaptogenic oils are Lavender, Geranium, Bergamot, and many others. When it comes to herbs like Ashwagandha (in EndoGize™ and PowerGize™), Turmeric (in AgilEase™), Licorice root (in FemiGen™), and even amino acids such as L-theanine (in KidScents® Unwind™), these all have the ability to help our bodies respond well to stress hormones. Our bodies work in synergy with plant life so it is no wonder that many will have adaptogenic abilities to help us adapt to both emotional and physical stress.

POSSIBLE REASONS FOR NEGATIVE REACTIONS

Is your body rejecting or responding in unusual ways to oils and/or natural supplements? Why do some people experience complete rejection of essential oils and natural supplements when previously they used them without issue?

When a person overuses an essential oil internally or over consumes a natural supplement (only you can determine if you are or not as each person is different) he or she may experience an odd reaction. This usually occurs after about two years of over consumption. Sometimes the body will start to reject them in the form of rashes or what seems like an allergic response. This person using essential oils may feel defeated because even simple topical or diffuser use can pose a problem.

The question to ask when someone is having these unusual responses is, "Are you under any abnormal stress lately?" Nine times out of ten the answer is "yes". For these people, the only recommendation is to calm down and try to manage your stress. CortiStop® and EndoGize™ are two helpful supplements.

When you are stressed out, your body creates more cortisol than normal. Your adrenals work overtime, and with larger amounts of cortisol coursing through your body, essential oils and natural supplements will try to help you out by attacking it. The result of their "help" is rapid and often rash-presenting detox.

Here is some advice if you find yourself having severe reactions to natural products when previously there were no negative responses. Try to manage the stress better. If you truly feel it is a response from the essential oils or the supplement and not an outside factor, such as stress or hormonal changes, you will need to stop using the item and possibly all essential oils for 120 days to fully reset your system, and then start again, slowly. Your blood recycles fully and is brand new every 120 days. This may seem extreme but this only applies to those having major reactions.

Please note, if you are having an essential oil response, any full essential oil supplements need to be stopped too. Powdered supplements with powdered oils are fine. You get about the same when you eat a salad. Essential oils are present in most raw plant foods we eat, but concentrated forms of essential oil from a bottle will be too much during your reset. When you start to reintroduce essential oils again it will be like you are new, so expect two weeks of normal detox, but after that, if you are still having reactions, then I'd say stop and consider the next potential issue.

If you think it is not an overuse response then you'll need to determine several factors. Rashes happen for any number of reasons and oftentimes people try to blame it on a topical application of some new deodorant, laundry detergent, or even natural essential oil. Topical responses to a topical application of a product is diagnosing the surface when we need to be looking at the root of the issue. It would be like wondering why a plant looks so unhealthy and trying to polish the leaves, when the soil is depleted. No amount of polishing will help the plant. Here are some questions to consider asking yourself:

1. Are you under abnormal stress?
2. Have you had an unusually long period of general stress? Loss of job, loss of marriage, loss of relationship, loss of a loved one to death, moved to a new town, change in career, etc.
3. Could you possibly be going through hormonal changes such as menopause, also known as perimenopause?
4. Have you started a new diet?
5. Have you started or stopped any major lifestyle habits? Exercise, hobbies, etc?
6. Could you possibly have come into contact with poison ivy or a plant protein that causes rashes?
7. Do you have an overgrowth of Candida? (Symptoms: tired all the time, thrush in your mouth, reoccurring urinary tract, sinus, or yeast infections, swollen and inflamed cuticles and fingernails, joint pain, and digestive issues.)
8. Is your body more acidic and you using natural supplements and oils?
9. Are you using natural supplements and oils alongside synthetic products?
10. Are you using natural supplements and oils and have not fully detoxed?

Find more info below if you are experiencing uncomfortable responses from essential oil use due to one of the last three items on the above list (number 8-10).

ACIDIC BODY

If your body is on the acidic side (bad) rather than pH neutral (better) or slightly alkaline (best) you may experience stronger than normal detox responses. The oils will react in abnormal ways in a body that is highly acidic. You'd need to determine that on your own by checking the following areas.

Factors that contribute to acidity in the body are smoking, prescription medications, high animal protein diets, drinking alcohol or coffee, eating anything processed, eating too many processed sugars, eating too much processed wheat (bread and pasta), getting little to no exercise, not sleeping enough, plus a whole host of other things. If your body is always acidic, then you will experience detox responses each time you use essential oils.

The number one goal of an essential oil is to seek and destroy oxidative stress, usually in the form of acid. They want to placate it first and then give you the action for which it is known. Essential oils will always work, but the more acidic you are, the more detox response you will have.

An interesting example of this is using lavender or other essential oils directly in your belly button. The "buttoning" method is highly effective for several reasons, such as better sleep and helping soothe stomach discomfort, but some people, when they try it, report a major rash on and around their belly button, often lasting for several days.

The belly button is a magnet for debris and build up of random toxins. Sunscreen, lotion, synthetic fibers from clothing are just a few invaders. There are thousands of bacteria found in belly buttons. The belly button is considered the "rainforest" of our body since there is such a random selection of bacteria present in each belly button.

A research team who studied belly buttons found a bacteria strain that is found only in the soil of Japan in one of their test subjects that had never been to Japan before. This goes to show you how international trade and possibly the clothing you buy from different countries can work like the earth's bacterial pollination playground. You can read the whole article here: **https://tinyurl.com/bellybuttonyuck**

My recommendation is to thoroughly clean out your belly button before trying this method and use a carrier oil such as grapeseed for the first few times.

SYNTHETIC PRODUCTS

This would also translate to the personal care products a person uses. If a person decides to use essential oils, but is unwilling to give up their Bath & Body Works® soaps and lotions (honestly, it took me a while to give those up) or their favorite face or body lotion, that person will need to be prepared for the oils to potentially react badly with the synthetic fragrances, synthetic preservatives, and other synthetic ingredients that are present in most store bought products.

TOXIC BODY

The issue, however, is not only with the products we are currently using, but the toxic build-up that has been going on in our bodies for decades. We have all grown up in a world that is so vastly different than even the one in which our parents lived. Processed synthetic greenwashing is happening all around us. Greenwashing is where a company tries to look healthy but is far from it. Our ancestral DNA does not know what to do with synthetics found in our processed foods, personal care products, household cleaning products, the plastics we type on, sit on, sleep on, and slather on, and so on and so forth; not to mention the unknown long-term damage all the electrical devices are doing to our bodies, in the form of electromagnetic radiation, that scientists have already determined to be a major cause of cancer. If your great grandparents could see us now, they would sit us all down in a corner with a great big "DUNCE" cap on.

All this to say, there could be any number of reasons someone has a negative reaction to all-natural essential oils, assuming they are, in fact, all natural, as many essential oils on the market contain synthetics as well.

The multi-billion dollar personal care industry would like us all to believe that essential oils are the problem. If we all would just use a little common sense and read the back of the labels to see what we are using, it may help clear up a lot of issues.

While this is not an exhaustive list of why you may be responding, and it may not encompass your specific issues, it may be helpful information for you to aid someone else down the line. Essential oils, herbs, and nature are God's gift to us, but sadly we can mess them up by contaminating them, overusing them, or stressing ourselves out so much that they just stop working the way in which they are designed.

allergies & notes

This list is not exhaustive. Please check with Young Living® Product Support. Products are often reformulated. The label on the bottle is always correct.

SUPPLEMENTS THAT MAY BE DUPLICATES

- Master Formula™ Duplicates may be Super B™, Super Vitamin D, Super C™ tablets, and MultiGreens™. Please determine your own personal needs.
- AgilEase™ was intended to replace BLM™ but many people wanted both.
- Super Cal™ Plus was intended to replace MegaCal™ but many people wanted both.
- Choose either PD 80/20™ or CortiStop®, do not take both at the same time.
- Allerzyme™ and Detoxzyme® are similar with slight differences.
- Life 9® and MightyPro™ are both probiotics. You may take both or just one.

SUPPLEMENTS THAT SHOULD NOT BE TAKEN TOGETHER

- Life 9® should be taken alone. Do not take with any essential oils.
- Super Cal™ Plus and MegaCal™ should not be taken together.
- Thyromin™ should be taken alone, at night, and on an empty stomach.
- ImmuPro™ and SleepEssence™ should not be taken together due to melatonin.

DO NOT USE WITH BLOOD THINNERS

MAY INTERACT WITH BLOOD THINNERS

- AgilEase™ (Turmeric)
- CardioGize™ (Coenzyme Q10)
- ComforTone® (Cayenne fruit)
- MindWise™ (Turmeric and Coenzyme Q10)
- OmegaGize3® (Coenzyme Q10)

CONTAINS CAFFEINE

SUPPLEMENTS THAT CONTAIN NATURAL CAFFEINE

- NingXia Nitro® (Green tea extract)
- NingXia Zyng® (White tea extract)
- Slique® CitriSlim™ (Guarana fruit extract)
- Slique® Shake (Guarana fruit extract)
- Slique® Tea (Jade Oolong Tea and Ecuadorian cacao powder)
- Master Formula™ (small amounts of Green tea)

CONTAINS NO OILS

SUPPLEMENTS WITHOUT ESSENTIAL OILS

- IlluminEyes™
- KidScents® MightyPro™
- KidScents® MightyVites™
- Life 9®
- PD 80/20™
- Sulfurzyme® Capsules
- Sulfurzyme® Powder

CONTAINS ALL OILS

SUPPLEMENTS THAT ARE MOSTLY ESSENTIAL OILS

- Digest & Cleanse®
- Inner Defense®
- Longevity™
- Master Formula™ liquid capsule (about half)
- ParaFree™
- Prostate Health™
- SleepEssence™
- Slique® CitriSlim™ liquid capsule

SUPPLEMENTS NOT ADVISED WHEN PREGNANT

CAUTION IF PREGNANT

- CardioGize™ - Dong Quai, Motherwort, and Cat's Claw are not advised.
- ComforTone® - Cascara Sagrada is not advised.
- CortiStop® - Black Cohosh, Clary Sage, and Fennel are not advised.
- Digest & Cleanse® - Excessive internal use of essential oils is not advised.
- EndoGize® - Ashwagandha is not advised.
- FemiGen™ - Black Cohosh, Dong Quai, and Licorice Root are not advised.
- Inner Defense® - Excessive internal use of essential oils is not advised.
- JuvaPower® - Anise and Slippery Elm can have estrogenic effects.
- JuvaTone® - Oregon Grape (Berberine) is not advised.
- ParaFree™ - Excessive internal use of essential oils is not advised.
- PowerGize™ - Ashwagandha is not advised.
- Rehemogen™ - Oregon Grape (Berberine) is not advised.
- SleepEssence™ - Rue is not advised.
- Slique® CitraSlim™ - Natural stimulants and internal use of oils is not advised.

SUPPLEMENTS THAT CONTAIN STEVIA LEAF EXTRACT

CONTAINS STEVIA

- AlkaLime®
- AminoWise®
- CBD Droppers
- ImmuPro™
- KidScents® MightyVites™
- KidScents® MightyZyme™
- MegaCal™
- NingXia Red®
- NingXia Zyng®
- Pure Protein™ Complete
- Slique® Essence Oil
- Slique® Shake
- Slique® Tea
- Sulfurzyme® Powder
- Super C™ Chewables

SUPPLEMENTS THAT CONTAIN XYLITOL

CONTAINS XYLITOL

- Balance Complete™
- KidScents® MightyPro™
- MegaCal™
- Slique® Gum

SUPPLEMENTS THAT CONTAIN CORN

CONTAINS CORN

- AgilEase™
- AlkaLime®
- Allerzyme™

SUPPLEMENTS THAT CONTAIN SOY

CONTAINS SOY

- CortiStop®
- EndoGize™
- Essentialzyme™
- MultiGreens™
- Slique® Gum

SUPPLEMENTS THAT CONTAIN BARLEY *(GLUTEN POTENTIAL)*

CONTAINS BARLEY

Barley Grass *(gluten cross-contamination may occur)*
- Allerzyme™
- Balance Complete™
- KidScents® MightyVites™
- Master Formula™
- MultiGreens™

Barley Sprouted Seed *(gluten cross-contamination may occur)*
- JuvaPower®

SUPPLEMENTS THAT CONTAIN NUTS

CONTAINS NUTS

- Slique® Bars (actual nuts)

Coconut and derivatives of coconut

- Digest & Cleanse®
- Inner Defense®
- Longevity™
- MindWise™
- SleepEssence™
- Slique® CitriSlim™

ALLERGY

NOT VEGAN

SUPPLEMENTS THAT ARE NOT VEGAN

- AgilEase™ (Chicken)
- Allerzyme™ (Milk derivative)
- Balance Complete™ (Dairy)
- BLM™ (Pork, Shellfish, Chicken)
- ComforTone® (Cow gelatin)
- CortiStop® (Cow gelatin)
- Detoxzyme® (Milk derivative)
- EndoGize™ (Cow gelatin)
- Essentialzyme™ (Pig/Cow)
- Essentialzymes-4™ (Cow, Bee Pollen)
- FemiGen™ (Cow gelatin)
- Inner Defense® (Fish gelatin)
- JuvaTone® (Bee Propolis)
- K & B™ (Royal Jelly)
- Mineral Essence™ (Bee Products)
- MultiGreens™ (Cow, Bee Pollen)
- NingXia Nitro® (Dairy)
- OmegaGize3® (Fish)
- PD 80/20™ (Cow gelatin)
- ParaFree™ (Fish gelatin)
- PowerGize™ (Dairy)
- Prostate Health™ (Pork gelatin)
- Pure Protein™ Complete (Egg, Dairy)
- Rehemogen™ (Royal Jelly)
- Slique® Bars (Eggs and Honey)
- Slique® CitriSlim™ (Cow)
- Super C™ Chewables (Dairy)
- Thyromin™ (Pork, Cow)

CONTAINS DAIRY

SUPPLEMENTS THAT CONTAIN DAIRY

- Allerzyme™
- Balance Complete™
- Detoxzyme®
- NingXia Nitro®
- PowerGize™
- Pure Protein™ Complete
- Super C™ Chewables

CONTAINS BEE PRODUCTS

SUPPLEMENTS THAT CONTAIN BEE PRODUCTS

- Essentialzymes-4™ (Bee Pollen)
- JuvaTone® (Bee Propolis)
- K & B™ (Royal Jelly)
- Mineral Essence™ (Royal Jelly and Honey)
- MultiGreens™ (Bee Pollen)
- Rehemogen™ (Royal Jelly)
- Slique® Bars (Honey)

CONTAINS SHELLFISH

SUPPLEMENTS THAT CONTAIN SHELLFISH

- BLM™ (ground up shrimp bodies for glucosamine)
- NOTE: AgilEase™ does not contain shellfish sourced glucosamine.

CONTAINS EGG

SUPPLEMENTS THAT CONTAIN EGG

- Pure Protein™ Complete

RELIGIOUS CONSIDERATION

SUPPLEMENTS OUTSIDE SPECIFIC RELIGIOUS LAWS
Possibly Not Kosher or Halal Friendly (see specific ingredients)

- BLM™ (Procine/pig/pork gelatin capsule, also contains shellfish)
- ComforTone® (Bovine/cow gelatin capsule)
- CortiStop® (Bovine/cow gelatin capsule)
- EndoGize™ (Bovine/cow source gelatin capsule)
- Essentialzyme™ (Pancreas from pigs)
- Essentialzymes-4™ (Bovine/cow gelatin capsule)
- FemiGen™ (Bovine/cow gelatin capsule)
- MultiGreens™ (Bovine/cow gelatin capsule)
- PD 80/20™ (Bovine/cow gelatin capsule)
- Prostate Health™ (Procine/pig/pork gelatin capsule)
- Slique® CitriSlim™ (Bovine/cow gelatin for liquid capsule)
- Thyromin™ (Gland powder from pig and cow)

OUT OF STOCK SUBSTITUTE GUIDE

AGILEASE™	**BLM™, SULFURZYME®, NATURE'S ULTRA CBD**
ALKALIME®	**SUPER C™ TABLETS** AND/OR **JUVAPOWER®**
ALLERZYME™	**DETOXZYME™**
AMINOWISE®	**MULTIGREENS™** AND/OR **MINERAL ESSENCE™**
BALANCE COMPLETE™	**PURE PROTEIN™ COMPLETE** OR **SLIQUE® SHAKE**
BLM™	**AGILEASE™** AND/OR **SULFURZYME®** AND/OR **NATURE'S ULTRA CBD**
CARDIOGIZE™	**MASTER FORMULA™**
COMFORTONE®	**ICP™** OR **REHEMOGEN™**
CORTISTOP®	**PD 80/20™**
DETOXZYME®	**ALLERZYME™**
DIGEST & CLEANSE®	**DIY CAPSULE:** 2 DROPS EACH OF PEPPERMINT, CARAWAY, GINGER, FENNEL, AND LEMON VITALITY™ IN CAPSULE TOPPED OFF WITH 4 DROPS CARRIER OIL.
ENDOGIZE™	**POWERGIZE™** OR **CORTISTOP®** OR **PD 80/20™**
ESSENTIALZYME™	**ESSENTIALZYMES-4™**
ESSENTIALZYMES-4™	**ESSENTIALZYME™**
FEMIGEN™	**CORTISTOP®** OR **PD 80/20™**
ICP™	**REHEMOGEN™** OR **COMFORTONE®**
ILLUMINEYES™	**MASTER FORMULA™**
IMMUPRO™	**SLEEPESSENCE™**
INNER DEFENSE®	**DIY CAPSULE:** 5 DROPS THIEVES®, 1 DROP EACH OREGANO, THYME AND LEMONGRASS VITALITY™ IN CAPSULE TOPPED OFF WITH 4 DROPS CARRIER OIL.
JUVAPOWER®	**JUVATONE®** OR **ALKALIME®**
JUVATONE®	**JUVAPOWER®**
K & B™	**JUVATONE®**
KIDSCENTS® MIGHTYPRO™	**LIFE 9®**
KIDSCENTS® MIGHTYVITES™	**TAKE ALL:** SUPER C™ CHEWABLES, SUPER VITAMIN D, MULTIGREENS™
KIDSCENTS® MIGHTYZYME™	**ESSENTIALZYME™ (CRUSHED)**
KIDSCENTS® UNWIND™	**CBD CALM**
LIFE 9®	**KIDSCENTS® MIGHTYPRO™**
LONGEVITY™	**DIY CAPSULE:** ADD 10 DROPS LONGEVITY VITALITY™ TO A CAPSULE AND TOP OFF WITH 4 DROPS CARRIER OIL.
MASTER FORMULA™	**TAKE ALL:** MULTIGREENS™, SUPER B™, SUPER VITAMIN D, SUPER C™ TABLETS, SUPER CAL™ PLUS, ILLUMINEYES™, MINERAL ESSENCE™,
MEGACAL™	**SUPER CAL™ PLUS**
MINDWISE™	**TAKE BOTH: OMEGAGIZE3®** AND **AGILEASE™**
MINERAL ESSENCE™	**NO SUBSTITUTE**
MULTIGREENS™	**MASTER FORMULA™**
NINGXIA NITRO®	**NINGXIA ZYNG®**
NINGXIA RED®	**NO SUBSTITUTE**
NINGXIA ZYNG®	**NINGXIA NITRO®**
OLIVE ESSENTIALS™	**NO SUBSTITUTE**
OMEGAGIZE3®	**NO SUBSTITUTE**
PD 80/20™	**CORTISTOP®**
PARAFREE™	**NO SUBSTITUTE. DO NOT ATTEMPT TO DIY ON THIS ONE.**
POWERGIZE™	**ENDOGIZE™**
PROSTATE HEALTH™	**NO SUBSTITUTE. MAIN INGREDIENT: SAW PALMETTO**
PURE PROTEIN™ COMPLETE	**BALANCE COMPLETE™** OR **SLIQUE® SHAKE**
REHEMOGEN™	**ICP™** OR **COMFORTONE®**
SLEEPESSENCE™	**IMMUPRO™**
SLIQUE® SHAKE	**BALANCE COMPLETE™** OR **PURE PROTEIN™ COMPLETE**
SLIQUE® BARS	**NO SUBSTITUTE**
SLIQUE® CITRISLIM™	**NO SUBSTITUTE**
SLIQUE® ESSENCE ESSENTIAL OIL	**CITRUS FRESH™ VITALITY™** ESSENTIAL OIL
SLIQUE® GUM	**NO SUBSTITUTE**
SULFURZYME® (CAPSULES & POWDER)	**SULFURZYME®** (CAPSULES & POWDER)
SUPER B™	**MASTER FORMULA™**
SUPER C™ (CHEWABLE)	**SUPER C™ (TABLET)**
SUPER C™ (TABLET)	**SUPER C™ (CHEWABLE)**
SUPER CAL™ PLUS	**MEGA CAL™**
SUPER VITAMIN D	**OMEGAGIZE3®**
THYROMIN™	**NO SUBSTITUTE**
YL VITALITY DROPS	**DASH OF PINK HIMALAYAN SALT WITH CITRUS FRESH™ VITALITY™**

CHARTS

WHEN TO TAKE CHART

	WHEN TO TAKE	FAT OR WATER SOLUBLE
AGILEASE™	ANYTIME - BEST WITH FOOD	FAT
ALKALIME®	1 HOUR BEFORE MEALS	WATER
ALLERZYME™	WITH MEALS	N/A
AMINOWISE®	ANYTIME	WATER
BALANCE COMPLETE™	ANYTIME	WATER & FAT (SELF CONTAINING)
BLM™	ANYTIME	WATER
CARDIOGIZE™	WITH FOOD	FAT
COMFORTONE®	ANYTIME	WATER
CORTISTOP®	BEFORE BREAKFAST	WATER
DETOXZYME®	BETWEEN MEALS	N/A
DIGEST & CLEANSE®	BEFORE MEALS	FAT (SELF CONTAINING)
ENDOGIZE™	ANYTIME	WATER
ESSENTIALZYME™	1 HOUR BEFORE MEALS	N/A
ESSENTIALZYMES-4™	WITH MEALS	N/A
FEMIGEN™	WITH FOOD	FAT
ICP™	ANYTIME	WATER
ILLUMINEYES™	WITH FOOD	FAT
IMMUPRO™	JUST BEFORE BED	WATER
INNER DEFENSE®	ANYTIME - BEST WITH FOOD	FAT (SELF CONTAINING)
JUVAPOWER®	SPRINKLE ON FOOD	N/A
JUVATONE®	BETWEEN MEALS	WATER
K & B™	ANYTIME	WATER
KIDSCENTS® MIGHTYPRO™	ANYTIME - BEST WITH FOOD	N/A
KIDSCENTS® MIGHTYVITES™	ANYTIME - BEST WITH FOOD	FAT & WATER
KIDSCENTS® MIGHTYZYME™	WITH MEALS	N/A
KIDSCENTS® UNWIND™	ANYTIME OR BEFORE BED	WATER
LIFE 9®	1 HOUR AFTER DINNER	N/A
LONGEVITY™	ANYTIME - BEST WITH FOOD	FAT (SELF CONTAINING)
MASTER FORMULA™	ANYTIME - BEST WITH FOOD	FAT & WATER
MEGACAL™	1 HOUR AFTER MEAL	FAT
MINDWISE™	ANYTIME - BEST WITH FOOD	FAT
MINERAL ESSENCE™	ANYTIME	WATER
MULTIGREENS™	ANYTIME (OR 1 HR BEFORE MEAL)	WATER
NINGXIA NITRO®	ANYTIME BEFORE 3PM	N/A
NINGXIA RED®	ANYTIME	N/A
NINGXIA ZYNG®	ANYTIME BEFORE 3PM	N/A
OLIVE ESSENTIALS™	ANYTIME	N/A
OMEGAGIZE3®	ANYTIME	FAT (SELF CONTAINING)
PD 80/20™	ANYTIME - BEST WITH FOOD	FAT
PARAFREE™	ANYTIME - BEST WITH FOOD	FAT (SELF CONTAINING)
POWERGIZE™	ANYTIME OR DURING EXERCISE	N/A
PROSTATE HEALTH™	ANYTIME - BEST WITH FOOD	FAT
PURE PROTEIN™ COMPLETE	ANYTIME	WATER
REHEMOGEN™	JUST BEFORE OR WITH MEAL	FAT
SLEEPESSENCE™	JUST BEFORE BED	FAT (SELF CONTAINING)
SLIQUE® SHAKE	ANYTIME	WATER & FAT (SELF CONTAINING)
SLIQUE® BARS	ANYTIME	N/A
SLIQUE® CITRISLIM™	MORNING THEN AGAIN BEFORE 3	N/A
SLIQUE® ESSENCE ESSENTIAL OIL	ANYTIME WITH WATER	N/A
SLIQUE® GUM	BETWEEN MEALS	N/A
SULFURZYME® (CAPSULES & POWDER)	ANYTIME OR BETWEEN MEALS	WATER
SUPER B™	MORNING OR BEFORE BREAKFAST	WATER
SUPER C™ (CHEWABLE)	ANYTIME	WATER
SUPER C™ (TABLET)	ANYTIME - BEST WITH FOOD	WATER
SUPER CAL™ PLUS	WITH FOOD	FAT
SUPER VITAMIN D	WITH FOOD	FAT
THYROMIN™	WITHOUT FOOD BEFORE BED	N/A
YL VITALITY DROPS	ANYTIME	WATER

These statements have not been evaluated by the Food and Drug Administration.
Young Living® products are not intended to diagnose, treat, cure, or prevent any disease.

MINIMUM AGE & DOSAGE CHART

CHARTS

	AGE	ADULT DOSAGE	4-11 CHILD DOSAGE
AGILEASE™	12+	2 CAPSULES PER DAY	½ OF ADULT DOSE
ALKALIME®	12+	1 PACK OR TSP. PER DAY	½ OF ADULT DOSE
ALLERZYME™	12+	1 CAPSULE 3 TIMES PER DAY	NONE - USE MIGHTYZYME™
AMINOWISE®	12+	1 SCOOP WITH WATER	½ OF ADULT DOSE
BALANCE COMPLETE™	1+	2 SCOOPS WITH WATER	SAME AS ADULT
BLM™	12+	1 CAPSULE 3-5 X PER DAY	½ OF ADULT DOSE
CARDIOGIZE™	18+	2 CAPSULES PER DAY	NONE
COMFORTONE®	12+	1 CAPSULE 3 TIMES PER DAY	NONE
CORTISTOP®	21+	2-4 CAPSULES PER DAY	NONE
DETOXZYME®	12+	1-2 CAPSULES 3 TIMES PER DAY	NONE - USE MIGHTYZYME™
DIGEST & CLEANSE®	12+	1 SOFTGEL 3 TIMES PER DAY	NONE
ENDOGIZE™	21+	1 CAPSULE 2 TIMES PER DAY	NONE
ESSENTIALZYME™	12+	1 CAPLET 1 HOUR BEFORE MEAL	NONE - USE MIGHTYZYME™
ESSENTIALZYMES-4™	12+	2 CAPSULES 2 TIMES PER DAY	NONE - USE MIGHTYZYME™
FEMIGEN™	21+	2-4 CAPSULES PER DAY	NONE
ICP™	12+	2 TSP. 1-3 TIMES PER DAY	NONE
ILLUMINEYES™	12+	1 CAPSULE PER DAY	¼ - ½ OF ADULT DOSE
IMMUPRO™	14+	1-2 TABLETS PER NIGHT	NONE
INNER DEFENSE®	14+	1 SOFTGEL 1-5 TIMES PER DAY	NONE
JUVAPOWER®	12+	1 TBS. 1-3 TIMES PER DAY	NONE
JUVATONE®	12+	2 TABLETS 2 TIMES PER DAY	¼ - ½ OF ADULT DOSE
K & B™	12+	3 ½ DROPPERS 3 TIMES PER DAY	½ OF ADULT DOSE
KIDSCENTS® MIGHTYPRO™	2+	1-2 PACKETS	1 PACKET
KIDSCENTS® MIGHTYVITES™	4+	8 TABLETS	4 TABLETS
KIDSCENTS® MIGHTYZYME™	2+	2 TABLETS 3 TIMES A DAY	1 TABLET 3 TIMES A DAY
KIDSCENTS® UNWIND™	4+	1 PACKET 1-2 TIMES A DAY	1 PACKET 1-2 TIMES A DAY
LIFE 9®	12+	1 CAPSULE PER NIGHT	NONE
LONGEVITY™	12+	1 SOFTGEL PER DAY	NONE
MASTER FORMULA™	12+	1 PACKET PER DAY	NONE - USE MIGHTYVITES™
MEGACAL™	12+	1 TSP. WITH WATER	¼ - ½ OF ADULT DOSE
MINDWISE™	12+	1 TBS. OR 1 SACHET	¼ - ½ OF ADULT DOSE
MINERAL ESSENCE™	12+	5ML 2 TIMES PER DAY	¼ - ½ OF ADULT DOSE
MULTIGREENS™	12+	3 CAPSULES 2 TIMES PER DAY	½ OF ADULT DOSE
NINGXIA NITRO®	14+	1 TUBE 1 TIME PER DAY	NONE
NINGXIA RED®	1+	1-2 OZ. 2 TIMES PER DAY	1-2 OZ. 1 TIME PER DAY
NINGXIA ZYNG®	18+	1 CAN AS DESIRED	NONE
OLIVE ESSENTIALS™	12+	1 CAPSULE PER DAY	½ OF ADULT DOSE
OMEGAGIZE3®	12+	2-4 CAPSULES 2 TIMES PER DAY	¼ - ½ OF ADULT DOSE
PD 80/20™	21+	1 CAPSULE PER DAY	NONE
PARAFREE™	18+	3 SOFTGELS 2 TIMES PER DAY	NONE
POWERGIZE™	18+	2 CAPSULES PER DAY	NONE
PROSTATE HEALTH™	21+	1 CAPSULE 2 TIMES PER DAY	NONE
PURE PROTEIN™ COMPLETE	1+	2 SCOOPS WITH WATER	½ OF ADULT DOSE
REHEMOGEN™	12+	3ML 3 TIMES PER DAY	¼ - ½ OF ADULT DOSE
SLEEPESSENCE™	18+	1-2 SOFTGELS PER NIGHT	NONE
SLIQUE® SHAKE	12+	1 PACKET PER DAY	½ OF ADULT DOSE
SLIQUE® BARS	2+	1-2 BARS PER DAY	SAME AS ADULT
SLIQUE® CITRISLIM™	14+	AM/PM REGIMEN	NONE
SLIQUE® ESSENCE ESSENTIAL OIL	6+	2-4 DROPS IN BEVERAGE	½ OF ADULT DOSE
SLIQUE® GUM	12+	1 TABLET BETWEEN MEALS	NONE
SULFURZYME® (CAPSULES)	12+	2 CAPSULES 3 TIMES PER DAY	¼ - ½ OF ADULT DOSE
SULFURZYME® (POWDER)	12+	½ TSP. 2 TIMES PER DAY	¼ - ½ OF ADULT DOSE
SUPER B™	12+	2 TABLETS PER DAY	¼ - ½ OF ADULT DOSE
SUPER C™ (CHEWABLE)	1+	1 TABLET 3 TIMES PER DAY	SAME AS ADULT
SUPER C™ (TABLET)	12+	1-2 TABLETS PER DAY	CRUSH OR TAKE CHEWABLE
SUPER CAL™ PLUS	12+	2 CAPSULES PER DAY	½ OF ADULT DOSE
SUPER VITAMIN D	12+	2 TABLETS PER DAY	¼ - ½ OF ADULT DOSE
THYROMIN™	19+	1 CAPSULE BEFORE BED	NONE
YL VITALITY DROPS	6+	1 SQUIRT PER 8 OZ. WATER	SAME AS ADULT

• *The dosage guidelines listed above are either found on the bottle or are based on medical dosing suggestions for adults and children based on specific ingredients within each supplement listed. When "none" is specified in the "4-11 Child Dosage" category, that is because there is a specific ingredient or ingredients that should not be taken by children under the age of 12.*
• *Hormone supplements should never be given to those under the age of 21 as their endocrine system is still developing.*
• *Products containing caffeine, melatonin, or all essential oils should be used with caution on those under 18.*

SUPPLEMENTS DESK REFERENCE BY JEN O'SULLIVAN

DIGESTIVE ENZYME USAGE GUIDE CHART

	ESSENTIALZYMES-4™	ESSENTIALZYME™	ALLERZYME™	DETOXZYME®	MIGHTYZYME™	ENDOGIZE™ (HORMONES & ENZYMES)	ICP™ (COLON & ENZYMES)
AMYLASE Breaks down starches, breads, and pastas.	√		√	√	√	√	
ALPHA-GALACTOSIDASE Breaks down foods that cause gas.			√	√			
BROMELAIN Breaks down protein and grains. Supports blood to help ease inflammation.	√	√	√	√	√		
CELLULASE Breaks down man-made fiber, plant fiber, fruits, and vegetables.	√		√	√	√	√	
DIASTASE (contains barley malt) Breaks down grain sugars and starch.			√				
GLUCOAMYLASE Breaks down starchy foods and cereals. Flushes body of dead white blood cells.				√		√	
INVERTASE Breaks down table sugar. Breaks the connection between fructose and glucose.			√	√			
LACTASE Breaks down dairy sugars. Helps with lactose intolerance.			√	√			
LIPASE Dietary fats and oils. Helps liver function.			√	√	√		√
PEPTIDASE Breaks down Protease. Supports immune system and helps ease inflammation.			√		√		√
PHYTASE Helps with bone health. Pulls needed minerals from grains.	√		√	√	√		√
PROTEASE 3.0 Supports blood circulation and toxicity. Breaks down animal protein.	√				√		√
PROTEASE 4.5 Helps digest protein. Has a lower acidity.	√			√	√		√
PROTEASE 6.0 Helps carry away toxins. Helps reduce pain and varicose veins. Least acidic.	√			√	√		√
PAPAIN Digestive aid to help break proteins down into peptides and amino acids.	√	√					
BETAINE HCL (Betaine hydrochloride) Promotes hydrochloric acid to help digestion. Helps absorb B12, Calcium, Iron, and Proteins.		√					
PANCRELIPASE (pancreas gland extract from pig) Combo of Lipase, Protease, and Amylase. Supports a poorly performing pancreas.		√					
PANCREATIN (pancreas from pigs or cows) Helps produce amylase, lipase, and protease. Supports a poorly performing pancreas.	√	√					
TRYPSIN Breaks down proteins. For muscle growth and hormone production.		√					

CHARTS

HORMONE SUPPORT USAGE GUIDE CHART

	FEMIGEN™	PD 80/20™	CORTISTOP®	ENDOGIZE™	THYROMIN™	PROSTATE HEALTH™	POWERGIZE™
ADRENAL FATIGUE				√			
APPETITE CONTROL	√					√	
ANIMAL GLAND EXTRACT - ADRENAL					√		
ANIMAL GLAND EXTRACT - PITUITARY					√		
ANIMAL GLAND EXTRACT - THYROID					√		
ANTIOXIDANT	√						
ANXIETY				√			√
BODY BUILDING				√			√
CIRCULATION				√	√		√
COGNITION	√	√	√	√		√	√
DEPRESSION	√	√	√	√	√	√	
DIGESTION	√			√		√	
DIGESTIVE ENZYME SUPPORT				√			
ENDURANCE	√						√
ENERGY	√	√	√	√			√
ERECTILE DYSFUNCTION				√			
FAT BURNING	√			√			
FERTILITY	√	√	√			√	
FLUID RETENTION	√						
GLUTATHIONE SUPPORT	√						
HOT FLASHES	√	√	√				
IMMUNE SYSTEM	√					√	√
INFLAMMATION				√		√	
INSULIN SUPPORT				√			
JOINT SUPPORT	√						√
LACTIC ACID FLUSHING	√						
LIBIDO	√	√	√	√			√
LIVER SUPPORT	√						
LOWERS BLOOD SUGAR				√			
MENOPAUSE	√	√	√		√		
MENSTRUAL BLOOD FLOW					√		
MEMORY	√	√	√	√		√	√
METABOLISM	√		√	√			
MOOD SWINGS	√	√	√	√		√	
MOTIVATION		√	√				√
MUSCLE AND BONE MASS		√	√	√			√
NATURAL ESTROGEN THERAPY		√	√				
PMS	√	√	√	√			
REDUCES CORTISOL LEVELS				√			
RENAL SYSTEM						√	√
STRESS	√	√	√	√		√	√
TESTOSTERONE SUPPORT FOR MEN		√	√	√		√	√
VAGINAL DRYNESS	√	√	√	√			
CONTAINS DHEA		√	√	√			
CONTAINS PREGNENOLONE		√	√				

VITALITY™ USAGE GUIDE CHART

	CALMING/SLEEP	CLARITY (MENTAL)	ENERGY	METABOLISM	WOMEN HORMONES	MOBILITY (MUSCLES/JOINTS)	BRAIN HEALTH	CIRCULATORY	DIGESTION (ENZYMES/GUT)	ENDOCRINE	IMMUNE	LYMPHATIC	LIVER	RENAL/URINARY	BLADDER	KIDNEY	NERVOUS	RESPIRATORY	HAIR, SKIN, NAILS
BASIL VITALITY™		√				√					√								
BERGAMOT VITALITY™	√				√					√	√								
BLACK PEPPER VITALITY™			√	√		√		√		√	√								
CARAWAY VITALITY™		√				√			√	√	√			√			√	√	√
CARDAMOM VITALITY™		√						√		√			√				√	√	
CARROT SEED VITALITY™										√			√	√					√
CELERY SEED VITALITY™						√				√			√	√					
CILANTRO VITALITY™										√	√		√						√
CINNAMON BARK VITALITY™		√		√				√	√	√	√								
CITRUS FRESH™ VITALITY™	√	√		√					√	√	√		√						
CLOVE VITALITY™						√		√	√	√	√			√	√				√
COPAIBA VITALITY™	√					√			√	√	√			√	√	√		√	√
CORIANDER VITALITY™	√								√		√		√	√					√
CUMIN VITALITY™								√	√		√		√	√		√			
DIGIZE™ VITALITY™				√					√		√								
DILL VITALITY™	√								√	√			√						
ENDOFLEX™ VITALITY™					√					√									
FENNEL VITALITY™			√	√					√	√	√		√						
FRANKINCENSE VITALITY™	√	√					√	√			√						√	√	√
GLF™ VITALITY™									√		√								
GERMAN CHAMOMILE VITALITY™	√								√				√						√
GINGER VITALITY™				√		√		√		√	√							√	
GRAPEFRUIT VITALITY™	√	√	√	√						√	√	√	√	√	√	√			
JADE LEMON™ VITALITY™		√	√						√		√	√	√	√	√	√	√		√
JUVACLEANSE® VITALITY™									√		√		√						
JUVAFLEX® VITALITY™									√		√		√						
LAURUS NOBILIS VITALITY™						√			√		√							√	
LAVENDER VITALITY™	√	√				√	√	√	√		√						√	√	√
LEMON VITALITY™		√	√					√	√		√	√	√	√	√	√			√
LEMONGRASS VITALITY™		√	√			√	√	√	√		√						√	√	
LIME VITALITY™	√			√				√	√	√	√		√	√				√	
LONGEVITY™ VITALITY™							√			√									
MARJORAM VITALITY™	√					√		√	√										
MOUNTAIN SAVORY VITALITY™		√							√		√			√	√				
NUTMEG VITALITY™		√	√			√	√	√	√	√	√								
ORANGE VITALITY™	√		√					√	√		√		√	√	√	√	√		√
OREGANO VITALITY™		√				√		√	√	√	√							√	
PARSLEY VITALITY™				√	√				√		√		√	√	√	√	√		
PEPPERMINT VITALITY™		√	√	√		√	√	√	√		√	√					√	√	√
ROSEMARY VITALITY™		√	√			√		√	√	√	√		√	√				√	√
SAGE VITALITY™		√	√	√	√				√	√									
SCLARESSENCE™ VITALITY™					√					√									
SPEARMINT VITALITY™		√	√			√		√	√										
TANGERINE VITALITY™	√		√					√	√		√			√	√			√	
TARRAGON VITALITY™	√							√	√		√		√						
THIEVES® VITALITY™			√	√		√		√	√	√	√			√				√	
THYME VITALITY™		√						√	√		√	√		√	√		√		

CHARTS

SUPPLEMENTS USAGE GUIDE CHART

	KID SAFE	MEN SPECIFIC	SLEEP	WEIGHT SUPPORT	ENERGY	HORMONES	MOBILITY (MUSCLES/JOINTS)	MILD LAXATIVE	BRAIN HEALTH	CIRCULATORY	DIGESTION (ENZYMES/GUT)	IMMUNE SYSTEM	RENAL/URINARY/LIVER	RESPIRATORY	HAIR, SKIN, NAILS	BONES	VEGAN	CONTAINS COW	CONTAINS PORK	CONTAINS SHELLFISH	CONTAINS DAIRY	CONTAINS BARLEY	CONTAINS CORN	CONTAINS SOY	CONTAINS BEE ITEMS	CONTAINS COCONUT	CONTAINS CAFFEINE
AGILEASE™							√					√			√									√			
ALKALIME®							√	√			√	√			√	√								√			
ALLERZYME™											√									√	√	√					
AMINOWISE®					√												√										
BALANCE COMPLETE™	√			√							√										√	√					
BLM™							√								√			√	√	√							
CARDIOGIZE™		√	√	√		√	√		√	√			√		√	√	√										
COMFORTONE®								√			√							√									
CORTISTOP®						√												√					√				
DETOXZYME®											√	√										√					
DIGEST & CLEANSE®											√	√	√				√									√	
ENDOGIZE™		√				√											√							√			
ESSENTIALZYME™											√	√							√								
ESSENTIALZYMES-4™											√	√					√						√				
FEMIGEN™				√		√											√										
ICP™								√			√						√										
ILLUMINEYES™									√			√			√		√										
IMMUPRO™			√									√					√										
INNER DEFENSE®											√	√		√												√	
JUVAPOWER®											√		√				√						√				
JUVATONE®											√		√													√	
K & B™											√		√													√	
KIDSCENTS® MIGHTYPRO™	√										√	√	√				√										
KIDSCENTS® MIGHTYVITES™	√											√					√						√				
KIDSCENTS® MIGHTYZYME™	√										√	√					√										
KIDSCENTS® UNWIND™	√		√			√			√								√										
LIFE 9®											√	√	√				√										
LONGEVITY™									√	√		√					√									√	
MASTER FORMULA™				√		√		√	√	√	√	√		√		√	√						√				√
MEGACAL™								√							√	√	√										
MINDWISE™				√					√	√							√									√	
MINERAL ESSENCE™			√											√	√	√							√				
MULTIGREENS™									√			√						√				√	√	√			
NINGXIA NITRO®				√					√	√													√				√
NINGXIA RED®	√			√					√	√	√	√	√	√	√		√										
NINGXIA ZYNG®				√					√	√							√										√
OLIVE ESSENTIALS™									√	√	√						√										
OMEGAGIZE3®									√	√		√			√	√											
PD 80/20™						√							√				√										
PARAFREE™												√	√														
POWERGIZE™		√								√				√			√							√			
PROSTATE HEALTH™		√				√														√							
PURE PROTEIN™ COMPLETE	√			√							√											√					
REHEMOGEN™							√																√				
SLEEPESSENCE™			√	√								√					√							√		√	
SLIQUE® SHAKE				√							√						√							√			√
SLIQUE® BARS	√			√																							
SLIQUE® CITRISLIM™				√																				√		√	√
SLIQUE® GUM				√													√							√	√		
SLIQUE® ESSENCE ESSENTIAL OIL				√													√										
SULFURZYME® (CAPSULES & POWDER)							√					√	√		√												
SUPER B™					√							√															
SUPER C™ (CHEWABLE)	√											√	√	√									√				
SUPER C™ (TABLET)												√	√	√	√												
SUPER CAL™ PLUS			√				√			√					√	√	√						√				
SUPER VITAMIN D	√				√							√		√	√	√											
THYROMIN™			√		√													√	√								
YL VITALITY DROPS	√			√	√							√					√										

SUPPLEMENTS 101 CLASS SCRIPT

PERSONAL PORTION: (about 20 minutes)

Welcome to the class! I am excited you are here and a little nervous to be teaching you all today. I would like to know how many of you are currently using a supplement to support your health? *[Ask them to raise their hands if they do.]*
Is anyone willing to share what they are currently using? Are they something you decided to take on your own or did a doctor recommend them? Did you know that most doctors recommend we take a multi-vitamin, B complex, omega, and possibly others depending on your health goals? Let me tell you a little about me and why I got started with Young Living® and why these supplements have completely transformed my life!
[Share your story on supplements for about 10-15 minutes. It is important to connect with your audience. Be passionate! Share the deep connection of your story. It is OK to share a moment in your life where you were really sick and decided to take your health regimen into your own hands. Be careful not to state that YL supplements are what cured or treated you. Share why they add vitality to your lifestyle now.]

EDUCATION PORTION: (about 20 minutes)
[You may read directly from this. People are OK with reading a script. You can even print this portion out and give it to them.]

We live in a world where supplementation is the norm. We take vitamin C in mass doses, get vitamin B injections, and swallow full-spectrum multivitamins by the handful. Dietary supplements were not a major thing until the U.S. Congress passed the Dietary Supplement and Health Education Act of 1994. After that, dietary supplement consumption skyrocketed. In the United States alone, the supplement market is a $31 billion dollar industry. Seventy-six percent of all adults in the United States take some form of dietary supplement, as of 2017. Just in this room alone _____ of you are taking supplements. It is estimated that there are 80 to 90 thousand dietary supplement products on the market, as of 2016 and since that time thousands more have been introduced.

The scary reality from the FDA, regarding all of these supplements, can be understood by the following quotes from the FDA.
- "Federal law does not require dietary supplements to be proven safe to FDA's satisfaction before they are marketed."
- "For most claims made in the labeling of dietary supplements, the law does not require the manufacturer or seller to prove to the FDA's satisfaction that the claim is accurate or truthful before it appears on the product."
- "Dietary supplement manufacturers do not have to get the agency's [meaning the FDA's] approval before producing or selling these products."

Supplements are exactly what the word means: to add an extra amount of what we are not getting in our nutrition. Whole-food nutrition is the most important aspect to proper health, and the goal is to get as much of that nutrition as possible from what God has created. The reality is, the food sources we currently have access to are very different from those that our grandparents, or even our parents, grew up consuming. We have massively depleted our soils, but more importantly, even if you are able to get organic, farmer's market type produce and proteins, they are usually picked far before they should be, or the animals are fed from sources that are not ideal such as GMO corn loaded with pesticides. Did you know most produce is picked about two weeks before it is ripe? Did you also know that often the most vital phytonutrients (plant nutrients) are developed during the last few days of ripening? It is unfortunate, but we do not get the right vitamins, minerals, micro minerals, and nutrients in the everyday food sources we eat. Supplementation is a great way to go, but sadly most supplements are synthetic or so isolated that your body does not know what to do with them, so you end up having the supplements you paid good money for go in one end and out the other, without even getting into your system to be used. The act of something going into your body and your body using it is called "bioavailability."

An article on Healthline states, "The majority of supplements available on the market today are made artificially." One study states 90% of all supplements are not fully bioavailable, because they are synthetic. The Organic Consumers Association states that they believe "95% of vitamins consist of some degree of synthetic." Artificial or synthetic nutrients are produced in a laboratory to mimic the effects of nature. Synthetic supplements are often less bioavailable than their natural counterpart. While science will tell you that your body will readily "absorb" synthetic versions just as well as it will absorb it in its natural form, they fail to tell you that your body won't readily recognize the synthetic version. Our ancestral DNA is programmed based on thousands of years of genetic code. Your body knows exactly what to do with the thousands of nutrients found in spinach. It gets a little confused when science isolates one vitamin or mineral and decides that is what you need. God created our food source to work synergistically. The entirety of the molecules together are what allow for greater bioavailability. Our bodies know what to do with the 10,000+ phytonutrients found in an apple, but isolating vitamin C and taking it at extremely high doses is something our bodies don't understand how to use, so you end up flushing the majority of your isolated vitamin C right down the toilet.

Isolated nutrients aside, the more frightening reality when it comes to supplements is the dangerous ingredients you may not even know you are consuming. Several dangerous ingredients found in supplements are artificial colors such as Blue #1, Red #40, and Yellow #5, hydrogenated oils such as partially hydrogenated soybean oil, lead, mercury, polychlorinated biphenyls (PBCs), talc as a cheap anti-caking substance, and titanium dioxide, all of which cause a myriad of illnesses and disease such as cancer, kidney damage, inflammation, heavy metal poisoning, heart disease and heart attack, autism, autoimmune diseases, and much more! With Young Living® you get naturally derived ingredients that your body knows exactly how to put to good use. There are many supplements available on the market today. Why should you consider Young Living® supplements over the sea of companies telling you theirs are better?

Young Living® is different for a couple of reasons. First, they use whole food sources in fruits, vegetables, herbs, and roots for their supplements. Second, they infuse many of their supplements with essential oils. Essential oils are extremely volatile and very small in their molecular structure, making them an excellent vehicle, or pathway, to increase the bioavailability of the supplements. The essential oils themselves are different than any you can purchase on the market because they are the true unaltered botanical, allowing for a true "entourage effect," which basically means that because the essential oil has not been modified, and the whole of the oil is used, there is much greater action, or synergy, that occurs within the oil, and therefore, within our bodies. Most companies practice what is called "fractional distillation" with their essential oils, simply because the final product smells better and is easier to market to the masses. With these two important factors in place — whole-plant nutrition infused with unaltered essential oils — you will get dietary supplementation through Young Living® that is second to none. Young Living® offers three types of nutritional supplements: Foundation, Cleansing, and Targeted.

Foundation Nutrition: Green labeled bottles. These products are the vitamins and minerals that support a healthy lifestyle.

Cleansing Nutrition: Blue labeled bottles. These products are specifically designed to support the detox and cleansing of the body.

Targeted Nutrition: Orange labeled bottles. These products are formulated with specific ingredients including powerful essential oils to support specific nutritional needs. These supplements target everything from gut, joint, heart, brain, and hormone health.

101 SCRIPT

SALES PORTION: (about 20 minutes)

Let's discuss how to get started… It is important to listen to your body. Start out slowly by taking ¼ to ½ the recommended daily dose. See how you feel. Each week moving forward, increase your dose to the recommended daily dose to figure out what amount is right for you. Once you feel you have the right amount, use that amount for 30 days. After 30 days, stop taking the supplement for 3-7 days to note how you feel, then resume if you determine the supplement is a fit for your needs.

Are you now worried about the supplements you are currently taking? May I ask what areas you would like supported? Let me give you some ideas!

[Ask them to say yes or nod yes or raise their hand at each question.]
- How would you like to have better and more sustained energy during the day? Yes!
- What about better focus and less squirrel moments? YES!
- How many of you would like a more restful night's sleep? YES!
- OK, we are all getting a little older, would you like to support your cognition and mental acuity? YES!
- What about gut health and immune support? Do you need help in those areas? YES!
- One area I love to support is my hair, skin, and nails. Is that something you would like to see improvement on? YES!
- All right, the last area that I want to cover today, how about emotions!? Do any of you deal with constant ups and downs? Would you like to regulate that a bit? YES!

I want to show you seven of my favorite Young Living® supplements that have helped transform my life! All of these help support what I just talked about. I want to also be up-front with you. This package is about $800! But before you get up and walk out the door, (laugh a bit), I want to be clear that when you use my Brand Partner number to sign up today, you can get them for about half of that price!

And, best of all, I am going to help you understand why a small investment of $400 will last you 2-3 months and will potentially save you thousands!

[Share a money saving story of your own about lessening your doctor visits or medical bills you had in the past. Share how many of the vitamins and supplements your doctor recommends you buy through a pharmacy that are just about the same price, if not higher, than these supplements and that these are far more bioavailable!]

Here are the top seven supplements to set you up with the perfect starter package today.
- NingXia Red®
- NingXia Nitro®
- Life 9®
- Super B™
- Essentialzymes-4™
- Sulfurzyme®
- OmegaGize3®

[Share your own personal stories on how these supplements help you.]
NingXia Red®: supports immune function, gut, brain, energy, and hair, skin, and nail growth.
NingXia Nitro®: supports energy, and brain cognition.
Life 9®: supports immune function and gut health
Super B™: supports energy, digestion, gut health, and hair, skin, and nail growth.
Essentialzymes-4™: supports digestion, immune function, and emotions
Sulfurzyme®: supports mobility, joints, and hair, skin, and nail growth.
OmegaGize3®: supports cognition, energy, healthy emotions, and hair, skin, and nail growth.

Once you get your kit, I will help you get started slowly and this package will last you anywhere from 2-3 months depending on your goals. I cannot wait to help you feel better and find transformation in your health. Who would like to get started today?

There are three ways you can get started.

1. You can simply order one or two items that I discussed that you feel would be a good "dip your toe in" way to start.
2. You can take advantage of the 50% discount and jump right in with the package.
3. You can get your starter package and then sign up with me to host your own class with your friends and I can show you how you can get all of your products for free! Yep, with only four friends diving into their health like you, I can help you get your $400 investment completely paid back with cash. That means you pay today, and in a month, with four friends signing up this month, you will get $400 back in a check from Young Living®! Don't you just love free stuff!?

HOW TO SIGN UP A NEW PERSON:

1. Go to YoungLiving.com.
2. Use your member number as enroller and sponsor (placement) or as you wish.
3. Select the NingXia Red® Starter Bundle.
4. Select Essential Rewards (Loyalty Rewards Program or Subscribe and Save) and go over a 50PV order for NEXT MONTH under CUSTOMIZE MONTHLY ORDER. Add supplements!
5. Under Continue Enrollment select the ADD MORE PRODUCTS link.
6. Add the following to their order which amounts to about a little over 200PV:
   - Life 9®
   - Super B™
   - Essentialzymes-4™
   - Sulfurzyme® Powder
   - OmegaGize3®

CONGRATULATE THEM ON BECOMING A YOUNG LIVING® MEMBER!

You did it! Schedule your next class or party and do it all over again and again!

Sources:
https://www.ncbi.nlm.nih.gov/books/NBK216048/
https://www.crnusa.org/resources/2017-crn-consumer-survey-dietary-supplements
https://www.pbs.org/wgbh/frontline/article/can-regulators-keep-up-with-the-supplements-industry/
https://www.fda.gov/consumers/consumer-updates/fda-101-dietary-supplements
https://myersdetox.com/90-of-vitamins-are-synthetic/
https://www.healthline.com/nutrition/synthetic-vs-natural-nutrients
https://www.organicconsumers.org/news/organic-consumers-association-takes-synthetic-vitamin-and-supplements-industry
https://www.scientificamerican.com/article/do-vitamins-in-pills-diff/
http://info.achs.edu/blog/dangerous-supplement-ingredients

PHOTO: ILLUMINEYES™ ON A MARIGOLD FLOWER

SECTION TWO
the protocols

DISCLAIMER

The protocols and supplement descriptions in this book are based on the usage descriptions from the Young Living® website and information readily available online. The amount and timing of each dosage is based on the label on each product. In some instances, lower doses are recommended in this book. When you start a new supplement regimen, it is important to start slowly and pay close attention to your body. Everyone's body is unique and will respond differently. When a product does not work for you, please try another one. Check with your doctor if you are taking prescription medications. Pharmaceutical drugs should not be consumed at the same time as natural supplements. It is best to give a four-hour buffer between them. Always consult your doctor when you start a new regimen. This book gives suggestions on how to support healthy systems. It is not intended to treat or diagnose existing conditions or illnesses. Each supplement consists of multiple ingredients. Each ingredient listed has a basic description of what it is commonly used for in the medical and holistic practice industries. Herbs and roots have been used for centuries and the traditionally studied uses for each are readily found on sources such as Science Direct, the National Center for Biotechnology Information, U. S. National Library of Medicine, PubMed, and the Food and Drug Administration websites. The content in this book has not been evaluated by the FDA and the supplements and protocols will not treat or cure any sickness or disease. The author is not a doctor and has published this book as a means to have a compilation of information, in one spot, to make it easier to understand the many supplements Young Living® carries.

PROTOCOLS

ESSENTIAL OIL PROTOCOLS USING VITALITY™ OILS

The Vitality™ line of essential oils through Young Living® is designed specifically for consumption. They are labeled as dietary supplements, in accordance with the FDA labeling regulations and guidelines. These oils are considered GRAS which means Generally Recognized (or Regarded) as Safe for consumption, which are known essential oils used in food additives and flavorings as well as for system function use. When consumed, essential oils support our body systems. The following body systems are supported by the internal use of essential oils labeled for consumption through the Young Living® Vitality™ line.

- Circulatory
- Digestive and Gut
- Endocrine
- Immune
- Integumentary
- Lymphatic
- Nervous
- Renal/Urinary
- Respiratory

You may use the Vitality™ line in capsules (preferred method), in liquids such as water or juice, as rectal (suppository), or vaginal (pessary) inserts. You may even add these oils to your food. To get the full supportive value from them, it is recommended that you use them in capsule form. There are two main types of capsules to consider: regular veggie capsules that dissolve in your stomach that you can buy directly from Young Living® or at a health food store, or a longer dissolving veggie capsule that dissolves in your stomach and intestines. The longer dissolving ones are harder to find. A good source is through AromaTools.com called "Design Release" capsules. Size 00 is larger and will hold around 14 drops of liquid. Size 0 is smaller and will hold around 10 drops.

There are two types of Vitality™ line essential oil capsules you may make: daily capsules and bomb capsules. Daily capsules may be created using around 3-5 drops of essential oil for daily support. Daily capsules may be created using around 8-10 drops to create a "bomb" for your system. A "bomb" is a stronger capsule intended to give you more aggressive support. Bombs should only be used 1-2 times over the course of 4-8 hours and only once per month. Please do not use bombs to treat sickness or disease, and always consult your doctor if you are sick. Daily capsules and bombs are meant to help support your terrain, meaning they strengthen your already healthy systems, protecting them from dipping below the wellness line. Lastly, do not take multiple capsules for multiple systems at the same time. Give at least four hours between capsules and do not take more than two per day.

It is best to create a synergy first of the recipe you would like to use by combining them into a clean dropper bottle. Use 5-10 times the recipe, swirl to blend, and let synergize for 24 hours before adding 4 drops of the synergy to the capsule with carrier oil. You should not take multiple recipes at the same time. Pay close attention to how your body responds. You may rotate these recipes or create your own. Always be your own best advocate for your health and consult your doctor if you choose to make any major adjustments in your health care regime.

CIRCULATORY SYSTEM CAPSULES

Circulatory System Daily Capsule Recipes Using Vitality™ Oils

GENERAL CIRCULATORY
- Recipe: 2 drops Cinnamon Bark, 1 drop Peppermint, 1 drop Lemon
- Recipe: 2 drops Orange, 1 drop Black Pepper, 1 drop Lemongrass
- Recipe: 1 drop Clove, 1 drop Rosemary, 1 drop Tangerine
- Recipe: 2 drops Marjoram, 1 drop Dill, 1 drop Fennel, 1 drop Oregano
- Recipe: 2 drops Lemongrass, 1 drop Tarragon, 1 drop Lavender
- Recipe: 2 drops Lavender, 1 drop Nutmeg, 1 drop Thyme

HEART HEALTH
- Recipe: 2 drops Orange, 1 drop Oregano, 1 drop Thyme

BLOOD HEALTH
- Recipe: 2 drops Tarragon, 1 drop Rosemary, 1 drop Orange
- Recipe: 2 drops Ocotea*, 1 drop Marjoram, 1 drop Lemon
  *Ocotea is not part of the Vitality™ line but is a GRAS oil by the FDA.
- Recipe: 1 drop Lemongrass, 1 drop Fennel, 1 drop Clove

Directions
Create a synergy first and then add 2-4 drops to a 0 or 00 size veggie capsule with carrier oil, or simply add the desired recipe, then top off with a minimum of 4 drops olive or grapeseed carrier oil. Consume with 4-8 oz. of water.

Storage
You may create multiple capsules ahead of time or create one each day.
Keep in the freezer in a labeled glass container.

How long should you use these capsules?
- Do not take multiple recipes at the same time. Use only one for a couple of days and then rotate through a few to see what works best for your body.
- There are two types of Vitality™ line essential oil capsules you may make: daily capsules and bomb capsules.
- Daily capsules may be created as the recipe states and used for daily support.
- Bomb capsules may be created using double or triple the recipes to create a "bomb" for your system. A "bomb" is a stronger capsule intended to give more aggressive support. Bombs should only be used 1-2 times over the course of 4-8 hours and only once per month. Please consult your doctor if you are sick.
- Daily capsules and bombs are meant to help support your terrain, meaning they strengthen your already healthy systems, protecting them from dipping below the wellness line.
- Do not take multiple capsules for multiple systems at the same time. Give at least four hours between capsules.

PROTOCOLS

DIGESTIVE SYSTEM CAPSULES

Digestive System Daily Capsule Recipes Using Vitality™ Oils

GENERAL DIGESTION
- Recipe: 3 drops DiGize™
- Recipe: 3 drops JuvaFlex®
- Recipe: 3 drops Juva Cleanse®

LIVER
- Liver Recipe: 2 drops Dill, 1 drop Cardamom, 1 drop Sage, 1 drop Coriander
- Liver Recipe: 3 drops Juva Cleanse®, 1 drop Rosemary
- Liver Recipe: 3 drops GLF™, 1 drop Carrot Seed
- Liver Recipe: 2 drops Rosemary, 1 drop Tangerine, 1 drop Celery Seed

GALLBLADDER
- Gallbladder Recipe: 2 drops Lemon, 1 drop Spearmint, 1 drop Oregano
- Gallbladder Recipe: 2 drops Lime, 1 drop Peppermint, 1 drop Jade Lemon™
- Gallbladder Recipe: 2 drops German Chamomile, 1 drop Lime

COLON
- Colon Recipe: 2 drops Thyme, 1 drop Fennel, 1 drop Cardamom
- Colon Recipe: 2 drops Tarragon, 1 drop Cinnamon Bark, 1 drop Peppermint

PANCREAS
- Pancreas Recipe: 2 drops Coriander, 1 drop Cinnamon Bark
- Pancreas Recipe: 1 drop Coriander, 1 drop Lemon, 1 drop Peppermint

Directions
Create a synergy first and then add 2-4 drops to a 0 or 00 size veggie capsule with carrier oil, or simply add the desired recipe, then top off with a minimum of 4 drops olive or grapeseed carrier oil. Consume with 4-8 oz. of water.

Storage
You may create multiple capsules ahead of time or create one each day.
Keep in the freezer in a labeled glass container.

How long should you use these capsules?
- Do not take multiple recipes at the same time. Use only one for a couple of days and then rotate through a few to see what works best for your body.
- There are two types of Vitality™ line essential oil capsules you may make: daily capsules and bomb capsules.
- Daily capsules may be created as the recipe states and used for daily support.
- Bomb capsules may be created using double or triple the recipes to create a "bomb" for your system. A "bomb" is a stronger capsule intended to give more aggressive support. Bombs should only be used 1-2 times over the course of 4-8 hours and only once per month. Please consult your doctor if you are sick.
- Daily capsules and bombs are meant to help support your terrain, meaning they strengthen your already healthy systems, protecting them from dipping below the wellness line.
- Do not take multiple capsules for multiple systems at the same time. Give at least four hours between capsules.

ENDOCRINE SYSTEM CAPSULES

Endocrine System Daily Capsule Recipes Using Vitality™ Oils

HORMONE HEALTH
- Recipe: 3 drops SclarEssence™
- Recipe: 2 drops Bergamot, 1 drop Nutmeg
- Recipe: 3 drops Lavender, 1 drop Sage, 1 drop Fennel

ENERGY SUPPORT
- Recipe: 2 drops Grapefruit, 1 drop Black Pepper, 1 drop Ginger
- Recipe: 2 drops Lemon, 1 drop Nutmeg, 1 drop Mountain Savory
- Recipe: 1 drop Lemongrass, 1 drop Jade Lemon™, 1 drop Peppermint

METABOLISM SUPPORT
- Recipe: 1 drop Grapefruit, 1 drop Cinnamon Bark
- Recipe: 1 drop Spearmint, 1 drop Lime, 1 drop Black Pepper

SLEEP & FOCUS SUPPORT
- Recipe: 2 drops Lavender, 1 drop Lime
- Recipe: 2 drops Frankincense, 2 drops Copaiba, 1 drop Tangerine

Directions
Create a synergy first and then add 2-4 drops to a 0 or 00 size veggie capsule with carrier oil, or simply add the desired recipe, then top off with a minimum of 4 drops olive or grapeseed carrier oil. Consume with 4-8 oz. of water.

Storage
You may create multiple capsules ahead of time or create one each day. Keep in the freezer in a labeled glass container.

How long should you use these capsules?
- Do not take multiple recipes at the same time. Use only one for a couple of days and then rotate through a few to see what works best for your body.
- There are two types of Vitality™ line essential oil capsules you may make: daily capsules and bomb capsules.
- Daily capsules may be created as the recipe states and used for daily support.
- Bomb capsules may be created using double or triple the recipes to create a "bomb" for your system. A "bomb" is a stronger capsule intended to give more aggressive support. Bombs should only be used 1-2 times over the course of 4-8 hours and only once per month. Please consult your doctor if you are sick.
- Daily capsules and bombs are meant to help support your terrain, meaning they strengthen your already healthy systems, protecting them from dipping below the wellness line.
- Do not take multiple capsules for multiple systems at the same time. Give at least four hours between capsules.

IMMUNE SYSTEM CAPSULES

Immune System Daily Capsule Recipes Using Vitality™ Oils
- Recipe: 3 drops Thieves®, 1 drop Oregano
- Recipe: 3 drops Frankincense, 1 drop Orange, 1 drop Lavender
- Recipe: 2 drops Lemongrass, 2 drops Copaiba, 1 drop Basil
- Recipe: 1 drop Cinnamon Bark, 1 drop Clove, 1 drop Bergamot
- Recipe: 2 drops Lavender, 1 drop Frankincense, 1 drop Oregano
- Recipe: 2 drops Bergamot, 1 drop Basil, 1 drop Thyme, 1 drop Lemon
- Recipe: 1 drop Rosemary, 1 drop Peppermint, 1 drop Black Pepper
- Recipe: 2 drops Clove, 1 drop Lemon, 1 drop Lavender

Directions
Create a synergy first and then add 2-4 drops to a 0 or 00 size veggie capsule with carrier oil, or simply add the desired recipe, then top off with a minimum of 4 drops olive or grapeseed carrier oil. Consume with 4-8 oz. of water.

Storage
You may create multiple capsules ahead of time or create one each day.
Keep in the freezer in a labeled glass container.

How long should you use these capsules?
- Do not take multiple recipes at the same time. Use only one for a couple of days and then rotate through a few to see what works best for your body.
- There are two types of Vitality™ line essential oil capsules you may make: daily capsules and bomb capsules.
- Daily capsules may be created as the recipe states and used for daily support.
- Bomb capsules may be created using double or triple the recipes to create a "bomb" for your system. A "bomb" is a stronger capsule intended to give more aggressive support. Bombs should only be used 1-2 times over the course of 4-8 hours and only once per month. Please consult your doctor if you are sick.
- Daily capsules and bombs are meant to help support your terrain, meaning they strengthen your already healthy systems, protecting them from dipping below the wellness line.
- Do not take multiple capsules for multiple systems at the same time. Give at least four hours between capsules.

PROTOCOLS

INTEGUMENTARY SYSTEM CAPSULES

Integumentary System Daily Capsule Recipes Using Vitality™ Oils

SKIN
- Recipe: 2 drops Carrot Seed, 1 drop Frankincense, 1 drop Lavender
- Recipe: 3 drops Orange, 1 drop German Chamomile, 1 drop Coriander
- Recipe: 2 drops Copaiba, 2 drops Clove

HAIR
- Recipe: 1 drop Frankincense, 1 drop Orange, 1 drop Peppermint
- Recipe: 2 drops Rosemary, 1 drop Lavender

NAILS
- Recipe: 2 drops Lemon, 1 drop Lavender, 1 drop Frankincense
- Recipe: 1 drop Copaiba, 1 drop Jade Lemon™, 1 drop Lavender

Directions
Create a synergy first and then add 2-4 drops to a 0 or 00 size veggie capsule with carrier oil, or simply add the desired recipe, then top off with a minimum of 4 drops olive or grapeseed carrier oil. Consume with 4-8 oz. of water.

Storage
You may create multiple capsules ahead of time or create one each day.
Keep in the freezer in a labeled glass container.

How long should you use these capsules?
- Do not take multiple recipes at the same time. Use only one for a couple of days and then rotate through a few to see what works best for your body.
- There are two types of Vitality™ line essential oil capsules you may make: daily capsules and bomb capsules.
- Daily capsules may be created as the recipe states and used for daily support.
- Bomb capsules may be created using double or triple the recipes to create a "bomb" for your system. A "bomb" is a stronger capsule intended to give more aggressive support. Bombs should only be used 1-2 times over the course of 4-8 hours and only once per month. Please consult your doctor if you are sick.
- Daily capsules and bombs are meant to help support your terrain, meaning they strengthen your already healthy systems, protecting them from dipping below the wellness line.
- Do not take multiple capsules for multiple systems at the same time. Give at least four hours between capsules.

PROTOCOLS

LYMPHATIC SYSTEM CAPSULES

Lymphatic System Daily Capsule Recipes Using Vitality™ Oils
- Recipe: 1 drop Thieves®, 1 drop Grapefruit
- Recipe: 2 drops Lemongrass, 1 drop Lime, 1 drop Lemon
- Recipe: 1 drop Nutmeg, 1 drop Lime
- Recipe: 1 drop Rosemary, 1 drop Grapefruit
- Recipe: 2 drops Peppermint, 1 drop Lemon, 1 drop Nutmeg
- Recipe: 2 drops Grapefruit, 1 drop Ginger

Directions
Create a synergy first and then add 2-4 drops to a 0 or 00 size veggie capsule with carrier oil, or simply add the desired recipe, then top off with a minimum of 4 drops olive or grapeseed carrier oil. Consume with 4-8 oz. of water.

Storage
You may create multiple capsules ahead of time or create one each day. Keep in the freezer in a labeled glass container.

How long should you use these capsules?
- Do not take multiple recipes at the same time. Use only one for a couple of days and then rotate through a few to see what works best for your body.
- There are two types of Vitality™ line essential oil capsules you may make: daily capsules and bomb capsules.
- Daily capsules may be created as the recipe states and used for daily support.
- Bomb capsules may be created using double or triple the recipes to create a "bomb" for your system. A "bomb" is a stronger capsule intended to give more aggressive support. Bombs should only be used 1-2 times over the course of 4-8 hours and only once per month. Please consult your doctor if you are sick.
- Daily capsules and bombs are meant to help support your terrain, meaning they strengthen your already healthy systems, protecting them from dipping below the wellness line.
- Do not take multiple capsules for multiple systems at the same time. Give at least four hours between capsules.

NERVOUS SYSTEM CAPSULES

Nervous System Daily Capsule Recipes Using Vitality™ Oils
GENERAL NERVOUS SYSTEM
- Recipe: 3 drops Orange, 1 drop Frankincense, 1 drop Lavender
- Recipe: 2 drops Lavender, 1 drop Peppermint

BRAIN
- Recipe: 1 drop Peppermint, 1 drop Thyme, 1 drop Cardamom
- Recipe: 2 drops Orange, 1 drop Lemongrass, 1 drop Lavender
- Recipe: 2 drops Frankincense, 2 drops Thyme

Directions
Create a synergy first and then add 2-4 drops to a 0 or 00 size veggie capsule with carrier oil, or simply add the desired recipe, then top off with a minimum of 4 drops olive or grapeseed carrier oil. Consume with 4-8 oz. of water.

Storage
You may create multiple capsules ahead of time or create one each day.
Keep in the freezer in a labeled glass container.

How long should you use these capsules?
- Do not take multiple recipes at the same time. Use only one for a couple of days and then rotate through a few to see what works best for your body.
- There are two types of Vitality™ line essential oil capsules you may make: daily capsules and bomb capsules.
- Daily capsules may be created as the recipe states and used for daily support.
- Bomb capsules may be created using double or triple the recipes to create a "bomb" for your system. A "bomb" is a stronger capsule intended to give more aggressive support. Bombs should only be used 1-2 times over the course of 4-8 hours and only once per month. Please consult your doctor if you are sick.
- Daily capsules and bombs are meant to help support your terrain, meaning they strengthen your already healthy systems, protecting them from dipping below the wellness line.
- Do not take multiple capsules for multiple systems at the same time. Give at least four hours between capsules.

RENAL SYSTEM CAPSULES

Renal System Daily Capsule Recipes Using Vitality™ Oils

RENAL SYSTEM GENERAL
- Recipe: 2 drops Carrot Seed, 2 drops Lemon, 1 drop Lavender
- Recipe: 1 drop Fennel, 1 drop Citrus Fresh™

KIDNEY
- Recipe: 2 drops Grapefruit, 1 drop Orange, 1 drop Copaiba
- Recipe: 2 drops Copaiba, 1 drop Jade Lemon™, 1 drop Tangerine

BLADDER
- Recipe: 1 drop Thyme, 1 drop Lime, 1 drop Copaiba, 1 drop Orange
- Recipe: 1 drop Clove, 1 drop Lemon, 1 drop Rosemary
- Recipe: 2 drops Mountain Savory, 1 drop Lemongrass, 1 drop Lavender

URINARY TRACT
- Recipe: 2 drops Celery Seed, 1 drop Tarragon, 1 drop Lemon
- Recipe: 2 drops Fennel, 1 drop Copaiba, 1 drop Lavender

Directions
Create a synergy first and then add 2-4 drops to a 0 or 00 size veggie capsule with carrier oil, or simply add the desired recipe, then top off with a minimum of 4 drops olive or grapeseed carrier oil. Consume with 4-8 oz. of water.

Storage
You may create multiple capsules ahead of time or create one each day.
Keep in the freezer in a labeled glass container.

How long should you use these capsules?
- Do not take multiple recipes at the same time. Use only one for a couple of days and then rotate through a few to see what works best for your body.
- There are two types of Vitality™ line essential oil capsules you may make: daily capsules and bomb capsules.
- Daily capsules may be created as the recipe states and used for daily support.
- Bomb capsules may be created using double or triple the recipes to create a "bomb" for your system. A "bomb" is a stronger capsule intended to give more aggressive support. Bombs should only be used 1-2 times over the course of 4-8 hours and only once per month. Please consult your doctor if you are sick.
- Daily capsules and bombs are meant to help support your terrain, meaning they strengthen your already healthy systems, protecting them from dipping below the wellness line.
- Do not take multiple capsules for multiple systems at the same time. Give at least four hours between capsules.

RESPIRATORY SYSTEM CAPSULES

Respiratory System Daily Capsule Recipes Using Vitality™ Oils
- Recipe: 2 drops Peppermint, 2 drops Frankincense, 1 drop Lavender
- Recipe: 2 drops Lavender, 2 drops Lemon, 2 drops Peppermint
- Recipe: 2 drops Thieves®, 1 drop Ginger, 1 drop Copaiba, 1 drop Peppermint
- Recipe: 2 drops Copaiba, 1 drop Laurus Nobilis, 1 drop Lemongrass
- Recipe: 2 drops Lemongrass, 1 drop Oregano, 1 drop Rosemary, 1 drop Lime
- Recipe: 2 drops Cardamom, 1 drop Lavender, 1 drop Peppermint

Directions
Create a synergy first and then add 2-4 drops to a 0 or 00 size veggie capsule with carrier oil, or simply add the desired recipe, then top off with a minimum of 4 drops olive or grapeseed carrier oil. Consume with 4-8 oz. of water.

Storage
You may create multiple capsules ahead of time or create one each day. Keep in the freezer in a labeled glass container.

How long should you use these capsules?
- Do not take multiple recipes at the same time. Use only one for a couple of days and then rotate through a few to see what works best for your body.
- There are two types of Vitality™ line essential oil capsules you may make: daily capsules and bomb capsules.
- Daily capsules may be created as the recipe states and used for daily support.
- Bomb capsules may be created using double or triple the recipes to create a "bomb" for your system. A "bomb" is a stronger capsule intended to give more aggressive support. Bombs should only be used 1-2 times over the course of 4-8 hours and only once per month. Please consult your doctor if you are sick.
- Daily capsules and bombs are meant to help support your terrain, meaning they strengthen your already healthy systems, protecting them from dipping below the wellness line.
- Do not take multiple capsules for multiple systems at the same time. Give at least four hours between capsules.

PROTOCOLS

PROTOCOLS

GENERAL HEALTH PROTOCOL

This protocol is a basic, healthy lifestyle protocol from which everyone 12 years and older can benefit. It covers all your bases for optimal dietary supplementation. You may add targeted nutrition items such as Sulfurzyme®, a hormone support like FemiGen™, or any other Young Living® supplement that is right for you.

SUPPLEMENTS FOR THIS PROTOCOL
- NingXia Red®
- Master Formula™
- MultiGreens™
- Life 9®
- OmegaGize3®
- Olive Essentials™
- Essentialzymes-4™ (or choose one of the digestive enzymes)
- Super Cal™ Plus (optional for additional plant derived calcium)
- Super B™ (optional for additional B support)

IDEAL SUPPLEMENT SCHEDULE

Breakfast
- NingXia Red® - Drink 1-2 oz. with breakfast.
- Master Formula™ - Take all 4 capsules with breakfast.
- OmegaGize3® - Take 2 capsules with breakfast.
- Olive Essentials™ - Take 1 capsule with breakfast.
- Super B™ - Take 1 tablet with breakfast.
- Super Cal™ Plus - Take 2 capsules with breakfast, or split the dose: one at breakfast, one at lunch or dinner.

Lunch
- Essentialzymes-4™ - Take 2 capsules (one dual dose blister pack) just before lunch.
- Super B™ - Take 1 tablet with lunch.
- MultiGreens™ - Take 3 capsules with lunch.

Dinner
- Essentialzymes-4™ - Take 2 capsules (one dual dose blister pack) just before dinner.
- MultiGreens™ - Take 3 capsules with dinner.
- OmegaGize3® - Take 2 capsules with dinner.

After Dinner
- Life 9® - Take 1 capsule 2-3 hours after dinner on an empty stomach. Do not take with any internal essential oils.

How long should you use this protocol?
Every person's needs are different and everyone's situation is different. Some may need to take this type of protocol every day for the rest of their lives, while others may only need it during certain seasons. Please be your own best advocate and always check with your doctor before starting or stopping any specific regimen.

These statements have not been evaluated by the Food and Drug Administration.
Young Living® products are not intended to diagnose, treat, cure, or prevent any disease.

AGING GRACEFULLY PROTOCOL

There are several things you can do to keep your systems working well if you are over 60. It is encouraged to also continue to move by getting 15-20 minutes of walking per day and eating lots of fruits and vegetables. If you are currently taking prescription drugs, make sure you check with your doctor before starting this protocol. It is recommended that you take natural supplements at a different time than your prescriptions. Give a minimum of four hours between them.

SUPPLEMENTS FOR THIS PROTOCOL
- NingXia Red®
- Super B™
- Super Cal™ Plus
- Super Vitamin D
- CardioGize™
- OmegaGize3®
- AgilEase™
- Sulfurzyme® capsules or powder
- Essentialzymes-4™
- IlluminEyes™
- Longevity™
- ImmuPro™

IDEAL SUPPLEMENT SCHEDULE
Breakfast
- Super B™ - Take 2 tablets before or with breakfast.
- NingXia Red® - Drink 1-2 oz. with breakfast.
- OmegaGize3® - Take 2 capsules with breakfast.
- Super Cal™ Plus - Take 2 capsules with breakfast.
- Super Vitamin D - Take 1-2 tablets with breakfast.
- CardioGize™ - Take 1 capsule with breakfast.

Between Breakfast and Dinner
- AgilEase™ - Take 2 capsules.
- Sulfurzyme® - Take 2-3 capsules or ½ tsp. powder with juice or water.

Lunch
- Essentialzymes-4™ - Take 2 capsules (one dual dose blister pack) just before lunch.
- Longevity™ - Take 1 capsule with lunch.

Dinner
- Essentialzymes-4™ - Take 2 capsules (one dual dose blister pack) just before dinner.
- IlluminEyes™ - Take 1 capsule with dinner.
- OmegaGize3® - Take 2 capsules with dinner.

Before Bed
- Life 9® - Take one capsule 1 hour before bed.
- ImmuPro™ - Chew 1 tablet just before bed.

How long should you use this protocol?
Every person's needs are different and everyone's situation is different. Some may need to take this type of protocol every day for the rest of their lives, while others may only need it during certain seasons. Please be your own best advocate and always check with your doctor before starting or stopping any specific regimen.

These statements have not been evaluated by the Food and Drug Administration.
Young Living® products are not intended to diagnose, treat, cure, or prevent any disease.

PROTOCOLS

BONE HEALTH PROTOCOL

As we age, bone density becomes more and more important to consider. There are multiple types of calcium and the key is to know what they are used for as well as how much calcium is actually in the supplement. The amount in each supplement is called Elemental Calcium. It can be a little confusing to figure out what is what in the world of calcium, but the key is to choose one based on your personal needs. Young Living® has products that contain calcium ascorbate, calcium carbonate, dicalcium phosphate, calcium fructoborate, and calcium citrate. The most common calcium supplements are calcium carbonate and calcium citrate.

- Calcium Carbonate is what is taken to help ease stomach acid. You find this in antacids to help with heartburn and stomach acid. It contains about 40% of elemental calcium. It is known to cause constipation.
- Calcium Citrate is what is used when stomach acid is low. It is a gentler form of calcium and is easier to absorb.
- Calcium Fructoborate is a natural derivative of boron. Boron is an important mineral to support bone density and reduce inflammation.
- Dicalcium Phosphate is not a technical source of calcium but is used by doctors and herbalists to help repair joints.
- Calcium Ascorbate is essentially vitamin C with about 10% calcium. People use this as it is a gentler form of calcium and will not cause gas. It is easily absorbed and you do not need to eat food with it. The downside is the small amount of calcium per serving.

While supplementation is often necessary, the best form of calcium comes from your diet. The most bioavailable forms are from non-animal sources such as seeds (poppy, sesame, and chia), beans, lentils, almonds, spinach, kale, seaweed, and figs. While these foods have a low RDI (recommended daily intake) of calcium, these sources are far more bioavailable than isolated supplements such as calcium carbonate and calcium citrate.

Another form of calcium, found in red algae is not often found in supplements, but is far more bioavailable than other forms of calcium. Super Cal™ Plus from Young Living® contains a synergistic blend of bioavailable calcium, magnesium, and trace minerals. These are derived from red algae that is harvested off the coast of Iceland. When you truly want to support your bones, you need to make sure you have calcium, magnesium, D3, and K2. Super Cal™ Plus has it all. For even more support, consider bumping up your mineral intake and also get some extra D3.

There are some lifestyle choices that can cause loss of calcium. Two factors that cause excess calcium elimination are caffeine and sodium. Limit these when using this protocol. Also, be sure to not take these natural supplements at the same time as pharmaceuticals. Give a four-hour buffer before or after.

These statements have not been evaluated by the Food and Drug Administration.
Young Living® products are not intended to diagnose, treat, cure, or prevent any disease.

SUPPLEMENTS FOR THIS PROTOCOL
- Super Cal™ Plus (for calcium, magnesium, D3, and K2)
- Mineral Essence™ (for magnesium and boron)
- Super Vitamin D (D3 for absorption)
- CardioGize™ (for K2)

IDEAL SUPPLEMENT SCHEDULE

Breakfast
- Super Cal™ Plus - Take 2 capsules with breakfast, or split the dose: one at breakfast, then one at lunch.
- Super Vitamin D - Take 2 capsules with breakfast, or split the dose: one at breakfast, then one at lunch.
- CardioGize™ - Take 2 capsules with breakfast, or split the dose: one at breakfast, then one at lunch.

Lunch
- Optional: Mineral Essence™ - Take 5 half-droppers (1ml each).

Dinner
- Mineral Essence™ - Take 5 half-droppers (1ml each) or put in 5 capsules.

How long should you use this protocol?
Every person's needs are different and everyone's situation is different. Some may need to take this type of protocol every day for the rest of their lives, while others may only need it during certain seasons. Please be your own best advocate and always check with your doctor before starting or stopping any specific regimen.

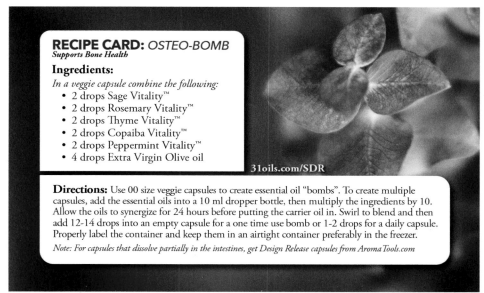

RECIPE CARD: *OSTEO-BOMB*
Supports Bone Health

Ingredients:
In a veggie capsule combine the following:
- 2 drops Sage Vitality™
- 2 drops Rosemary Vitality™
- 2 drops Thyme Vitality™
- 2 drops Copaiba Vitality™
- 2 drops Peppermint Vitality™
- 4 drops Extra Virgin Olive oil

31oils.com/SDR

Directions: Use 00 size veggie capsules to create essential oil "bombs". To create multiple capsules, add the essential oils into a 10 ml dropper bottle, then multiply the ingredients by 10. Allow the oils to synergize for 24 hours before putting the carrier oil in. Swirl to blend and then add 12-14 drops into an empty capsule for a one time use bomb or 1-2 drops for a daily capsule. Properly label the container and keep them in an airtight container preferably in the freezer.
Note: For capsules that dissolve partially in the intestines, get Design Release capsules from AromaTools.com

BRAIN HEALTH AND COGNITION PROTOCOL

The brain is a complex organ that should not be overlooked when considering your overall health. Our memory, thought process, ability to move and think, sight, speech, emotions, and logic all rely on the brain. Loss of any one of these functions would be catastrophic for most of us, yet we often take them for granted until they are gone. Support your brain naturally by eating a diet rich in omega-3s, such as salmon and tuna, antioxidant-rich berries like blueberries and strawberries, broccoli, nuts, avocados, and other healthy items rich in antioxidants and healthy fats. Also, make sure to get at least 15-30 minutes of exercise at least five times a week. The added benefits to your brain when you simply take a walk every day are exceptionally powerful. There are also some things to stay away from, such as processed sugar, alcohol, processed foods, and interestingly, staying up late and not getting enough sleep. Out of all of these, getting enough sleep is the most important thing to help support your brain. Most people need 7-9 hours of sleep per night, and the average American gets 6.8 hours of sleep. Over time, this will compound upon itself causing sleep deprivation. Sleep deprivation causes memory loss and a slower functionality rate in motor skills. It is important to consider these tips when working on improving your brain health. The Brain Health and Cognition Protocol features products known to help support cardiovascular and cognitive health. The ingredients in this protocol support memory function, focus, and overall brain health.

SUPPLEMENTS FOR THIS PROTOCOL
- MindWise™ Sachets
- OmegaGize3®
- Super B™
- CardioGize™ (do not use if you are on blood thinners)
- Olive Essentials™
- NingXia Red®
- NingXia Nitro®

IDEAL SUPPLEMENT SCHEDULE

Breakfast
- CardoGize™ - Take 2 capsules before breakfast.
- NingXia Red® - Drink 1-2 oz. with breakfast.
- OmegaGize3® - Take 2 capsules with breakfast.
- Super B™ - Take 1 tablet with breakfast.
- Olive Essentials™ - Take 1 capsule with breakfast.
- MindWise™ Sachets - Take 1 sachet just after breakfast.

Lunch
- NingXia Red® - Drink 1-2 oz. with lunch.
- NingXia Nitro® - Drink 1 tube with lunch. (optional as needed)
- Super B™ - Take 1 tablet with lunch.
- OmegaGize3® - Take 2 capsules with lunch.

How long should you use this protocol?
Every person's needs are different and everyone's situation is different. Some may need to take this type of protocol every day for the rest of their lives, while others may only need it during certain seasons. Please be your own best advocate and always check with your doctor before starting or stopping any specific regimen.

These statements have not been evaluated by the Food and Drug Administration.
Young Living® products are not intended to diagnose, treat, cure, or prevent any disease.

BUDGET FRIENDLY PROTOCOL

The supplements in this protocol are well rounded and at a lower cost, plus many of them are able to be split up and spread out over a longer amount of time. Going slow with supplements is a good way to get the benefits on a tight budget. Most of these will last two or more months. The most expensive one is Sulfurzyme® but you can make that last for up to five months making it only $12.30 per month! Read up on what each supplement does to choose what is right for you. The baseline supplement protocol would include Super Cal™ Plus, Super B™, Super Vitamin D, and Sulfurzyme®, three of Young Living's® most popular supplements at only $44.30 per month. It is important to listen to your body and increase or decrease supplements based on how you are feeling. Some may need more than is posted in this protocol, while others may need less.

SUPPLEMENTS FOR THIS PROTOCOL
- Super Cal™ Plus ($27.50 wholesale for 60 capsules)
  Take 1 per day to last two months.
- Super B™ ($21 wholesale for 60 capsules)
  Take 1 per day to last two months.
- Super Vitamin D ($31 wholesale for 120 tablets)
  Take 1 every day to last four months.
- Sulfurzyme® Capsules ($61.50 wholesale for 300 capsules)
  Take 2 per day to last five months.

IDEAL SUPPLEMENT SCHEDULE

Breakfast
- Super B™ - Take 1 tablet with breakfast.
- Super Cal™ Plus - Take 1 capsule with breakfast.
- Super Vitamin D - Take 1 tablet with breakfast

Between Breakfast and Lunch
- Sulfurzyme® - Take 2 capsules.

Other Supplements to consider when on a tight budget
- AlkaLime™ ($31 wholesale for 30 servings)
  Take 1 every other day to last two months.

- FemiGen™ ($24.25 wholesale for 60 capsules)
  Take 1 per day to last two months.

- Inner Defense® ($28.50 wholesale for 30 softgels)
  Take 1 twice a week or as needed to last 3-4 months.

- Super C™ Chewables ($34 wholesale for 90 tablets)
  Take 1 per day for three months.

CHOLESTEROL SUPPORT PROTOCOL

Cholesterol is a waxy particle found in the blood. There is good and bad cholesterol. The liver creates 75% of cholesterol we have in our body, while 25% comes from food sources. Cholesterol is necessary for healthy cells and to help the cells do their job correctly.

Good cholesterol (HDL) is responsible for taking cholesterol from the cells to the liver. The liver will then break down the cholesterol and pass it out of the body in the feces. Bad cholesterol (LDL) takes cholesterol from the liver back into the cells. While cholesterol in the cells is necessary, a build up can cause health issues such as a restriction of blood and oxygen to the organs.

The liver cleans toxins from our body and eliminates them through urine from the kidneys. In the case of cholesterol, the liver eliminates it through the colon. Supporting the liver and the digestive process through a diet high in fiber-rich vegetables, good fats, such as nuts and avocados, along with the use of digestive enzymes high in Lipase and Protease, omega-3 fatty acids high in DHA, magnesium, and probiotics can improve proper cholesterol levels.

SUPPLEMENTS FOR THIS PROTOCOL

- JuvaTone® (for general liver support)
- Essentialzymes-4™ (for Lipase & Protease)
  Alternative: Allerzyme™ or Detoxzyme®
- Mineral Essence™ (for magnesium)
- OmegaGize3® (for DHA)
- Olive Essentials™ (supports blood)
- Life 9® (supports gut health)
- JuvaPower® (optional - for liver support)
- Daily capsule: Happy Blood Capsule

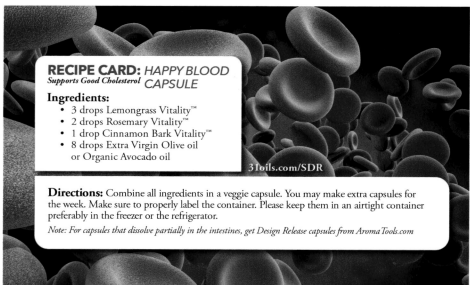

RECIPE CARD: *HAPPY BLOOD*
Supports Good Cholesterol *CAPSULE*

Ingredients:
- 3 drops Lemongrass Vitality™
- 2 drops Rosemary Vitality™
- 1 drop Cinnamon Bark Vitality™
- 8 drops Extra Virgin Olive oil
  or Organic Avocado oil

31oils.com/SDR

Directions: Combine all ingredients in a veggie capsule. You may make extra capsules for the week. Make sure to properly label the container. Please keep them in an airtight container preferably in the freezer or the refrigerator.

Note: For capsules that dissolve partially in the intestines, get Design Release capsules from AromaTools.com

IDEAL SUPPLEMENT SCHEDULE

Before Breakfast
- Take 1 "Happy Blood Capsule". Use a veggie capsule filled with 3 drops Lemongrass Vitality™, 2 drops Rosemary Vitality™, 1 drop Cinnamon Bark Vitality™ with 8 drops olive or avocado oil. Take with 4-8 oz. of water.

Breakfast
- Mineral Essence™ - Add 5 half-droppers (1 ml each) as a shot or with juice.
- OmegaGize3® - Take 2 capsules with breakfast.
- Olive Essentials™ - Take 1 capsule with breakfast.

Between Breakfast and Lunch
- JuvaTone® - Take 2 tablets.

Before Lunch
- Essentialzymes-4™ - Take 2 capsules (one dual dose blister pack) before lunch.

Between Lunch and Dinner
- JuvaTone® - Take 2 tablets.

Before Dinner
- Essentialzymes-4™ - Take 2 capsules (one dual dose blister pack) before dinner.

Dinner
- OmegaGize3® - Take 2 capsules with dinner.

After Dinner
- Life 9® - Take 1 capsule 2-3 hours after dinner, on an empty stomach. Do not take with any internal essential oils.

How long should you use this protocol?
Every person's needs are different and everyone's situation is different. Some may need to take this type of protocol every day for the rest of their lives, while others may only need it during certain seasons. Please be your own best advocate and always check with your doctor before starting or stopping any specific regimen.

These statements have not been evaluated by the Food and Drug Administration. Young Living® products are not intended to diagnose, treat, cure, or prevent any disease.

PROTOCOLS

PROTOCOLS

COLON CLEANSE PROTOCOL

Our intestines are home to a whole host of potential issues. Waste can pile up and depending on your age and size, you are storing anywhere from 5-20 pounds of fecal matter in your body at any given time. If not eliminated correctly, it can cause health issues. The large intestine is your colon and measures at about five feet long. The small intestine comes in at a whopping 20 feet long, making the combined length of your intestines 25 feet. Colon cleansing can improve your health by removing unwanted toxins from your gastrointestinal tract. It can improve your immune system, as well as help to improve your overall energy levels. You may take other supplements with this protocol, such as Master Formula™ and NingXia Red®.

SUPPLEMENTS FOR THIS PROTOCOL
- NingXia Red® (for antioxidant support)
- ICP™ (laxative, intestinal tract support)
- ComforTone® (mild laxative, intestinal tract support)
- JuvaTone® (liver support with dandelion)
- CardioGize™ (supports the cardiovascular system)
- Digest & Cleanse® (supports digestion) see sub option if out of stock.
- Essentialzyme™ (supports digestion)
- Life 9® (supports gut health)

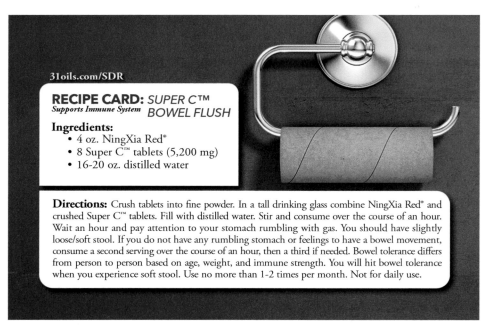

31oils.com/SDR

RECIPE CARD: *SUPER C™*
Supports Immune System *BOWEL FLUSH*

Ingredients:
- 4 oz. NingXia Red®
- 8 Super C™ tablets (5,200 mg)
- 16-20 oz. distilled water

Directions: Crush tablets into fine powder. In a tall drinking glass combine NingXia Red® and crushed Super C™ tablets. Fill with distilled water. Stir and consume over the course of an hour. Wait an hour and pay attention to your stomach rumbling with gas. You should have slightly loose/soft stool. If you do not have any rumbling stomach or feelings to have a bowel movement, consume a second serving over the course of an hour, then a third if needed. Bowel tolerance differs from person to person based on age, weight, and immune strength. You will hit bowel tolerance when you experience soft stool. Use no more than 1-2 times per month. Not for daily use.

Digest + Cleanse™ Substitute:
Add 2 drops each Peppermint, Caraway, Ginger, Fennel, and Lemon Vitality™ essential oils, topped off with 4 drops carrier oil to a veggie capsule.

IDEAL SUPPLEMENT SCHEDULE

1 Hour Before Breakfast
- Digest & Cleanse® - Take 1 capsule.

Breakfast
- NingXia Red® - Drink 1-2 oz. with breakfast.
- CardioGize™ - Take 2 capsules just before breakfast.
- ICP™ - Mix 2 rounded teaspoons with at least 8 oz. of juice or water.
- ComforTone® - Take 1 capsule.

1 Hour After Breakfast
- JuvaTone® - Take 2 tablets.

1 Hour Before Lunch
- Essentialzyme™ - Take 1 tablet.

Lunch
- ComforTone® - Take 1 capsule.

1 Hour After Lunch
- JuvaTone® - Take 2 tablets.

1 Hour Before Dinner
- Digest & Cleanse® - Take 1 capsule.

Dinner
- ICP™ - Mix 2 rounded teaspoons with at least 8 oz. of juice or water.
- ComforTone® - Take 1 capsule.

After Dinner
- Life 9® - Take 1 capsule 2-3 hours after dinner, on an empty stomach. Do not take with any internal essential oils.

Note: Do not take CardioGize™ if you are on blood thinning medication.

How long should you use this protocol?
This is recommended as a 4-7 day protocol. Every person's needs are different and everyone's situation is different. Please be your own best advocate and always check with your doctor before starting or stopping any specific regimen.

DIGESTIVE, GUT, AND COLON HEALTH PROTOCOL

Gut health seems to be on the top of everyone's mind. A quick look at Google trends and you will find that the search term "best foods for gut health" had a 350% increase from 2012 to 2017 in the USA. More and more people are learning that healing our gut will go a long way in healing our various ailments. It has been studied that simply improving the gut bacteria in a patient can help support the health of diabetics, heart health, IBS, obesity, autoimmune disorders, ADHD, as well as healthy emotions and peace.

Our gut is often referred to as our little brain or second brain. The technical term for it is the enteric nervous system, or ENS. It is comprised of two thin layers that contain more than 100 million nerve cells that line your entire GI (gastrointestinal) tract, from your esophagus all the way down to your rectum. While most focus on only the intestinal tract, it is important to realize that a healthy gut starts in your mouth with your saliva enzymes.

Probiotics are the healthy or good bacteria in your gut. When you are sick, it usually means there is more bad bacteria than good bacteria. Eating foods rich in probiotics is a great way to support the healthy or good bacteria in your gut. Yogurt, kefir, and sauerkraut are excellent sources, but many people need to supplement with a broader spectrum of healthy probiotics. One of the best broad-spectrum probiotics on the market is Life 9® from Young Living®.

Another option would be KidScents® MightyPro™, which contains broad-spectrum probiotics along with prebiotics. When you feel like the bad bacteria has overtaken the good bacteria, it is helpful to dose, using Life 9® for 1-2 days, taking 2-6 times the recommended dose on an empty stomach, just before bed. Only do this for one or two days, maximum, then resume your normal one capsule per day.

SUPPLEMENTS FOR THIS PROTOCOL
- Life 9® and/or KidScents® MightyPro™ (probiotics)
- NingXia Red® (contains prebiotics and L-Glutamine Amino Acid)
- OmegaGize³® (for D3 and omegas)
- Super B™ (supports digestion and gut health)
- AminoWise® (contains L-Glutamine Amino Acid)
- FemiGen™ (contains Licorice Root)
- Essentialzyme™ (contains Betaine hydrochloride)

IDEAL SUPPLEMENT SCHEDULE

Breakfast
- KidScents® MightyPro™ - Take 1 packet with breakfast.
- NingXia Red® - Drink 1-2 oz. with breakfast.
- Super B™ - Take 1 tablet with breakfast.
- OmegaGize3® - Take 2 capsules with breakfast.
- FemiGen™ - Take 1 capsule with breakfast.

Lunch
- Super B™ - Take 1 tablet with lunch.
- OmegaGize3® - Take 2 capsules with lunch.
- FemiGen™ - Take 1 capsule with lunch.

Between Lunch and Dinner or During Exercise
- AminoWise® - Mix 1 scoop with 8 oz. of water and consume after lunch or during or after exercise.

Before Dinner
- Essentialzyme™ - Take 1 capsule one hour before dinner.

After Dinner
- Life 9® - Take 1 capsule 2-3 hours after dinner on an empty stomach. Do not take with any internal essential oils.

How long should you use this protocol?
Every person's needs are different and everyone's situation is different. Some may need to take this type of protocol every day for the rest of their lives, while others may only need it during certain seasons. Please be your own best advocate and always check with your doctor before starting or stopping any specific regimen.

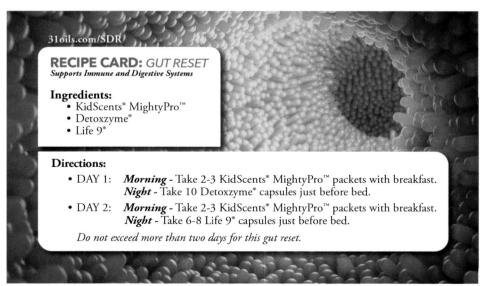

31oils.com/SDR

RECIPE CARD: *GUT RESET*
Supports Immune and Digestive Systems

Ingredients:
- KidScents® MightyPro™
- Detoxzyme®
- Life 9®

Directions:
- DAY 1: *Morning* - Take 2-3 KidScents® MightyPro™ packets with breakfast.
  Night - Take 10 Detoxzyme® capsules just before bed.
- DAY 2: *Morning* - Take 2-3 KidScents® MightyPro™ packets with breakfast.
  Night - Take 6-8 Life 9® capsules just before bed.

Do not exceed more than two days for this gut reset.

ENERGY SUPPORT PROTOCOL

We often find ourselves overworked, overwhelmed, and over everything. Energy levels drop and so does our motivation to get anything done. Supporting your digestive, immune, and endocrine systems are important to sustained energy.

SUPPLEMENTS FOR THIS PROTOCOL
- Super B™ (for energy)
- EndoGize™ (for Ashwagandha)
- Essentialzymes-4™ (for digestive enzyme)
- NingXia Red® (for immune system)
- NingXia Nitro® (for energy)

IDEAL SUPPLEMENT SCHEDULE

Breakfast
- NingXia Red® - Drink 1-2 oz. with breakfast.
- Super B™ - Take 1 tablet with breakfast.
- EndoGize™ - Take 1 capsule with breakfast. Use daily for four weeks. Discontinue for two weeks before resuming.

Lunch
- Essentialzymes-4™ - Take 2 capsules (one dual dose blister pack) before lunch.
- Super B™ - Take 1 tablet with lunch.
- NingXia Nitro® - Drink 1 tube after lunch. (optional)

Dinner
- Essentialzymes-4™ - Take 2 capsules (one dual dose blister pack) before dinner.
- EndoGize™ - Take 1 capsule with dinner. Use daily for four weeks. Discontinue for two weeks before resuming.

How long should you use this protocol?
Every person's needs are different and everyone's situation is different. Some may need to take this type of protocol every day for the rest of their lives, while others may only need it during certain seasons. Please be your own best advocate and always check with your doctor before starting or stopping any specific regimen.

EMOTIONAL SUPPORT PROTOCOL

Emotional states can vary drastically from day to day, moment by moment, and person to person. If you feel like your emotions are out of control, you are going through too many bouts of low or sad feelings, or you are going through hormone changes, there are several things you will want to consider. First, take a look at this list of food items that can wreak havoc on your emotions. Some you may know already, but some may be shocking. If you are dealing with sadness or are in a constant slump, this list may just change your life.

Foods to stay away from when feeling blue: gluten, soda - both regular and diet, coffee - both regular and decaf, all processed sugar, processed juice, like orange or apple juice, processed meats, like lunch meats, pepperoni, sausage, and jerky, high fructose corn syrup, energy drinks, alcohol - even wine, stay away from it, and trans fat found in frosting and many processed items. Below is a list of supplements to use to support healthy emotions. Please do not go off any medications unless you consult with your doctor. If you are taking pharmaceuticals, please do not take them at the same time as natural supplements.

SUPPLEMENTS FOR THIS PROTOCOL
- OmegaGize³® (for healthy omegas needed for the brain)
- Super B™ (for natural energy support)
- Super Vitamin D (for emotional health)
- NingXia Red® (for antioxidant support)
- NingXia Nitro® (for additional energy without the fall)
- ImmuPro™ (for zinc and better sleep)
- FemiGen™ (when needed for hormonal emotions)

IDEAL SUPPLEMENT SCHEDULE
Breakfast
- NingXia Red® - Drink 1-2 oz. with breakfast.
- Super B™ - Take 1 tablet with breakfast.
- Super Vitamin D - Take 2 tablets with breakfast.
- OmegaGize³® - Take 2 capsules with breakfast.
- FemiGen™ - Take 1 capsule with breakfast. (women only)

Lunch
- Super B™ - Take 1 tablet with lunch.
- OmegaGize³® - Take 2 capsules with lunch.
- FemiGen™ - Take 1 capsule with lunch. (women only)
- NingXia Nitro® - Drink 1 tube after lunch. (optional)

Before Bedtime
- ImmuPro™ - Take 1-2 chewable tablets just before bed.

How long should you use this protocol?
Every person's needs are different and everyone's situation is different. Some may need to take this type of protocol every day for the rest of their lives, while others may only need it during certain seasons. Please be your own best advocate and always check with your doctor before starting or stopping any specific regimen.

These statements have not been evaluated by the Food and Drug Administration.
Young Living® products are not intended to diagnose, treat, cure, or prevent any disease.

GLUCOSE SUPPORT PROTOCOL

To help control sugar, consider the following regimen. This is for both men and women. You may continue taking other foundation nutrition supplements, if you are taking them, such as Mineral Essence™ (recommended), MultiGreens™, Life 9®, and Master Formula™. Combine this protocol with exercise and plenty of water. Drink a minimum of 10 cups of water per day. Get more fiber by adding dark leafy greens to your diet, as well as good fats, such as avocados and unsalted raw nuts. Limit red meat consumption. Limit processed carbohydrates, like pasta, bread, and foods that are high in sugar.

SUPPLEMENTS FOR THIS PROTOCOL
- Balance Complete™
- NingXia Red®
- Slique® Tea - Ocotea Oolong
- Detoxzyme®
- OmegaGize3®
- Super B™
- Super Vitamin D
- Super Cal™ Plus
- EndoGize™

IDEAL SUPPLEMENT SCHEDULE

Breakfast
- Detoxzyme® - Take 2 capsules before breakfast.
- Balance Complete™ Shake - One shake for breakfast as a meal replacement.
- OmegaGize3® - Take 2 capsules with breakfast.
- Super B™ - Take 1 tablet with breakfast.
- Super Vitamin D - Take 1 tablet with breakfast.
- Super Cal™ Plus - Take 1 capsule with breakfast.
- NingXia Red® - Drink 1-2 oz. with breakfast.
- Slique® Tea - Ocotea Oolong - Drink 1 cup with breakfast (1 bag makes 2-4 cups). Note: if out of stock: use 1 drop Ocotea in warm or cold water 1-2 times per day.

Between Breakfast and Lunch
- EndoGize™ - Take 1 capsule between breakfast and lunch.

Lunch
- Detoxzyme® - Take 2 capsules before lunch.
- OmegaGize3® - Take 2 capsules with lunch.
- Super B™ - Take 1 tablet with lunch.
- Super Vitamin D - Take 1 tablet with lunch.
- Super Cal™ Plus - Take 1 capsule with lunch.
- Slique® Tea - Ocotea Oolong - Drink 1 cup with lunch (1 bag makes 2-4 cups).

Between Lunch and Dinner
- EndoGize™ - Take 1 capsule between lunch and dinner.

Dinner
- Detoxzyme® - Take 2 capsules before dinner.
- OmegaGize3® - Take 2 capsules with dinner.

How long should you use this protocol?
Every person's needs are different and everyone's situation is different. Some may need to take this type of protocol every day for the rest of their lives, while others may only need it during certain seasons. Please be your own best advocate and always check with your doctor before starting or stopping any specific regimen.

These statements have not been evaluated by the Food and Drug Administration. Young Living® products are not intended to diagnose, treat, cure, or prevent any disease.

GLUTEN SUPPORT PROTOCOL

Gluten sensitivity and intolerance can vary greatly from person to person. Gluten allergies or sensitivities are manifested in several ways, from headaches, swelling, bloating, gas, acne, and even intense bouts of emotional instability from anger to extreme sadness. Note: if you are diagnosed with Celiac Disease, do not use this protocol and do not consume any forms of wheat, gluten, or many grains.

Many people have sensitivities to gluten and may not know it. The only real way to find relief is to not consume any gluten. Gluten is found in anything containing American grain wheat, barley grass, and rye. It turns up in soy sauce, salad dressings, and even French fries that have been fried in oil that was previously used for something such as battered onion rings.

People with gluten intolerances absolutely must check every label and take extra precautions when eating out. Even the smallest particle will cause a response. The following protocol is not meant to help you eat gluten. It is a means to help your body process it through your system if you are eating something that could have cross contamination. This usually happens when eating at a friend's home or out at a restaurant. Digestive enzymes are a key support to help your body digest gluten.

SUPPLEMENTS FOR THIS PROTOCOL
- Essentialzymes-4™
- Allerzyme™

IDEAL SUPPLEMENT SCHEDULE

Take 10 minutes before eating a meal that may contain gluten
- Essentialzymes-4™ - Take 2-4 capsules (1-2 dual dose blister pack).
- Allerzyme - Take 2-4 capsules.

Note on Allerzyme™: While this supplement is noted to contain Barley grass, which is a possible contaminant, the Barley grass itself does not contain any gluten. The only way to have a gluten response from Barley grass is if the production of the grass was contaminated with the Barley seed, which contains gluten. Young Living's® Allerzyme™ contains clean Barley grass, however it is up to each individual to decide if they are going to try this supplement. Allerzyme™ is specifically noted to help support the proper digestion of wheat products.

How long should you use this protocol?
It is not recommended to use this protocol as an excuse to eat gluten. Gluten and lectins are very hard on the digestive system. It is best to stay away from gluten, and only use this when you think you might be eating something that could be cross-contaminated or when you're unsure if it's gluten-free. This protocol is not for those with Celiac Disease. Please be your own best advocate and always check with your doctor before starting or stopping any specific regimen.

PROTOCOLS

HEALTHY HAIR, SKIN, AND NAILS PROTOCOL

Having great hair, skin, and nails is something most women desire. Men too, but women especially. The three keys to a healthy integumentary system are: eat a diet rich in a colorful array of vegetables, drink lots of water, and find daily peace. Stress is one of the most prevalent causes of hair loss, brittle nails, and skin conditions such as rashes and blemishes. One of the best things you can do for your integumentary system is to relax, and drink a tall glass of water. Taking a walk daily that gets your heart pumping and skin sweating is helpful too, in order to stimulate your circulatory system and lymphatic system which is needed to help flush toxins from your skin.

Your hair, skin, and nails may also be compromised, or go through health fluctuations due to hormonal changes. By monitoring your hormones and taking the necessary precautions to keep your body healthy, you can mitigate many of the issues that arise from hormonal shifts. See the next section called "Hormone Support Protocols Introduction" for details on how to keep your endocrine system working at its best.

The most common supplements to support the largest organ in the body, also known as the integumentary system (your hair, skin, nails, and exocrine glands), are antioxidants in the form of vitamins A, C, and E, Coenzyme Q10, fatty acids found in fish oils, all the B vitamins, D3, K2, calcium, MSM, magnesium, and small amounts of selenium. This protocol is designed to help support your entire integumentary system.

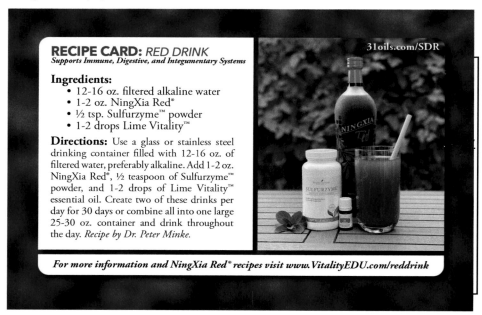

RECIPE CARD: *RED DRINK*
Supports Immune, Digestive, and Integumentary Systems

Ingredients:
- 12-16 oz. filtered alkaline water
- 1-2 oz. NingXia Red®
- ½ tsp. Sulfurzyme™ powder
- 1-2 drops Lime Vitality™

Directions: Use a glass or stainless steel drinking container filled with 12-16 oz. of filtered water, preferably alkaline. Add 1-2 oz. NingXia Red®, ½ teaspoon of Sulfurzyme™ powder, and 1-2 drops of Lime Vitality™ essential oil. Create two of these drinks per day for 30 days or combine all into one large 25-30 oz. container and drink throughout the day. *Recipe by Dr. Peter Minke.*

31oils.com/SDR

For more information and NingXia Red® recipes visit www.VitalityEDU.com/reddrink

SUPPLEMENTS FOR THIS PROTOCOL

- NingXia Red® (antioxidant)
- Sulfurzyme® (MSM to strengthen hair and nails)
- AgilEase™ (collagen for glowing skin)
- OmegaGize3® (Vitamin D3 for hair loss, Coenzyme Q10 for free radicals, and EPA for wrinkles and acne)
- Super Cal™ Plus (calcium for hair loss, magnesium for wrinkles and strong nails, D3 for hair, K2 for aging and skin)
- Super C™ Chewables and Tablets (antioxidant)
- Super B™ (a must for glowing skin and strong nails)
- Super Vitamin D (D3 for hair strength)
- Mineral Essence™ (magnesium for wrinkles and strong nails, selenium for hair)
- IlluminEyes™ (supports eyes, hair, skin, and nails)

IDEAL SUPPLEMENT SCHEDULE

Breakfast

- Super C™ - Take 1-2 tablets before breakfast.
- NingXia Red® - Drink 1-2 oz. with breakfast.
- OmegaGize3® - Take 2 capsules with breakfast.
- Super Cal™ Plus - Take 2 capsules with breakfast.
- Super B™ - Take 1 tablet with breakfast.
- Super Vitamin D - Take 2 tablets with breakfast.
- IlluminEyes™ - Take 1 capsule with breakfast.

Between Breakfast and Lunch

- Sulfurzyme® - Take 2-3 capsules or ½ tsp. powder with juice or water. You may also make yourself the "Red Drink." (see recipe on page 62)

Lunch

- OmegaGize3® - Take 2 capsules with lunch.
- AgilEase™ - Take 2 capsules with lunch.
- Super B™ - Take 1 tablet with lunch.
- Super C™ Chewables - Take 1 chewable tablet with lunch.
- Mineral Essence™ - Take 5 half-droppers (1 ml each) with breakfast. You may use five 00 veggie capsules.

Between Lunch and Dinner

- Sulfurzyme® - Take 2-3 capsules or ½ tsp. powder with juice or water.

Dinner

- Mineral Essence™ - Take 5 half-droppers (1 ml each) with dinner. You may use five 00 veggie capsules.
- Super C™ Chewables - Take 1 chewable tablet with dinner.

How long should you use this protocol?

Every person's needs are different and everyone's situation is different. Some may need to take this type of protocol every day for the rest of their lives, while others may only need it during certain seasons. Please be your own best advocate and

HORMONE SUPPORT PROTOCOLS INTRODUCTION

Our hormones come from our endocrine system. It is comprised of 10 glands, nine for each sex. The eight glands common to both sexes are the hypothalamus, pineal, pituitary, thyroid, parathyroid, thymus, adrenals, and pancreas. For men, they also have testes (testicles), and for women, ovaries. These glands secrete various hormones into the body using the bloodstream to help the body maintain homeostasis or balance within the body systems. The hormones support how we grow and develop, our metabolism and energy levels, our stress response, our wake and sleep patterns, the reproductive systems, and a whole host of other functions. It is important to have healthy blood and a healthy supply of it since blood is the carrier of all hormones.

There are four outside factors that can drastically affect your hormones positively or negatively. These factors are stress levels, sleep patterns, diet, and exercise habits. If you are experiencing changes in your hormones, consider these simple (or possibly not so simple) modifications to your lifestyle to support the needs of your body. Work on one or two at a time over the course of 30 days. Once you feel good about that change, try tackling another one for the next 30 days. Monitor how you feel and any positive changes you see.

1. **Drink more water.** Increasing your water consumption will help your circulation and improve not only your blood flow, but also your ability to remove waste from your body. Try drinking half of your body weight in ounces of water. As an example, if you weigh 200 pounds, you need 100 ounces of water. If you weigh 150 pounds, you need 75 ounces of water. Another method is 1 liter per 50 pounds of body weight.

2. **Add greens.** Add 1-2 more servings of dark green vegetables or leafy greens. This will help rid your body of oxidative stress and will help your blood and hormones work better. We are supposed to get at least 3-4 servings of vegetables per day, but many of consume much less than that.

3. **Get more sleep.** Go to bed one hour earlier than normal. Sleep is such an important factor when supporting your hormones. When you are sleep deprived (less than seven hours of sleep per night) your hormones become uncoordinated. Here are a couple of reasons to get more sleep if you still aren't convinced:
   #1 - Lack of sleep increases your hunger hormone. When you are awake, your brain will tell you to eat more, even if you don't need to.
   #2 - Lack of sleep causes your fat storage to get out of whack. Not getting enough sleep increases insulin resistance, essentially contributing to weight gain and obesity.

4. **Go on a walk.** Walking increases oxygen to your blood and brain, which is paramount for hormones to travel where they need to go. It is like traveling on a winding dirt road as opposed to a freshly paved straight highway. Try to take a 15-30 minute walk at least five times a week.

5. Create space. We tend to say "yes" to too many things. Start saying no, and create more white space on your calendar and your daily to-do list. This will give you some much needed downtime. Every time someone asks you to do something, consider if it is the best thing for you to do. Not every need is a calling. It is important to not overwhelm yourself helping everyone but you.

6. Take a nap. When you have an overwhelming number of items on your to-do list, you may feel guilty taking a nap. Don't worry about what others might think. Just do it. Taking a 30-minute nap, or even a 10-minute power nap when you are able to, will help your energy levels and motivation throughout the day. Because sleep is important to hormone production, a nap will give your body a quick refueling.

7. Limit noise. While social media has allowed us to seemingly get a lot more done and stay connected to a lot more people, it has also very successfully added loads of stress to our lives. Stress from social media comes from many angles: FOMO (fear of missing out), keeping up with the Jones's, people-pleasing, and time-sucking. It is the ultimate distraction and the ultimate relationship blocker. Next time you go to a restaurant, take a look around. Most parties are all on their cell phones. I recommend leaving your phone in the car when you are eating out, or leave your cell phone in the kitchen when you go to bed. Having a cell phone in your bedroom can damage your sleep patterns because of the incessant need to check it, but also because of the electromagnetic radiation that emits from cell phones that is poisoning your ability to sleep soundly. When you need your phone in your bedroom, simply shut the entire thing down at a specific time, at least one hour before bedtime.

8. Limit coffee and alcohol. Coffee and alcohol are both endocrine disruptors. This means they mess with your hormones. Coffee tells your adrenal glands that they can take a break. You've got it covered so the adrenals do not need to produce any "wake up" hormone (cortisol). Even one cup is damaging to your endocrine system. Alcohol dumps massive amounts of sugar into your system. Alcohol also imposes damaging effects on growth, metabolism, energy storage, bones, blood pressure, and the ability to get pregnant (this goes for both sperm count in men, and ovulation in women).

9. Ditch white sugar. Sugar in the form of table sugar and refined carbohydrates, such as bread and pasta, are a major insulin hormone disruptor also known as endocrine disruptor. Insulin is a highly connected hormone to all the other hormones and can directly affect a woman's estrogen levels and a man's testosterone levels. It is one of the hardest things to do, but going on a sugar moratorium for 30 days, and then hopefully longer, will go a long way in supporting healthy hormones. A sugar moratorium (aka no sugar, aka death to sugar) means not eating processed sugar. You will want to stay away from items with high glycemic indexes such as bread, muffins, cookies, and anything containing white sugar and/or wheat.

10. **Limit junk.** Both fast food and processed food contain hormone disrupting ingredients in the form of GMOs, preservatives, additives, synthetic flavoring, and other nasty things. Processed foods are notorious for messing with our bodies. A simple trip to any country outside of the USA, that has not adopted USA food practices, and you will find a much healthier nation with far less obesity, heart disease, and osteoporosis. Start by changing one meal that is usually processed or from a fast food establishment to a meal that is made with real ingredients. Some sneaky forms of processed foods to stay away from are: sandwiches, any processed meats such as sausage, pepperoni, and deli meats, milk (unless you live on a farm, do not consume processed milk), store-bought orange juice, sports drinks (while these seem like they replenish your body, all they are doing is flooding your system with sugar and salt), and bacon. Bacon? Noooooo! OK I hear you, but seriously, bacon is one of the worst foods you can eat. That is unless, of course, you own some pigs and are able to make your own. Otherwise, most bacon is filled with preservatives, nitrates, and hormones that you do NOT want in your system. Visit **www.endo180.com** for more tips on resetting your endocrine system through your diet.

11. **Ditch and switch.** Get rid of all the synthetic products in your home and replace them with synthetic-free versions. Petrochemicals are considered the worst invader on your endocrine system. They make up the majority of the plastics and synthetic molecules in many of the household and personal care products on the market today. Consider all areas such as cleaning supplies, laundry detergent, fabric softener, dish washing detergent, air fresheners, candles, facial wash and lotions, body lotions, toothpaste, deodorant, makeup, hand soap, hand sanitizer, shampoo, conditioner, body wash, etc.

While making lifestyle changes takes time, and in some cases can be next to impossible, because you know we are, after all, only human, I encourage you to consider adding some healthful supplements to your daily regimen. The following protocols cover various hormone needs. You will find six protocols: general hormone health for men, general hormone health for women, fertility support, adrenal support, menopause support, and thyroid support.

HORMONES (MEN) - GENERAL PROTOCOL

The below protocol is for general hormone health for men. It is important to monitor yourself to see how you feel. Note: While EndoGize™ states it is a women's supplement, that is only because the majority of customers in Young Living® are women. Please refer to the write up on EndoGize™ and you will see how powerful this supplement is for men specifically.

SUPPLEMENTS FOR THIS PROTOCOL
- EndoGize™
- Prostate Health™ (optional)
- OmegaGize3® (D3, Omegas)
- PowerGize™ (Fenugreek)
- JuvaPower® (Ginger root)

IDEAL SUPPLEMENT SCHEDULE

Breakfast
- EndoGize™ - Take 1 capsule with breakfast. Use daily for four weeks. Discontinue for two weeks before resuming.
- OmegaGize3® - Take 2 capsules with breakfast.
- JuvaPower® - Sprinkle 1 Tbsp. onto food, mix into shake mix or 4 oz. of water.

Between Breakfast and Lunch
- Prostate Health™ (optional) - Take 1 capsule between meals.

Lunch
- PowerGize™ - Take 2 capsules with lunch.
- JuvaPower® - Sprinkle 1 Tbsp. onto food, mix into shake mix or 4 oz. of water.

Between Lunch and Dinner
- Prostate Health™ (optional) - Take 1 capsule between meals.

Dinner
- EndoGize™ - Take 1 capsule with dinner. Use daily for four weeks. Discontinue for two weeks before resuming.
- OmegaGize3® - Take 2 capsules with dinner.
- JuvaPower® - Sprinkle 1 Tbsp. onto food, mix into shake mix or 4 oz. of water.

How long should you use this protocol?
EndoGize™ should be used daily for four weeks. Discontinue for two weeks before resuming. For the whole protocol, every person's needs are different and everyone's situation is different. Some may need to take this protocol every day for the rest of their lives, while others may only need it during certain seasons. Please be your own best advocate and always check with your doctor before starting or stopping any specific regimen.

These statements have not been evaluated by the Food and Drug Administration. Young Living® products are not intended to diagnose, treat, cure, or prevent any disease.

HORMONES (WOMEN) - MENOPAUSE PROTOCOL

As we age, our hormone production changes. We still have and need our hormones, but in some areas, such as reproduction, these hormones are not as necessary. This shift in hormones can cause undesirable effects in our body, such as night sweats, temperature regulation from hot to cold, and erratic mood swings. The supplements in this protocol will help regulate this process. It is important to note, women who are desiring to get pregnant may also follow this protocol. If you are going through menopause, and do not wish to become pregnant, please use precautions. This protocol effectively regulates and restores your reproductive system. During menopause, this protocol will slow down the process, and you could get pregnant. Synthetic fragrances and petrochemicals (plastics) in your products you use around the home can cause a major shift in your hormones. It is important to clean up as many synthetic items in your home as possible.

NOTE: This protocol is the same for those wanting to get pregnant. If you are going through perimenopause, use caution as this may also help your fertility.

SUPPLEMENTS FOR THIS PROTOCOL
- Progessence Plus™
- FemiGen™
- PD 80/20™
- Master Formula™ (vitamins A, B, D, E)

IDEAL SUPPLEMENT SCHEDULE

Before Breakfast
- Progessence Plus™ - Rub 1 drop on each inner arm, from the inner elbow to the inner wrist, when you wake up. You may rotate application sites. Other areas to apply: back of neck, front of neck, on the bottom of your feet, or on your inner thighs.

Breakfast
- FemiGen™ - Take 1 capsule with breakfast.
- PD 80/20™ - Take 1 capsule with breakfast.
- Master Formula™ - Take full packet with breakfast.

Before Bedtime
- Progessence Plus™ - Rub 1 drop on each inner arm, from the inner elbow to the inner wrist, when you wake up. You may rotate application sites. Other areas to apply: back of neck, front of neck, on the bottom of your feet, or on your inner thighs.

How long should you use this protocol?
Every person's needs are different and everyone's situation is different. Some may need to take this type of protocol every day for the rest of their lives, while others may only need it during certain seasons. Please be your own best advocate and always check with your doctor before starting or stopping any specific regimen.

These statements have not been evaluated by the Food and Drug Administration.
Young Living® products are not intended to diagnose, treat, cure, or prevent any disease.

HORMONES (WOMEN) - POST-MENOPAUSE PROTOCOL

The below protocol is for general hormone health in women who are post-menopause. Take note of how you feel and what amount works best for your needs.

SUPPLEMENTS FOR THIS PROTOCOL
- FemiGen™ (vaginal dryness, mood swings, metabolism)
- OmegaGize3® (heart and mood health)
- Super B™ (for folate and B12 for immune support and energy)
- Super Vitamin D (immune support and bone health)
- Super Cal™ Plus (immune support and bone health)
- Mineral Essence™ (boron and minerals for bone health)
- CardioGize™ (heart and bone health)
- Essentialzymes-4™ (digestive enzymes)

IDEAL SUPPLEMENT SCHEDULE

Breakfast
- Super B™ - Take 1 tablet with breakfast.
- Super Vitamin D - Take 1 tablet with breakfast.
- OmegaGize3® - Take 2 capsules with breakfast.
- Super Cal™ Plus - Take 1 capsule with breakfast.
- CardioGize™ - Take 1 capsule with breakfast.
- FemiGen™ - Take 1 capsule with breakfast.

Lunch
- Essentialzymes-4™ - Take 2 capsules (one dual dose blister pack) just before lunch.
- Super B™ - Take 1 tablet with lunch.
- Super Vitamin D - Take 1 tablet with lunch.
- OmegaGize3® - Take 2 capsules with lunch.
- Super Cal™ Plus - Take 1 capsule with lunch.
- CardioGize™ - Take 1 capsule with lunch.
- FemiGen™ - Take 1 capsule with lunch.

Dinner
- Essentialzymes-4™ - Take 2 capsules (one dual dose blister pack) just before lunch.
- Mineral Essence™ - Add 5 half-droppers (1 ml each) as a shot or with juice.

How long should you use this protocol?
Every person's needs are different and everyone's situation is different. Some may need to take this type of protocol every day, while others may only need it during certain seasons. Please be your own best advocate and always check with your doctor before starting or stopping any specific regimen.

PROTOCOLS

HORMONES - ADRENAL SUPPORT PROTOCOL

The adrenal glands are a part of your endocrine system, regulating energy output in the form of adrenaline and cortisol. When you are stressed out or get scared, your adrenals release hormones to help get you through the experience. It is commonly referred to as the "fight or flight" response. When you go through long periods of heightened stress, your body will produce more cortisol and adrenaline than normal for an extended period. This effectively wears out your adrenals and this could lead to what is called adrenal fatigue.

This protocol is not a treatment for adrenal fatigue. It is meant to help you manage stressful seasons so you do not get to the point of adrenal fatigue. If you are planning a move, switching careers, working through grief and loss, or anything that you know would cause longer periods of stress, you will want to consider this protocol. It is also important to protect your cells during times of stress by reducing the amount of processed sugar and increasing the amount of water you consume. Also, try to get 1-2 hours of extra sleep. While this may sound impossible during stressful times of your life, it is better to get some extra sleep than to binge watch television.

There are two different supplements from which to choose. CortiStop® would be selected when you are under mild stress, and EndoGize™ would be selected when you are under severe stress. Please note: EndoGize™ is only to be taken daily for four weeks and then you must discontinue for two weeks before resuming. Mineral Essence™ may be taken once or twice a day. Super B™ may be taken as one dose of 2 tablets with breakfast, but it is recommended to space out the 2 tablets for more prolonged energy support benefits. Super C™ is a completely different supplement compared to Super C™ Chewables. Super C™ regular tablets are the ones you want for this protocol.

SUPPLEMENTS FOR THIS PROTOCOL
- CortiStop® (mild)
- EndoGize™ (severe)
- Super B™
- Super C™
- Mineral Essence™ (for magnesium)

NOTE: There are two protocols to consider. One uses CortiStop® and one uses EndoGize™. Please see individual supplement write-ups to determine which is right for your needs.

IDEAL SUPPLEMENT SCHEDULE USING CORTISTOP®

Before Breakfast
- Super C™ - Take 1-2 tablets before breakfast.
- CortiStop® - Take 1-2 capsules before breakfast.

Breakfast
- Super B™ - Take 1 tablet with breakfast.
- Mineral Essence™ - Take 5 half-droppers (1 ml each) with breakfast. You may use five 00 veggie capsules.

Lunch
- Super B™ - Take 1 tablet with lunch.
- Mineral Essence™ - Take 5 half-droppers (1 ml each) with lunch. You may use five 00 veggie capsules.

Before Bedtime
- CortiStop® - Take 1-2 capsules before bedtime.

IDEAL SUPPLEMENT SCHEDULE USING ENDOGIZE™

Before Breakfast
- Super C™ - Take 1-2 tablets before breakfast.

Breakfast
- EndoGize™ - Take 1 capsule with breakfast. Use daily for four weeks. Discontinue for two weeks before resuming.
- Super B™ - Take 1 tablet with breakfast.
- Mineral Essence™ - Take 5 half-droppers (1 ml each) with breakfast. You may use five 00 veggie capsules.

Lunch
- Super B™ - Take 1 tablet with lunch.

Dinner
- EndoGize™ - Take 1 capsule with dinner. Use daily for four weeks. Discontinue for two weeks before resuming.
- Mineral Essence™ - Take 5 half-droppers (1 ml each) with dinner. You may use five 00 veggie capsules.

How long should you use this protocol?
EndoGize™ should be used daily for four weeks. Discontinue for two weeks before resuming. For the whole protocol, every person's needs are different and everyone's situation is different. Some may need to take this protocol every day for the rest of their lives, while others may only need it during certain seasons. Please be your own best advocate and always check with your doctor before starting or stopping any specific regimen.

PROTOCOLS

HORMONES - FERTILITY SUPPORT PROTOCOL

This protocol uses herbal supplements to help regulate your reproductive system. During normal reproductive years, this protocol will support a healthy system. If you are trying to get pregnant, please remove all synthetic toxins from your surroundings to the very best of your ability. This includes synthetic ingredients found in your makeup, personal care products, synthetic supplements, and toxic cleaning supplies. Consider all areas such as cleaning supplies, laundry detergent, fabric softener, dish washing detergent, air fresheners, candles, facial wash and lotions, body lotions, toothpaste, deodorant, makeup, hand soap, hand sanitizer, shampoo, conditioner, body wash, etc. Try to remove actual plastics as well. Memory foam is a massive petrochemical and should be avoided. Memory foam is found in many mattresses, pillows, running and walking shoes, and other items. Plastic shower curtains and pool blow up toys should not be used. If you can smell the plastic, that is the bad kind. Consider eliminating plastic water bottles and opt instead to use filtered water that you drink out of a glass or stainless steel container.

SUPPLEMENTS FOR THIS PROTOCOL
- Progessence Plus™
- PD 80/20™
- Master Formula™

IDEAL SUPPLEMENT SCHEDULE

Before Breakfast
- Progessence Plus™ - Rub 1 drop on each inner arm, from the inner elbow to the inner wrist, when you wake up. You may rotate application sites such as the back of neck, front of neck, on the bottom of your feet, or on your inner thighs.

Breakfast
- PD 80/20™ - Take 1 capsule with breakfast.
- Master Formula™ - Take full packet with breakfast.

Before Bedtime
- Progessence Plus™ - Rub 1 drop on each inner arm, from the inner elbow to the inner wrist, in the evening before you go to sleep. You may rotate application sites. Other areas to apply: back of neck, front of neck, on the bottom of your feet, or on your inner thighs.

How long should you use this protocol?
Every person's needs are different and everyone's situation is different. Some may need to take this type of protocol every day for the rest of their lives, while others may only need it during certain seasons. Please be your own best advocate and always check with your doctor before starting or stopping any specific regimen.

These statements have not been evaluated by the Food and Drug Administration.
Young Living® products are not intended to diagnose, treat, cure, or prevent any disease.

HORMONES - THYROID SUPPORT PROTOCOL

Supporting your thyroid can help increase energy, improve digestion and metabolism, help with mood swings, and supports healthy bones. It is important to consider dietary changes as well, like eating more vegetables and going on a daily walk to increase circulation. Please consult your doctor if you are currently on a thyroid supporting regimen. It is best to bring in the labels for each of the below supplements so he or she can see what they contain.

SUPPLEMENTS FOR THIS PROTOCOL
- Thyromin™ (natural thyroid support with pig and cow gland extracts)
- MultiGreens™ (contains Eleuthero to support the thyroid)
- JuvaTone® (contains Echinacea to support the thyroid)

IDEAL SUPPLEMENT SCHEDULE

Between Breakfast and Lunch
- JuvaTone® - Take 2 tablets between meals.

Lunch
- MultiGreens™ - Take 3 capsules with lunch.

Between Lunch and Dinner
- JuvaTone® - Take 2 tablets between meals.

Dinner
- MultiGreens™ - Take 3 capsules with dinner.

Before Bedtime
- Thyromin™ - Take 1-2 capsules, just before bed, on an empty stomach.

How long should you use this protocol?
Every person's needs are different and everyone's situation is different. Some may need to take this type of protocol every day for the rest of their lives, while others may only need it during certain seasons. Please be your own best advocate and always check with your doctor before starting or stopping any specific regimen.

PROTOCOLS

PROTOCOLS

HORSE HEALTH

The following are supplements safe to use with your horse. Please consult with your veterinary doctor prior to starting a new regimen.

SUPPLEMENTS TO CONSIDER

- NingXia Red® (immune system and gut health) - 1-4 oz. per day straight, in their water, or mixed into their feed.
- Detoxzyme® (digestive enzyme) - may use up to 20 capsules per day.
- Sulfurzyme® powder (joint support) - add 1-2 Tbsp to their feed per day.
- K&B™ Tincture (kidney and bladder support) - 10-15 drops in bottom lip gum area morning and night.
- Life 9® (probiotic for immune system and gut health) - 2-4 capsules in their feed per day or as needed.
- DiGize™ Vitality™ (digestive support) - 10 drops in bottom lip gum area.
- Thieves® Vitality™ (immune system support) - 5 drops with equal parts carrier in bottom lip gum area.

How should I approach my horse with these supplements?
Every horse is different. Pay close attention to your horse's behavior when introducing supplements. Check with your veterinary doctor before starting or stopping any specific regimen.

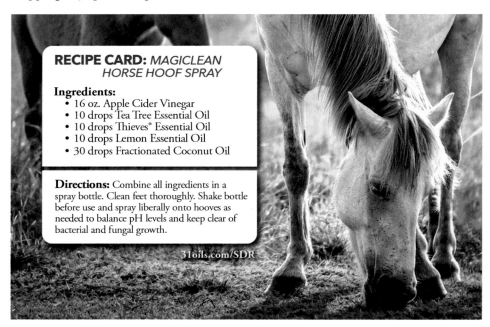

RECIPE CARD: *MAGICLEAN HORSE HOOF SPRAY*

Ingredients:
- 16 oz. Apple Cider Vinegar
- 10 drops Tea Tree Essential Oil
- 10 drops Thieves® Essential Oil
- 10 drops Lemon Essential Oil
- 30 drops Fractionated Coconut Oil

Directions: Combine all ingredients in a spray bottle. Clean feet thoroughly. Shake bottle before use and spray liberally onto hooves as needed to balance pH levels and keep clear of bacterial and fungal growth.

31oils.com/SDR

These statements have not been evaluated by the Food and Drug Administration.
Young Living® products are not intended to diagnose, treat, cure, or prevent any disease.

IMMUNE SYSTEM SUPPORT PROTOCOL

When you ask a doctor, "What is the most important function in our body?" They will tell you that your immune system is the thing to keep strong. Our immune system is supported by our blood, lymph nodes, and gut. Supplements high in antioxidants are a must, but also a good diet, exercise, and getting enough sleep are important in supporting your immune system. The following is recommended to support all areas of your immune system. You may add additional supplements to this protocol, such as Super Cal™ Plus, Super B™, and Essentialzymes-4™, or any that you are already taking.

SUPPLEMENTS FOR THIS PROTOCOL
- NingXia Red®
- Super C™ Tablets
- Super C™ Chewables
- Super Vitamin D
- Olive Essentials™
- Inner Defense®
- Life 9®
- ImmuPro™

NOTE: Both Super C™ supplements are needed for this protocol. They are not the same.

IDEAL SUPPLEMENT SCHEDULE

Before Breakfast
- Inner Defense® - Take 1 capsule at least 20 minutes before breakfast.

Breakfast
- NingXia Red® - Drink 1-2 oz. with breakfast.
- Super C™ Tablets - Take 1-2 tablets with breakfast.
- Super Vitamin D - Take 2 tablets with breakfast
- Olive Essentials™ - Take 1 capsule with breakfast.

Lunch
- NingXia Red® - Drink 1-2 oz. with lunch or in the afternoon.

Dinner
- Super C™ Chewables - Take 1 chewable tablet with dinner.

After Dinner
- Life 9® - Take 1 capsule 2-3 hours after dinner, on an empty stomach. Do not take with any internal essential oils.
- ImmuPro™ - Take 1 chewable tablet 30 minutes before bed and at least an hour after taking Life 9®.

How long should you use this protocol?
Every person's needs are different and everyone's situation is different. Some may need to take this type of protocol every day for the rest of their lives, while others may only need it during certain seasons. Please be your own best advocate and always check with your doctor before starting or stopping any specific regimen.

PROTOCOLS

JOINT AND MOBILITY HEALTH PROTOCOL

As we age, our mobility declines. Our connective tissue is not as strong and our joints can become inflamed. This is also true of athletes who are putting extra pressure and continual strain on the joints. For those of you who are not aggressive athletes, it is always recommended to stretch every day, as well as get a minimum of 30 minutes of exercise per day. A walk around the block can sometimes be the best remedy. This will get your lymphatic and circulatory systems moving, to help rid waste and oxygenate your cells.

It is important to also drink plenty of water when desiring the support of healthy joints, ligaments, bones, and muscles. Simply drink half of your body weight number in ounces. For example: if you are 200 pounds, you would strive to drink 100 ounces of water per day.

Another often misunderstood area of concern, when it comes to joint and mobility health, is our diet. Many foods can cause inflammation in our bodies and the removal of these items can help tremendously. Consider lowering the intake of, or eliminating altogether, processed meats (sliced sandwich meats or canned meats), gluten (anything containing flour, such as breads and pasta), soybean and vegetable oils, processed foods such as chips and crackers, sodas, sugary drinks such as alcohol, trans fats found in fried foods, dairy such as cheese and milk, aspartame (sugar substitute), and all items containing corn such as popcorn, chips, corn tortillas, many cereals, and items where corn is hiding, such as salad dressings, chewing gum, peanut butter, soft drink sweeteners (corn syrup), etc. To find a great meal plan, go to **www.endo180.com** to help you take charge of the inflammatory response in your body. If you have a hard time with food elimination, please consider taking a digestive enzyme. The one recommended below is Allerzyme™.

Supplementation can help support in many ways. Using products with MSM, turmeric, omega-3 fatty acids, and spirulina may help improve mobility in both athletes and people who need additional support. It is also important to support your overall immune system and gut health.

SUPPLEMENTS FOR THIS PROTOCOL
- CBD by Nature's Ultra
- Life 9® and/or KidScents® MightyPro™
- NingXia Red®
- OmegaGize3®
- Sulfurzyme® (capsules or powder drink mix)
- AgilEase™
- MultiGreens™
- Allerzyme™ (optional)

IDEAL SUPPLEMENT SCHEDULE

Before Breakfast
- CBD by Nature's Ultra Dropper (flavor of your choice) - Place 0.5 to 1.0 ml on desired area.

Breakfast
- Allerzyme™ (optional) - Take 1 capsule just prior to breakfast.
- KidScents® MightyPro™ - Take 1 packet with breakfast.
- NingXia Red® - Drink 1-2 oz. with breakfast.
- OmegaGize3® - Take 2 capsules with breakfast.
- AgilEase™ - Take 2 capsules with breakfast.

Between Breakfast and Lunch
- Sulfurzyme® - Take 2-3 capsules or ½ tsp powder with juice or water.

Lunch
- Allerzyme™ (optional) - Take 1 capsule just prior to lunch.
- OmegaGize3® - Take 2 capsules with lunch.
- MultiGreens™ - Take 3 capsules with lunch.

Between Lunch and Dinner
- Sulfurzyme® - Take 2-3 capsules or ½ tsp powder with juice or water.

Dinner
- Allerzyme™ (optional) - Take 1 capsule just prior to dinner.
- MultiGreens™ - Take 3 capsules with dinner.

After Dinner
- Life 9® - Take 1 capsule, 2-3 hours after dinner, on an empty stomach. Do not take with any internal essential oils.

Before Bed
- CBD by Nature's Ultra Dropper (flavor of your choice) - Place 0.5 to 1.0 ml on desired area.

How long should you use this protocol?
Every person's needs are different and everyone's situation is different. Some may need to take this type of protocol every day for the rest of their lives, while others may only need it during certain seasons. Please be your own best advocate and always check with your doctor before starting or stopping any specific regimen.

These statements have not been evaluated by the Food and Drug Administration.
Young Living® products are not intended to diagnose, treat, cure, or prevent any disease.

PROTOCOLS

RECIPE CARD: *NINGXIA GUMMIES*
Supports Immune System

Ingredients:
- 8 oz. NingXia Red®
- 1 ½ tsp. Agar Agar powder
- 1 Tbsp. local organic Honey or Agave syrup
- 5 drops Tangerine Vitality™ oil
- 3 drops Lime Vitality™ oil
- 2 drops Lemon Vitality™ oil

Directions: Combine first three ingredients into a saucepan and heat on medium until fully dissolved, stirring continually. Once it begins to boil, remove from heat and continue to stir. Allow to cool while stirring, add the essential oils, then pour into silicone molds and place in the fridge to set. Pop out of molds and place in a jar. Keep them in the fridge or a cool place.

31oils.com/SDR

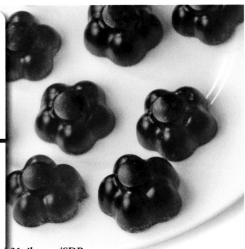

KID'S HEALTH PROTOCOL - GENERAL HEALTH SUPPORT

For kids 4 years and older.

SUPPLEMENTS FOR THIS PROTOCOL
- NingXia Red® (immune system support)
- KidScents® MightyZyme™ (digestive enzymes)
- KidScents® MightyVites™ (full-spectrum vitamin)
- KidScents® MightyPro™ (prebiotics and probiotics)
- Super C™ Chewables (antioxidants and immune system support)
- Super Vitamin D (respiratory and immune system support)

IDEAL SUPPLEMENT SCHEDULE

Breakfast
- KidScents® MightyVites™ - Take 2 chewable tablets.
- KidScents® MightyZyme™ - Take 1 chewable tablet.
- KidScents® MightyPro™ - Take 1 sachet.
- Super C™ Chewables - Take 1 chewable tablet.
- NingXia Red® - Drink 1-2 oz. with breakfast.
- Super Vitamin D - Take 1 tablet with breakfast.

Dinner
- KidScents® MightyVites™ - Take 2 chewable tablets.
- KidScents® MightyZyme™ - Take 1 chewable tablet.
- Super C™ Chewables - Take 1 chewable tablet.

How long should you use this protocol?

Pay close attention to your child and how they respond as they may not be able to tell you, or simply won't tell you. Keep track of their bowel movements and adjust accordingly. Please be your child's best advocate and always check with your doctor before starting or stopping any specific regimen.

These statements have not been evaluated by the Food and Drug Administration.
Young Living® products are not intended to diagnose, treat, cure, or prevent any disease.

KID'S HEALTH PROTOCOL - IMMUNE SYSTEM SUPPORT (4 DAYS)

For kids 4 years and older to be taken only for 1-4 days maximum.

SUPPLEMENTS FOR THIS PROTOCOL

- NingXia Red® (immune system support)
- KidScents® MightyPro™ (prebiotics and probiotics)
- Super C™ Chewables (immune system support)
- Super Vitamin D (respiratory and immune system support)
- Thieves® Vitality™ (immune system support)
- Frankincense Vitality™ (immune system support)

IDEAL SUPPLEMENT SCHEDULE

Breakfast

- KidScents® MightyPro™ - Take 1 sachet.
- Super C™ Chewables - Take 1 chewable tablet.
- Super Vitamin D - Take 1 tablet with breakfast.
- NingXia Red® - Drink 1-2 oz. with optional 1 drop only Thieves® Vitality™.

Afternoon

- NingXia Red® - Drink 1-2 oz. with 1-2 drops Frankincense Vitality™.

Dinner

- KidScents® MightyPro™ - Take 1 sachet.
- Super C™ Chewables - Take 1 chewable tablet.

How long should you use this protocol?

This protocol is meant to be used for only 1-4 days maximum. It is to rapidly support your child's immune system. Please be your child's best advocate and always check with your doctor before starting or stopping any specific regimen.

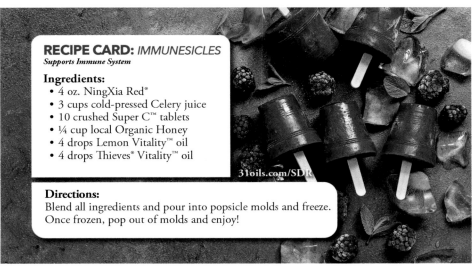

RECIPE CARD: *IMMUNESICLES*
Supports Immune System

Ingredients:
- 4 oz. NingXia Red®
- 3 cups cold-pressed Celery juice
- 10 crushed Super C™ tablets
- ¼ cup local Organic Honey
- 4 drops Lemon Vitality™ oil
- 4 drops Thieves® Vitality™ oil

31oils.com/SDR

Directions:
Blend all ingredients and pour into popsicle molds and freeze. Once frozen, pop out of molds and enjoy!

These statements have not been evaluated by the Food and Drug Administration. Young Living® products are not intended to diagnose, treat, cure, or prevent any disease.

PROTOCOLS

KID'S HEALTH PROTOCOL - INFANT TO TODDLER (AGE 1-4)

For kids ages 1-4 years.

SUPPLEMENTS FOR THIS PROTOCOL
- NingXia Red® (immune system support)
- Super C™ Chewables (antioxidants and immune system support)
- KidScents® MightyPro™ (optional for those 2 and older)

IDEAL SUPPLEMENT SCHEDULE

Breakfast
- Super C™ Chewables - Crush 1 chewable tablet and mix into applesauce.
- NingXia Red® - Drink 1 oz. with breakfast.
- KidScents® MightyPro™ - Take 1 sachet every other day. (2 years and older)

Dinner
- Super C™ Chewables - Crush 1 chewable tablet and mix into applesauce.

Optional (use discretion)

- MultiGreens™ - For toddlers able to eat solid food and yet are having a hard time getting vegetables in their diet, you may open 1-2 capsules of MultiGreens™ and mix the powder into some applesauce. Cinnamon flavored applesauce will help make the powder taste better. Make sure your child is drinking plenty of fluids. Water is always best.

How long should you use this protocol?
Pay close attention to your child and how they respond as they may not be able to tell you. Keep track of their bowel movements and adjust accordingly. Please be your child's best advocate and always check with your doctor before starting or stopping any specific regimen.

PROTOCOLS

KID'S HEALTH PROTOCOL - SCHOOL FOCUS SUPPORT
For kids 4 years and older.

SUPPLEMENTS FOR THIS PROTOCOL
- NingXia Red® (antioxidants)
- KidScents® Unwind™ (helps to increase GABA for better focus)
- KidScents® KidPower™ (encourages focus)

IDEAL SUPPLEMENT SCHEDULE

Breakfast
- NingXia Red® - Drink 1-2 oz. with breakfast.
- KidScents® Unwind™ - Take 1 sachet mixed with 4 oz. of cold water.
- KidScents® KidPower™ - Apply one drop to the back of the neck and wrists.

How long should you use this protocol?
You may use this protocol daily along with the Sleep protocol below. Pay close attention to your child and how they respond as they may not be able to tell you. Please be your child's best advocate and always check with your doctor before starting or stopping any specific regimen.

These statements have not been evaluated by the Food and Drug Administration. Young Living® products are not intended to diagnose, treat, cure, or prevent any disease.

PROTOCOLS

KID'S HEALTH PROTOCOL - SLEEP SUPPORT
For kids 4 years and older.

SUPPLEMENTS FOR THIS PROTOCOL
- KidScents® Unwind™ (supports natural melatonin in low light environments)
- KidScents® Sleepyize™ (encourages a more restful sleep)

IDEAL SUPPLEMENT SCHEDULE

Before Bed
- KidScents® Unwind™ - Take 1 sachet mixed with 4 oz. of water before bed.
- KidScents® SleepyIze™ - Apply one drop or with a roller fitment roll on to the back of the neck, on big toes, or in belly button.

How long should you use this protocol?
You may use this protocol nightly along with the School Focus protocol. Pay close attention to your child and how they respond as they may not be able to tell you. Please be your child's best advocate and always check with your doctor before starting or stopping any specific regimen.

These statements have not been evaluated by the Food and Drug Administration. Young Living® products are not intended to diagnose, treat, cure, or prevent any disease.

LIVER SUPPORT PROTOCOL

The liver is about the size of a football and sits on the right side of the belly inside the rib cage. It filters blood from the digestive system. It is the detox center of your body. Support your liver by eating a healthy diet high in vegetables and fiber, exercise regularly, don't drink alcohol that often, and try to avoid synthetics in the form of processed foods. This protocol is used for general liver support.

SUPPLEMENTS FOR THIS PROTOCOL
- AgilEase™ (turmeric is a powerful liver detoxifier)
- JuvaTone® (for overall liver support with high protein diets)
- JuvaPower® (for general liver and intestine support)
- Juva Cleanse® Vitality™ capsule (supports liver)
- JuvaFlex® Vitality™ capsule (supports liver and digestion)
- GLF™ Vitality™ capsule (supports gallbladder and liver)

IDEAL SUPPLEMENT SCHEDULE

Before Breakfast
- Juva Cleanse® Vitality™ - Add 2 drops Juva Cleanse® Vitality™ to a veggie capsule, top off with grapeseed or olive oil, and take with 8 oz. of water.

Breakfast
- JuvaPower® - Sprinkle 1 Tbsp. onto food, mix into shake mix or 4 oz. of water.
- AgilEase™ - Take 2 capsules with breakfast.

Between Breakfast and Lunch
- JuvaTone® - Take 2 tablets between meals.

Lunch
- JuvaPower® - Sprinkle 1 Tbsp. onto food, mix into shake mix or 4 oz. of water.
- JuvaFlex® Vitality™ - Add 2 drops JuvaFlex Vitality™ to a veggie capsule, top off with grapeseed or olive oil, and take with at least 8 oz. of water.

Between Lunch and Dinner
- JuvaTone® - Take 2 tablets between meals.

Dinner
- JuvaPower® - Sprinkle 1 Tbsp. onto food, mix into shake mix or 4 oz. of water.

Before Bedtime
- GLF™ Vitality™ - Add 2 drops GLF™ Vitality™ to a veggie capsule, top off with grapeseed or olive oil, and take with at least 8 oz. of water.

How long should you use this protocol?
Take this for a 3-4 day liver support or for up to one month. This is not recommended for 365 day use. Every person's needs are different and everyone's situation is different. Some may need to take this type of protocol every day for the rest of their lives, while others may only need it during certain seasons. Please be your own best advocate and always check with your doctor before starting or stopping any specific regimen.

These statements have not been evaluated by the Food and Drug Administration. Young Living® products are not intended to diagnose, treat, cure, or prevent any disease.

PROTOCOLS

LYMPHATIC SUPPORT PROTOCOL

The lymphatic system is directly connected to your immune system. Its job is to rid the body of toxic waste and transport immune supporting white blood cells throughout the body. The lymphatic system is stimulated by movement. If you have swelling in your fingers, cold hands and feet, brain fog, bloating, chronic fatigue, depression, and a feeling of stiffness or soreness when you wake in the morning, you may have a sluggish lymphatic or clogged immune system. Make sure you give your lymphatic system all the support it needs by using the right supplements, exercising, using lymphatic drainage techniques, and drinking plenty of water.

SUPPLEMENTS FOR THIS PROTOCOL
- AgilEase™ (turmeric is a powerful detoxifier)
- ComforTone® (for echinacea, garlic, and ginger)
- Super C™ Chewables (for citrus bioflavinoids)
- Cilantro Vitality™ (supports lymphatic drainage)
- Parsley Vitality™ (supports lymphatic drainage)
- Ginger Vitality™ (supports lymphatic drainage)
- GLF™ Vitality™ (supports lymphatic drainage)

IDEAL SUPPLEMENT SCHEDULE

Before Breakfast
- Lymph Capsule - Add 2 drops each of Cilantro, Parsley, and Ginger Vitality™ to a veggie capsule, top off with grapeseed or olive oil, and take with 8 oz. of water.

Breakfast
- Super C™ Chewable - Take 1 with breakfast.
- ComforTone® - Take 1 capsule with breakfast.

Lunch
- Super C™ Chewable - Take 1 with lunch.
- ComforTone® - Take 1 capsule with lunch.

Dinner
- Super C™ Chewable - Take 1 with dinner.
- ComforTone® - Take 1 capsule with dinner.

Before Bedtime
- AgilEase™ - Take 2 capsules before bed.
- GLF™ Vitality™ - Add 2 drops GLF™ Vitality™ to a veggie capsule, top off with grapeseed or olive oil, and take with at least 8 oz. of water.

How long should you use this protocol?
Do not use if pregnant. Take this for a 3-4 day lymphatic support protocol. This is not recommended for 365 day use. Every person's needs are different and everyone's situation is different. Some may need to take this type of protocol every day for the rest of their lives, while others may only need it during certain seasons. Please be your own best advocate and always check with your doctor before starting or stopping any specific regimen.

These statements have not been evaluated by the Food and Drug Administration. Young Living® products are not intended to diagnose, treat, cure, or prevent any disease.

PROTOCOLS

METAL DETOX PROTOCOL

Small amounts of metals are needed for our health, such as zinc, copper, and iron to name a few, but when there is too much, we can experience diarrhea, chills, weakness, vomiting, pain, and nausea. Both chelation and metabolism play a role in how our bodies rid itself of metal toxins. Chelation is when a substance binds or grabs toxins for removal. There are many natural chelators found in foods. Good fats such as nuts and avocados, garlic, onions, dark leafy greens, chlorella, and food-grade activated charcoal are all excellent chelators. Your metabolism and the metabolic function of plants play a significant role in helping to flush your body of toxins as well. Exercise, dry-brushing, and drinking a lot of water helps metabolize toxins from your body.

SUPPLEMENTS FOR THIS PROTOCOL
- NingXia Red® (supports flushing of toxins)
- Sulfurzyme® (supports the liver to help flush toxins)
- AgilEase™ (turmeric is an excellent natural chelator)
- MultiGreens™ (dark greens are natural chelators)
- Super C™ (high antioxidant and helps flush toxins)
- AminoWise® (amino acids support metal chelation)
- KidScents® MightyPro™ (probiotics help support immune function)
- Inner Defense® (helps support immune function and flushing)

IDEAL SUPPLEMENT SCHEDULE

Breakfast
- NingXia Red® - Drink 2 oz. with breakfast.
- AgilEase™ - Take 2 capsules with breakfast.
- MultiGreens™ - Take 3 capsules with breakfast.
- Super C™ - Take 1-2 chewables or tablets with breakfast
- KidScents® Mighty Pro™ - Take 1 packet with breakfast

Between Breakfast and Lunch
- Red Drink - 1-2 oz. NingXia Red® with 1/2 tsp. Sulfurzyme® in 16 oz. water.

Lunch
- MultiGreens™ - Take 3 capsules with lunch.
- AminoWise® - Use one scoop in 8 oz. of water with lunch.

Before Bedtime
- Inner Defense® - Take 1 softgel before bed.
- Super C™ - Take 1-2 chewables or tablets before bed.

How long should you use this protocol?
Take this for a seven day detox support then stop for at least seven days before resuming for a total of two months chelation. This is not recommended for 365 day use. Every person's needs are different and everyone's situation is different. Please be your own best advocate and always check with your doctor before starting or stopping any specific regimen.

PET - CAT HEALTH PROTOCOL

There are not many supplements that a cat will readily take. Most vitamins and minerals are found in cat food. Omega-3 supplements are helpful for shedding and a shiny coat. Probiotics are helpful to keep their gut and overall immune system healthy. The following protocol is worth trying with your cat, but in the end, remember to allow your cat to choose. If they do not accept the supplements, then by all means, leave them alone and do not force them.

SUPPLEMENTS FOR THIS PROTOCOL
- OmegaGize3®
- Life 9®

IDEAL SUPPLEMENT SCHEDULE

Breakfast
- OmegaGize3® - 1 capsule in their food bowl.

Dinner
- Life 9® - 1 capsule sprinkled in their food bowl.

How long should you use this protocol?
Every cat is different. Pay close attention to their behavior when introducing supplements. Please consider weight and activity level. Check with your veterinary doctor before starting or stopping any specific regimen.

NOTE ON ESSENTIAL OILS USE WITH CATS

Many cats (not all) lack the enzyme glucuronyl transferase which is an important liver metabolism catalyst for cytochrome P450. Without this enzyme, cats are open to potential toxicity from plants such as aloe, lilies, onions, and garlic; chocolates, pesticides, lead, zinc, caffeine, aspirin, ibuprofen, and essential oils high in phenols and terpenes. Below is a list of oils to avoid using or use highly diluted around cats.

- Phenols: Clove, Oregano, Cinnamon Bark, Tea Tree, Basil, Fennel, Oregano, Peppermint, Thyme, and Wintergreen
- Terpenes: Tea Tree, Citrus

The best way to approach cats with oils is to allow them to tell you what they like and don't like. They are super smart and usually come near with an oil they like or flee with an oil they don't like.

PROTOCOLS

PET - DOG HEALTH PROTOCOL - DIGESTIVE SUPPORT

SUPPLEMENTS FOR THIS PROTOCOL
- NingXia Red®
- Essentialzyme™
- K & B™ Tincture
- Life 9®

IDEAL SUPPLEMENT SCHEDULE

Breakfast
- NingXia Red® - 1 capful in water bowl with water.
- Essentialzyme™ - ½ tablet in food bowl.

Dinner
- K & B™ Tincture -
  5 drops for small dogs. Half dropper for large dogs in food.
- Life 9® - 1 capsule after dinner or sprinkled in food bowl.

How long should you use this protocol?
Every dog is different. Pay close attention to their behavior when introducing supplements. Please consider weight and activity level. Check with your veterinary doctor before starting or stopping any specific regimen.

These statements have not been evaluated by the Food and Drug Administration. Young Living® products are not intended to diagnose, treat, cure, or prevent any disease.

PET - DOG HEALTH PROTOCOL - HEALTHY COAT

SUPPLEMENTS FOR THIS PROTOCOL
- NingXia Red®
- Sulfurzyme® (capsules only)
- OmegaGize3®
- Mineral Essence™

IDEAL SUPPLEMENT SCHEDULE

Breakfast
- NingXia Red® - 1 capful in their water.
- OmegaGize3® - 1-2 capsules in their food bowl.
- Sulfurzyme® - 1 capsule opened and sprinkled into the food bowl.
  NOTE: You may use Sulfurzyme® powdered drink mix, but please pay close attention to their bowel movements. Too much stevia can cause diarrhea in dogs.

Dinner
- Mineral Essence™ - ½ dropper in food bowl.

How long should you use this protocol?
Every dog is different. Pay close attention to their behavior when introducing supplements. Please consider weight and activity level. Check with your veterinary doctor before starting or stopping any specific regimen.

These statements have not been evaluated by the Food and Drug Administration. Young Living® products are not intended to diagnose, treat, cure, or prevent any disease.

PET - DOG HEALTH PROTOCOL - MOBILITY SUPPORT

Depending on the size of your dog you may do this as a morning and evening regimen or only in the morning.

SUPPLEMENTS FOR THIS PROTOCOL
- NingXia Red®
- AgilEase™
- Sulfurzyme® (capsules only)

IDEAL SUPPLEMENT SCHEDULE

Breakfast
- NingXia Red® - 1 capful in water bowl with water.
- AgilEase™ - 1 capsule opened and sprinkled into the food bowl.
- Sulfurzyme® - 1 capsule opened and sprinkled into the food bowl.
  NOTE: You may use Sulfurzyme® powdered drink mix, but please pay close attention to their bowel movements. Too much stevia can cause diarrhea in dogs.

Dinner
- NingXia Red® - 1 capful in water bowl with water.
- AgilEase™ - 1 capsule opened and sprinkled into the food bowl.
- Sulfurzyme® - 1 capsule opened and sprinkled into the food bowl.
  NOTE: You may use Sulfurzyme® powdered drink mix, but please pay close attention to their bowel movements. Too much stevia can cause diarrhea in dogs.

How long should you use this protocol?
Every dog is different. Pay close attention to their behavior when introducing supplements. Please consider weight and activity level. Check with your veterinary doctor before starting or stopping any specific regimen.

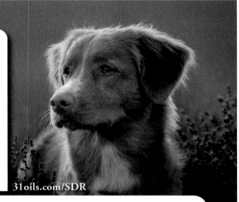

RECIPE CARD: *NINGXIA DOG TREATS*

Ingredients:
- 1 ¾ cups YL Einkorn Berries *(ground)* *(or 2 ½ cups Einkorn flour)*
- 1 large Egg
- ⅓ cup NingXia Red®
- ⅔ cup organic canned Pumpkin
- 3 Tbsp. organic Nut Butter of choice
- 1 mashed organic Banana
- 1 drop Cinnamon Vitality™
- ½ tsp. Salt
- ½ tsp. ground Cinnamon

31oils.com/SDR

Directions: Preheat oven to 300° Fahrenheit. Combine all ingredients and mix/mash using your hand. Dough will be thick and sticky. Roll out onto a lightly oiled baking sheet until ¼-½ inch thick. Score with pizza cutter to make ½ inch cubes. Bake for 40 minutes or until hard (or slightly soft for a chewy treat!) Cool completely then snap off pieces and store in an airtight container. Makes 400 treats. *Note: Cinnamon bark essential oil at this dose is not toxic to dogs.*

PREGNANCY AND BREASTFEEDING PROTOCOL

Pregnancy and breastfeeding pose specific health concerns for each individual mother. Please do your own research and consult with your doctor before starting any protocol. The following is a protocol that is a basic starting point for pregnant moms, followed by a list of supplements that are generally recognized as safe for pregnancy based on their ingredients. You will also see a list of supplements to use with caution and ones to avoid all together.

SUPPLEMENTS FOR THIS PROTOCOL
- NingXia Red® (for immune system support)
- Master Formula™ (for iron and nutrients)
- MultiGreens™ (for immune system support and nutrients)
- OmegaGize3® (for DHA and D3)
- Super Cal™ Plus (for building bones)
- Super Vitamin D (for immune and bone health)
- Super B™ (for folate)
- NingXia Nitro® (for energy support) - use sparingly
- Life 9® (for immune system support and gut health)
- Optional: Sulfurzyme® and one digestive enzyme - see Digestive Enzyme Usage Guide chart to select the one that is right for you.

IDEAL SUPPLEMENT SCHEDULE
Breakfast
- NingXia Red® - Drink 1-2 oz. with breakfast.
- Master Formula™ - Take all 4 capsules with breakfast.
- OmegaGize3® - Take 2 capsules with breakfast.
- Super B™ - Take 1 tablet with breakfast.
- Super Cal™ Plus - Take 2 capsules with breakfast, or split the dose: one at breakfast, one at lunch or dinner.
- Super Vitamin D - Take 2 tablets with breakfast.

Lunch
- Super B™ - Take 1 tablet with lunch.
- MultiGreens™ - Take 3 capsules with lunch.
- NingXia Nitro® - Drink 1 tube with lunch if needed (do not take after 3pm).

Dinner
- MultiGreens™ - Take 3 capsules with dinner.
- OmegaGize3® - Take 2 capsules with dinner.

After Dinner
- Life 9® - Take 1 capsule 2-3 hours after dinner on an empty stomach. Do not take with any internal essential oils.

How long should you use this protocol?
Every person's needs are different and everyone's situation is different. Some may need to take this type of protocol every day for the duration of their pregnancy and while breastfeeding. Please monitor yourself closely and consult your doctor. Please be your own best advocate and always check with your doctor before starting or stopping any specific regimen.

These statements have not been evaluated by the Food and Drug Administration.
Young Living® products are not intended to diagnose, treat, cure, or prevent any disease.

PREGNANCY AND BREASTFEEDING USAGE GUIDE

SAFE TO USE DURING PREGNANCY AND BREASTFEEDING

- AgilEase™
- AlkaLime®
- Allerzyme™
- AminoWise®
- Balance Complete™
- BLM™
- CBD by Nature's Ultra
- Detoxzyme®
- Essentialzyme™
- Essentialzymes-4™
- ICP™
- IlluminEyes™
- KidScents® - All
- Life 9®
- Master Formula™
- MindWise™
- Mineral Essence™
- MultiGreens™
- NingXia Red®
- Olive Essentials™
- OmegaGize3®
- PD 80/20™
- Pure Protein™ Complete
- Sulfurzyme®
- Super B™
- Super C™ Tablets and Chewables
- Super Cal™ Plus
- Super Vitamin D
- Slique® Bars
- Slique® Gum
- Slique® Shakes
- YL Vitality Drops

USE ONLY AS NEEDED DURING PREGNANCY (BREASTFEEDING IS OPTIONAL)

- Inner Defense® - OK for short term use - 1 capsule every so often as needed.
- ImmuPro™ - Melatonin is considered safe for occasional use but not daily use.
- K & B™ - Clove and Fennel should be used with caution in blends.
- Longevity™ - Internal use of essential oils should be used with caution.
- MegaCal™ - May cause constipation, which is not good for pregnancy.
- NingXia Nitro® - OK to use once per day or only when necessary.
- NingXia Zyng® - Limit the use of caffeine.
- Slique® Essence - Internal use of essential oils should be used with caution.
- Slique® Tea - Caffeine and natural stimulants are to be limited during pregnancy.
- Thyromin™ - Consult your doctor when using this supplement.

NOT ADVISED DURING PREGNANCY (BREASTFEEDING IS OPTIONAL)

- ComforTone® - Cascara Sagrada is not advised.
- JuvaTone® - Oregon Grape (Berberine) is not advised.
- Digest & Cleanse® - Excessive internal use of essential oils is not advised.
- ParaFree™ - Excessive internal use of essential oils is not advised.
- JuvaPower® - Anise and Slippery Elm can have estrogenic effects.
- CardioGize™ - Dong Quai, Motherwort, and Cat's Claw are not advised.
- CortiStop® - Black Cohosh, Clary Sage, and Fennel are not advised.
- EndoGize™ - Ashwagandha is not advised.
- FemiGen™ - Black Cohosh, Dong Quai, and Licorice Root are not advised.
- PowerGize™ - Ashwagandha is not advised.
- Rehemogen™ - Oregon Grape (Berberine) is not advised.
- SleepEssence™ - Rue is not advised.
- Slique® CitraSlim™ - Natural stimulants and internal use of oils is not advised.

PROTOCOLS

STRESS AND SLEEP SUPPORT PROTOCOL

When you are not getting enough sleep, your response to stress gets compromised. When you are stressed out, your ability to sleep well gets compromised. It is a terrible lose-lose cycle. Most people need 7-9 hours of sleep per night, and the average American gets 6.8 hours of sleep. Over time, this will compound upon itself, causing sleep deprivation. Sleep deprivation causes memory loss and a slower functionality rate in motor skills. Lack of sleep increases your hunger hormone, so when you are awake, your brain will tell you to eat more, even if you don't need to. Lack of sleep also causes your fat storage to get out of whack. Not getting enough sleep increases insulin resistance, essentially contributing to weight gain and obesity. Here are some supplements that may help you get a more restful night's sleep.

SUPPLEMENTS FOR THIS PROTOCOL
- Super B™ (for stress)
- CBD by Nature's Ultra Dropper (for stress and sleep)
- Mineral Essence™ (for magnesium)
- CardioGize™ (for resilience)
- ImmuPro™ or (for melatonin and immune system)
- Sleep Essence™ (for melatonin and immune system)

IDEAL SUPPLEMENT SCHEDULE

Before Breakfast
- CBD by Nature's Ultra Dropper (flavor of your choice) - Place 0.5 to 1.0 ml on desire area.

Breakfast
- CardioGize™ - Take 2 capsules before breakfast.
- Super B™ - Take 2 tablets with breakfast or split dosage with lunch.
- Mineral Essence™ - Take 5 half-droppers (1 ml each) with breakfast. You may use five 00 veggie capsules.

Dinner
- Mineral Essence™ - Take 5 half-droppers (1 ml each) with dinner. You may use five 00 veggie capsules.

Before Bedtime
- CBD by Nature's Ultra Dropper (flavor of your choice) - Place 0.5 to 1.0 ml on desired area.
- ImmuPro™ or Sleep Essence™ - Take 1-2 tablets or softgels just before bed.

How long should you use this protocol?
Every person's needs are different and everyone's situation is different. Some may need to take this type of protocol every day for the rest of their lives, while others may only need it during certain seasons. Please be your own best advocate and always check with your doctor before starting or stopping any specific regimen.

These statements have not been evaluated by the Food and Drug Administration.
Young Living® products are not intended to diagnose, treat, cure, or prevent any disease.

SYNTHETIC DETOX PROTOCOL

Many processed foods and pharmaceuticals contain harmful synthetics. Even some shots and inoculations contain synthetics and preservatives that are not healthful. Anytime you need to have a surgery or use pharmaceuticals, consider doing this detox before, during, and after. This will not guard you from mRNA changes or issues with injections that could cause permanent genetic damage. Please be your own best advocate!

LIFESTYLE THINGS TO CONSIDER:

- **Food:** For 1-2 weeks before and after any shot, try to eat as clean as possible. Eat little to no processed sugar or grains.
  Consider eating from the **www.Endo180.com** diet.

- **Water:** Drink at least half your body weight in ounces or 1 liter per 50 pounds. Example: if you weigh 200 pounds, drink 100 ounces or 4 liters of water per day.

- **Sweat:** Sweat it out by doing cardio exercise that is sweat inducing for at least 30 minutes a day for 2-3 days directly after getting the shot.

- **Bath:** Take an Epsom Salt bath after getting the shot. Use 4 cups of salt in a warm to hot bath and soak for 20 minutes.

SUPPLEMENTS TO CONSIDER USING:

- NingXia Red® (supports flushing of toxins)
- Sulfurzyme® (supports the liver to help flush toxins)
- AgilEase™ (turmeric is an excellent natural chelator)
- MultiGreens™ (dark greens are natural chelators)
- Super C™ (to bowel tolerance see Bowel Flush on page 54 - high antioxidant and helps flush toxins)
- MightyPro™ and/or Life 9® (probiotics help support immune function)
- Inner Defense® (helps support immune function and flushing)
- JuvaCleanse® Vitality™ essential oil (Use sublingual 20 minutes before event)
- Thieves® essential oil (use directly on site application both before and after)
- Additional: Organic Chlorella powder (rapidly flushes system)
- Additional: Activated Charcoal (rapidly flushes heavy metals)
- Additional: Cold Pressed Green Juice (use celery, cucumber chard, kale, spinach, parsley, cilantro)
- Additional: Fresh Crushed Garlic (natural detoxifier and chelator)

These statements have not been evaluated by the Food and Drug Administration.
Young Living® products are not intended to diagnose, treat, cure, or prevent any disease.

TEEN PROTOCOL

For teens (and adults) who don't like swallowing pills and who only have a one-minute attention span in the morning before school or work.

SUPPLEMENTS FOR THIS PROTOCOL

- NingXia Red®
- Super C™ Chewables
- Super Vitamin D
- Sulfurzyme® Capsules or Powder
- KidScents® MightyPro™
- KidScents® MightyVites™

IDEAL SUPPLEMENT SCHEDULE

Breakfast
- NingXia Red® - Drink 1-2 oz. with breakfast.
- Super C™ Chewables - Take 1-2 chewable tablets with breakfast.
- Super Vitamin D - Take 1 tablet with breakfast.
- Sulfurzyme® Capsules or Powder - Take 1 capsule or ¼ teaspoon mixed into NingXia Red® with breakfast.
- KidScents® MightyPro™ - Eat 1 packet with breakfast.
- KidScents® MightyVites™ - Eat 4-6 tablets with breakfast.

How long should you use this protocol?
Every person's needs are different and everyone's situation is different. Some teens may need to take this type of protocol every day, while others may only need it during certain seasons. Please be your own best advocate and always check with your doctor before starting or stopping any specific regimen.

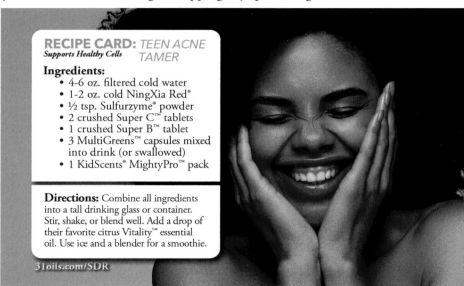

RECIPE CARD: *TEEN ACNE TAMER*
Supports Healthy Cells

Ingredients:
- 4-6 oz. filtered cold water
- 1-2 oz. cold NingXia Red®
- ½ tsp. Sulfurzyme® powder
- 2 crushed Super C™ tablets
- 1 crushed Super B™ tablet
- 3 MultiGreens™ capsules mixed into drink (or swallowed)
- 1 KidScents® MightyPro™ pack

Directions: Combine all ingredients into a tall drinking glass or container. Stir, shake, or blend well. Add a drop of their favorite citrus Vitality™ essential oil. Use ice and a blender for a smoothie.

31oils.com/SDR

These statements have not been evaluated by the Food and Drug Administration. Young Living® products are not intended to diagnose, treat, cure, or prevent any disease.

URINARY SUPPORT PROTOCOL

The urinary system, or renal system, is made up of the kidneys, ureters, bladder, and the urethra. It is important to support your urinary system by drinking lots of fluids. Water is best, and it is recommended that you get at least 80-100 ounces of water per day; more if you are excessively sweating or exercising.

SUPPLEMENTS FOR THIS PROTOCOL
- K & B™
- CardioGize™
- ComforTone®
- Super C™ Tablets
- NingXia Red®

IDEAL SUPPLEMENT SCHEDULE

Before Breakfast
- CardioGize™ - Take 2 capsules.
- Super C™ Tablets - Take 1-2 tablets.

Breakfast
- K & B™ - Take 3 half droppers in distilled water.
- NingXia Red® - Drink 1-2 oz. with breakfast.
- ComforTone® - Take 1 capsule.

Lunch
- K & B™ - Take 3 half droppers in distilled water.

Between Lunch and Dinner
- JuvaTone® - Take 2 tablets between meals.

Dinner
- K & B™ - Take 3 half droppers in distilled water.
- ComforTone® - Take 1 capsule.

Note: Do not take CardioGize™ if you are on blood thinning medication.

How long should you use this protocol?
Every person's needs are different and everyone's situation is different. Some may need to take this type of protocol every day for the rest of their lives, while others may only need it during certain seasons. Please be your own best advocate and always check with your doctor before starting or stopping any specific regimen.

These statements have not been evaluated by the Food and Drug Administration. Young Living® products are not intended to diagnose, treat, cure, or prevent any disease.

PROTOCOLS

WEIGHT SUPPORT PROTOCOL

Maintaining a healthy weight becomes more challenging as we grow older and our metabolism slows down. This protocol works well when you combine it with healthy eating and a daily exercise routine.

SUPPLEMENTS FOR THIS PROTOCOL
- Slique® Shake
- Slique® CitraSlim™
- Slique® Tea
- Slique® Bars
- Slique® Chewing Gum
- Peppermint, Lemon, Grapefruit , and Thieves® Vitality™

IDEAL SUPPLEMENT SCHEDULE

Before Breakfast
- Slique® CitraSlim™ - Take 2 powder capsules with 8 oz. of water.

Breakfast
- Slique® Shake - Drink one as a meal replacement for breakfast.
- Slique® Tea - Drink and add 1 drop of Thieves® Vitality™.

Between Breakfast and Lunch
- Infused Water - Drink 20+ oz. of water with 1 drop Peppermint Vitality™ and 1-2 drops each of Lemon Vitality™ and Grapefruit Vitality™.
- Slique® Bar - Eat one as a snack.

Lunch
- Eat a sensible, healthy lunch.

Between Lunch and Dinner
- Slique® CitraSlim™ - Take 1 powder capsule and 1 Slique® CitraSlim™ liquid capsule in the afternoon before 3pm.
- Infused Water - Drink 20+ oz. of water with 1 drop Peppermint Vitality™ and 1-2 drops each of Lemon Vitality™ and Grapefruit Vitality™.
- Slique® Tea - Drink in the afternoon.
- Eat a healthy snack or one Slique® Bar.
- Slique® gum - Chew 1 tablet to help hunger cravings.

Dinner
- Eat a sensible healthy dinner.

Exercise
- Get in a minimum of five 30-minute walks per week.

How long should you use this protocol?
30-90 days at a time. Every person's needs are different and everyone's situation is different. Please be your own best advocate and always check with your doctor before starting or stopping any specific regimen.

These statements have not been evaluated by the Food and Drug Administration. Young Living® products are not intended to diagnose, treat, cure, or prevent any disease.

BONUS: D. GARY YOUNG'S "HAPPY" & "GREAT DAY" PROTOCOLS

GREAT DAY PROTOCOL
Step 1: Use the "Happy" protocol every day.
This protocol was shared by D. Gary Young at a class in Wyoming in 1994. Slight modifications have been made based on new products.

"HAPPY" PROTOCOL
- Valor® - Apply on the bottoms of the feet, or a single drop on one wrist and hold the other wrist to it for a few moments to balance the entire system.
- Harmony™ - Use a single drop, over the solar plexus (above the belly button).
- Joy™ - Apply a single drop over the heart.
- White Angelica™ - Apply a single drop in one hand, rub hands together, and brush over the head, face, chest, shoulders, down the body, right over the clothes, as though applying an angelic shield.

Step 2: Drink 1-6 oz. of NingXia Red® every day.

Step 3: Take a Longevity™ capsule every day.

Step 4: Keep Stress Away™ in your pocket and use it anytime during the day.

Step 5: Take Master Formula™ every day.

Step 6: Take 1-3 MultiGreens™ capsules once or twice a day.

Step 7: Apply Thieves® and Peppermint on the bottom of your feet every day.

Step 8: Take SleepEssence™ (or ImmuPro™) before bed.

Step 9: Take Detoxzyme® before bed to help break down foods left in your system.

Step 10: Swap out all your household products for Thieves® Household Products for extra health benefits.

"Live every day in joy, gratitude, and appreciation!"
~ D. Gary Young

PROTOCOLS

This book gives suggestions on how to support healthy systems. It is not intended to treat or diagnose existing conditions or illnesses. Each supplement consists of multiple ingredients. Each ingredient listed has a basic description of what it is commonly used for in the medical and holistic practice industries. Herbs and roots have been used for centuries and the traditionally studied uses for each are readily found on sources such as Science Direct, the National Center for Biotechnology Information, U. S. National Library of Medicine, PubMed, and the Food and Drug Administration websites.

The content in this book has not been evaluated by the FDA and the supplements and protocols will not treat or cure any sickness or disease. The author is not a doctor and has published this book as a means to have a compilation of information, in one spot, to make it easier to understand the many supplements Young Living® carries.

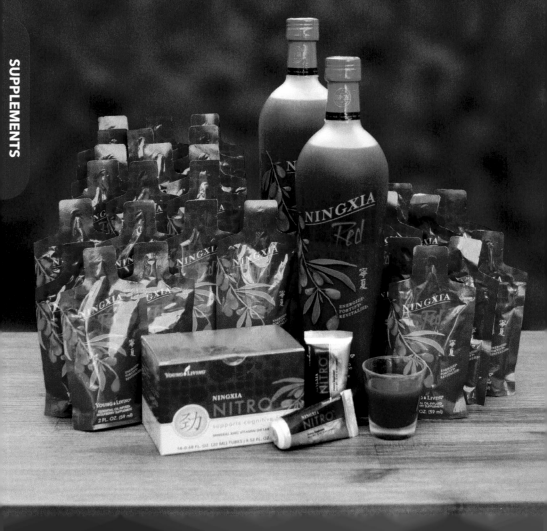

SUPPLEMENTS

SECTION THREE

the supplements

There are several types of supplements you will find through Young Living®. The mainstay of Young Living® is essential oils. The foundation of Young Living® is a healthy lifestyle. The founder, D. Gary Young, understood how important it was to not only have the best essential oils available to consumers, but also the best, most bioavailable herbal supplements as well. It took years of commitment and research to find exactly the right sources and synergies for the supplements Young Living® carries. There are several things that set Young Living's® supplement line high above the rest: commitment to purity, commitment to research backed ingredients with proven efficacy, and the main key: infusion of essential oils into powdered herbal supplements.

For many years, the Young Living® supplement line was above average with better ingredients and better synergies of those ingredients. It was not until several years later, after many studies and tests, that Young Living® discovered infusing herbal supplements with a powdered form of essential oils made the supplements far more efficacious and bioavailable. This was a ground-breaking discovery by Gary Young that makes the Young Living® supplement line something that no other company on the planet today is able to match or even come close to. For this very reason, we will start the supplement section with the Vitality™ Line of essential oils that are specifically designed to be consumed. They are considered by the FDA as GRAS.

As stated by the FDA, "'GRAS' is an acronym for the phrase Generally Recognized As Safe. Under sections 201(s) and 409 of the Federal Food, Drug, and Cosmetic Act, any substance that is intentionally added to food is a food additive, that is subject to premarket review and approval by FDA, unless the substance is generally recognized, among qualified experts, as having been adequately shown to be safe under the conditions of its intended use, or unless the use of the substance is otherwise excepted from the definition of a food additive."

You can find a complete list of GRAS essential oils at https://tinyurl.com/GRAS-EO

VITALITY™ LINE ESSENTIAL OIL SUPPLEMENTS

VEGAN — ALL OILS — MINIMUM AGE 6+

Young Living® carries a full line of consumable essential oils in the USA called Vitality™ that are labeled as dietary supplements, in accordance with the FDA labeling regulations and guidelines. These oils are considered GRAS which means Generally Recognized (Regarded) As Safe for consumption. In the UK these oils are called the Plus Oil Range line. These are known essential oils used in food additives and flavorings as well as for system function use. You are consuming essential oils practically every day without even knowing it. Soda pop, mints, lemon zest, orange juice, concentrated lemon juice, lemon slices in your water, spearmint gum, even eating a salad gives you essential oils.

Dr. Cole Woolley once stated that Pepsi® and Coca-Cola® use essential oils in massive amounts to flavor their products. Dr. Woolley stated, "I know the owner of a company that sells $50 million dollars of orange oil, lemon oil, tangerine oil, cinnamon oil, nutmeg oil, mandarin oil and grapefruit oil to Pepsi® and Coca-Cola® companies. He knows they go into their drinks."

This may be fascinating, but how does this help us understand the system function use of these oils outside of simple flavoring agents? Let's go back to how essential oils work. Essential oils are the life-force of plants. They help the plant to regulate itself and add health and overall wellness to the cells and structure of the plant as well as act as an aroma or pheromone to attract or detract insects or invaders. These oils can work in much the same way for us as humans.

When consumed, essential oils work on our body systems. The following body systems are supported by internal use of essential oils labeled for consumption through the Vitality™ line as per the FDA guidelines. Plus Oil Range for the UK are regulated as only for food flavoring so they will not be mentioned further.

- Circulatory
- Digestive and Gut
- Endocrine (hormones, sleep, energy, metabolism, etc)
- Immune
- Integumentary
- Lymphatic
- Nervous
- Renal and Urinary
- Respiratory
- Skeletal (Bones)

On the following pages is each system along with the essential oils that can help support that system when used internally as a dietary supplement. Please only use essential oils from the Vitality™ line. For the best results, use an essential oil single, blend, or blend 2-3 singles from the same category to create your own blend, then add 1-2 drops of the essential oils to a capsule and top off with a carrier oil such as organic olive or grapeseed oil.

CIRCULATORY SYSTEM

- Black Pepper Vitality™
- Caraway Vitality™
- Cinnamon Bark Vitality™
- Clove Vitality™
- Cumin Vitality™
- Dill Vitality™
- Fennel Vitality™
- Lavender Vitality™
- Lemon Vitality™
- Lemongrass Vitality™
- Marjoram Vitality™
- Nutmeg Vitality™
- Orange Vitality™
- Oregano Vitality™
- Peppermint Vitality™
- Rosemary Vitality™
- Tangerine Vitality™
- Tarragon Vitality™
- Thyme Vitality™

DIGESTIVE SYSTEM

- Caraway Vitality™ (digestion)
- Cardamom Vitality™ (liver, colon, digestion)
- Carrot Seed Vitality™ (liver, digestion)
- Celery Seed Vitality™ (liver, digestion)
- Cilantro Vitality™ (liver, digestion)
- Cinnamon Bark Vitality™ (digestion, colon)
- Coriander Vitality™ (pancreas, liver, digestion)
- Cumin Vitality™ (digestion, liver)
- DiGize™ Vitality™ blend (digestion)
- Dill Vitality™ (liver, digestion)
- Fennel Vitality™ (colon, digestion)
- GLF™ Vitality™ blend (gallbladder, liver, digestion)
- German Chamomile Vitality™ (gallbladder, liver, digestion)
- Ginger Vitality™ (digestion)
- Jade Lemon™ Vitality™ (gallbladder, liver, digestion)
- Juva Cleanse® Vitality™ blend (liver, digestion)
- JuvaFlex® Vitality™ blend (digestion)
- Lemon Vitality™ (liver, gallbladder, digestion)
- Lemongrass Vitality™ (digestion)
- Lime Vitality™ (liver, gallbladder, digestion)
- Marjoram Vitality™ (digestion)
- Nutmeg Vitality™ (liver, digestion)
- Orange Vitality™ (liver, digestion)
- Oregano Vitality™ (liver, gallbladder, colon, digestion)
- Parsley Vitality™ (digestion, liver)
- Peppermint Vitality™ (liver, gallbladder, colon, digestion)
- Rosemary Vitality™ (liver)
- Sage Vitality™ (liver)
- Spearmint Vitality™ (gallbladder, digestion)
- Tangerine Vitality™ (liver, digestion)
- Tarragon Vitality™ (colon, digestion)
- Thyme Vitality™ (colon)

VITALITY™ SUPPLEMENTS

ENDOCRINE SYSTEM (hormones)
- Black Pepper Vitality™ (energy, metabolism)
- Cinnamon Bark Vitality™ (energy, metabolism)
- Citrus Fresh™ Vitality™ blend (energy, metabolism)
- Clove Vitality™ (thyroid, energy)
- Copaiba Vitality™ (sleep, emotions, focus)
- EndoFlex™ Vitality™ blend (hormones)
- Fennel Vitality™ (metabolism, hormones, PMS)
- Frankincense Vitality™ (sleep, emotions, focus)
- Grapefruit Vitality™ (energy, metabolism)
- Lavender Vitality™ (sleep, focus, emotions, hormones, PMS)
- Lemongrass Vitality™ (thyroid)
- Lime Vitality™ (metabolism, sleep, focus)
- Mountain Savory Vitality™ (energy)
- Nutmeg Vitality™ (adrenals, energy)
- Oregano Vitality™ (prostate)
- Parsley Vitality™ (hormones)
- Peppermint Vitality™ (thyroid, energy, focus, emotions)
- Sage Vitality™ (prostate, hormones, metabolism, PMS)
- SclarEssence™ Vitality™ blend (hormones, PMS)
- Spearmint Vitality™ (thyroid, metabolism)
- Tangerine Vitality™ (sleep, emotions, focus)
- Tarragon Vitality™ (emotions, PMS)
- Thieves® Vitality™ blend (emotions)
- Thyme Vitality™ (prostate)

IMMUNE SYSTEM
- Basil Vitality™
- Bergamot Vitality™
- Black Pepper Vitality™
- Caraway Vitality™
- Cilantro Vitality™
- Cinnamon Bark Vitality™
- Citrus Fresh™ Vitality™ blend
- Clove Vitality™
- Copaiba Vitality™
- Cumin Vitality™
- Frankincense Vitality™
- GLF™ Vitality™ blend
- Ginger Vitality™
- Jade Lemon™ Vitality™
- Juva Cleanse® Vitality™ blend
- JuvaFlex® Vitality™ blend
- Laurus Nobilis Vitality™
- Lavender Vitality™
- Lemon Vitality™
- Lemongrass Vitality™
- Lime Vitality™
- Longevity™ Vitality™ blend
- Mountain Savory Vitality™
- Nutmeg Vitality™

The statements about essential oils have not been evaluated by the Food and Drug Administration. Young Living® products and oils are not intended to diagnose, treat, cure, or prevent any disease.

IMMUNE SYSTEM (continued)
- Orange Vitality™
- Oregano Vitality™
- Parsley Vitality™
- Peppermint Vitality™
- Rosemary Vitality™
- Sage Vitality™
- Spearmint Vitality™
- Tangerine Vitality™
- Thieves® Vitality™ blend
- Thyme Vitality™

INTEGUMENTARY SYSTEM
- Caraway Vitality™ (skin)
- Carrot Seed Vitality™ (skin)
- Cilantro Vitality™ (skin)
- Clove Vitality™ (skin)
- Copaiba Vitality™ (skin, nails)
- Coriander Vitality™ (skin)
- Frankincense Vitality™ (skin, hair, nails)
- German Chamomile Vitality™ (skin)
- Jade Lemon™ Vitality™ (nails)
- Lavender Vitality™ (skin, hair, nails)
- Lemon Vitality™ (nails)
- Orange Vitality™ (skin, hair)
- Peppermint Vitality™ (hair)
- Rosemary Vitality™ (hair)

LYMPHATIC SYSTEM
- Grapefruit Vitality™
- Jade Lemon™ Vitality™
- Lemon Vitality™
- Lemongrass Vitality™
- Lime Vitality™
- Nutmeg Vitality™
- Peppermint Vitality™
- Rosemary Vitality™
- Thieves® Vitality™ blend

NERVOUS SYSTEM
- Caraway Vitality™ (general)
- Cardamom Vitality™ (brain)
- Frankincense Vitality™ (brain, general)
- Lavender Vitality™ (brain, general)
- Lemongrass Vitality™ (brain)
- Orange Vitality™ (general)
- Parsley Vitality™ (general)
- Peppermint Vitality™ (brain)
- Thyme Vitality™ (brain)

VITALITY™ SUPPLEMENTS

RENAL/URINARY SYSTEM
- Caraway Vitality™ (general)
- Carrot Seed Vitality™ (general)
- Celery Seed Vitality™ (general)
- Citrus Fresh™ Vitality™ (general)
- Clove Vitality™ (bladder)
- Copaiba Vitality™ (kidney, bladder)
- Cumin Vitality™ (kidney, bladder)
- Fennel Vitality™ (general)
- Grapefruit Vitality™ (kidney, bladder)
- Jade Lemon™ Vitality™ (kidney)
- Lavender Vitality™ (general)
- Lemon Vitality™ (kidney, bladder)
- Lemongrass Vitality™ (bladder)
- Lime Vitality™ (bladder)
- Mountain Savory Vitality™ (bladder)
- Orange Vitality™ (kidney, bladder)
- Parsley Vitality™ (kidney, bladder)
- Rosemary Vitality™ (bladder)
- Tangerine Vitality™ (kidney, bladder)
- Tarragon Vitality™ (general)
- Thieves® Vitality™ blend (general)
- Thyme Vitality™ (bladder)

RESPIRATORY
- Caraway Vitality™
- Cardamom Vitality™
- Copaiba Vitality™
- Frankincense Vitality™
- Ginger Vitality™
- Laurus Nobilis Vitality™
- Lavender Vitality™
- Lemongrass Vitality™
- Lime Vitality™
- Oregano Vitality™
- Peppermint Vitality™
- Rosemary Vitality™
- Tangerine Vitality™
- Thieves® Vitality™ blend

SKELETAL (specifically bone health)
- Copaiba Vitality™
- Frankincense Vitality™
- Lemongrass Vitality™
- Peppermint Vitality™
- Rosemary Vitality™
- Sage Vitality™
- Thyme Vitality™

BONUS: HOW TO MAKE "BOMB" RECIPES

CAPSULES   VEGAN   ALL OILS   MINIMUM AGE 12+

Creating "bomb" recipes is a good way to boost your health in a specific area. A normal daily capsule would have 1-4 drops of essential oil and the rest carrier oil. A bomb would have 10-12 drops of essential oils with only 4 drops of carrier oil. The purpose of a bomb is to give your system more essential oils than normal for a short amount of time; usually only once a day for up to three days. A typical immune system bomb would be taken just before bed so that you wake up refreshed and ready for the day. It is not wise to do a full bomb every single day, nor is it wise to do the same bomb every day.

To make a bomb you will want to alternate by picking three or five essential oils from one body system category. Using an odd number allows the synergy to be more integrative. Choose different essential oils each time you do a bomb. This will help your body more than if you did the same recipe each time. This is because we are constantly changing, and are in a state of homeodynamics. Essential oils are not meant to work like pharmaceuticals, so it's important not to use them that way.

Choose essential oils that compliment each other. For instance, if you look in the Immune System category you will find more intense oils such as Clove and Oregano along with some calming oils like Lavender and Frankincense. You will also find most citrus oils in the Immune System category. Choose 1-2 from each sub category. Sub categories would be protecting/stimulating, calming, and uplifting. An example immune system bomb would be:

IMMUNE SYSTEM BOMB
- 2 drops Oregano Vitality™
- 2 drops Clove Vitality™
- 2 drops Frankincense Vitality™
- 2 drops Lavender Vitality™
- 2 drops Bergamot Vitality™
- 4 drops carrier oil of choice

You may pre-mix a synergy, or simply put 2 drops of five essential oils into a veggie capsule. Put your finger over the top and shake up the oils then add a minimum of 4 drops carrier oil. Remember, this is for a one time bomb. It is not something you should do as a daily capsule. To do a daily capsule, you can make a synergy of five essential oils then put only 2 drops of the synergy into a capsule and top off with carrier oil. Bombs should only be taken once a day for up to three days then stop.

VITALITY™ SUPPLEMENTS

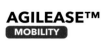

TAKE ANYTIME | BEST WITH FOOD | NOT VEGAN | CONTAINS CORN | MINIMUM AGE 12+ | ½ DOSAGE IF UNDER 12 | DON'T USE WITH BLOOD THINNERS

This delightful little gem in the supplement lineup is no joke! If you need a little (or a lot) of extra help with healthy mobility, then AgilEase™ is the one for you! This supplement is perfect if you're a gym rat, love to run or walk daily, are an athlete, or are in the middle-aged or elderly category. I'm guessing that's most of us! It supports the natural, acute inflammation response in joints after exercise. AgilEase™ helps to promote joint and cartilage health, along with more healthful mobility and flexibility through a reduction of inflammation. If you're looking for a supplement that contains Turmeric along with black pepper extract to help make the main active ingredient, curcumin, in Turmeric more bioavailable, then AgilEase™ is the best choice. Here are a few of the excellent ingredients in AgilEase™ and what they support.

INGREDIENTS
AgilEase™ Blend – 537.5 mg
- Frankincense (*Boswellia sacra*) resin powder
- Calcium fructoborate (from plant minerals)
- Curcuminoids complex - Turmeric (*Curcuma longa*) rhizome extract
- Piperine whole fruit extract from Black Pepper (*Piper nigrum*)
- Collagen (with undenatured type II collagen)
- Glucosamine sulfate (not derived from shellfish)
- Hyaluronic acid (Sodium hyaluronate)

Essential Oils - Wintergreen (*Gaultheria procumbens*) leaf oil, Copaiba (*Copaifera reticulata*) wood oil (oleoresin), Clove (*Syzygium aromaticum*) flower bud oil, Northern Lights Black Spruce™ (*Picea mariana*) whole tree oil

Other Ingredients - Rice Flour, Hypromellose, Silicon Dioxide, Potassium Chloride

WHAT THE INGREDIENTS DO
- Frankincense resin powder - anti-inflammatory and anti-arthritis properties.
- Calcium fructoborate - helps ease inflammation of the mucous membranes, discomfort and stiffness.
- Turmeric rhizome extract - high antioxidant and anti-inflammatory properties. Also helps increase brain function.
- Piperine extract - protects liver function and helps promote the bioavailability of other supplements (helps other ingredients to absorb properly).
- UC-II undenatured collagen - protects tissue in aging joints and helps by absorbing physical impact.
- Glucosamine sulfate - occurs naturally in the human body as fluid surrounding the joints. In supplements it is often from ground up shells from shellfish. The source used for AgilEase™ is from non-GMO fermented corn.

The statements about the supplement and the ingredients have not been evaluated by the Food and Drug Administration. Young Living® products are not intended to diagnose, treat, cure, or prevent any disease.

AGILEASE™

WHAT THE INGREDIENTS DO (continued)
- Hyaluronic acid - for joint pain in osteoarthritis.
- Wintergreen, Copaiba, Clove, and Northern Lights Black Spruce™ - known for their joint supporting properties.

Other Ingredients - Rice Flour, Hypromellose, Silicon Dioxide, Potassium Chloride - capsule base and substrate.

COMMENTS FROM YOUNG LIVING®
"Especially beneficial for athletes, as well as middle-aged and elderly people who may experience a natural, acute inflammation response in their joints after exercise, AgilEase™ is a joint health supplement that's perfect for healthy individuals who are looking to gain greater mobility and flexibility through the reduction of inflammation. We used unique and powerful ingredients such as frankincense powder, UC-II undenatured collagen, hyaluronic acid, calcium fructoborate, and a specially formulated proprietary essential oil blend of Wintergreen, Copaiba, Clove, and Northern Lights Black Spruce – oils that are known for their joint health benefits. Take AgilEase™ to support joint health or as a preventative measure to protect joint and cartilage health."

YOUNG LIVING STATED BENEFITS
- Supports and protects joint and cartilage health.
- Beneficial for athletes and active individuals of all ages who want to support and protect their joints and cartilage.
- Perfect companion to an active lifestyle, promoting healthy joint function and supporting cartilage health.
- Supports the body's response to acute inflammation in healthy individuals.
- Helps support healthy joint flexibility and mobility.
- Formulated with ingredients and essential oils for healthy joint support.
- Helps ease acute joint discomfort to improve quality of life.

DIRECTIONS FOR USE
For best results, take 2 capsules daily for joint support.
You may take this anytime of the day or with a meal containing fat. While the instructions on the bottle say take anytime, and that is technically correct, the Turmeric in AgilEase™ is better absorbed when taken with fat. Piperine extract is already in this supplement so this is the best Turmeric supplement you can find. NOTE: Do not take turmeric with blood thinners such as Coumadin® or other blood thinners. Turmeric can magnify the effect of anti-clotting medications.

AGILEASE™

The statements about the supplement and the ingredients have not been evaluated by the Food and Drug Administration. Young Living® products are not intended to diagnose, treat, cure, or prevent any disease.

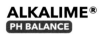

ALKALIME®
PH BALANCE

TAKE 1 HOUR BEFORE MEAL | VEGAN | CONTAINS STEVIA | CONTAINS CORN | MINIMUM AGE 12+ | 1/2 DOSAGE IF UNDER 12

AlkaLime® is a must for most people. It helps maintain the proper pH balance in the body. Formulated with Lemon and Lime essential oils, organic lemon powder, and biochemical mineral cell salts, this effervescent supplement formula starts working right away to soothe the occasional upset stomach. The citrus notes are sure to brighten your mood, and the mineral cell salts help support optimal pH balance in the stomach. Store a few packs in your purse or backpack and enjoy them on those hurried or stressful days when acidity soars.

INGREDIENTS
- Calories - 10
- Total Carbohydrate - 3 g
- Calcium (Calcium carbonate, Dicalcium phosphate, Calcium sulfate) - 201 mg (15% DV)
- Sodium (Sodium bicarbonate, Disodium phosphate, Sodium sulfate) 505 mg (22% DV)
- Potassium (Potassium bicarbonate, Tripotassium phosphate, Potassium sulfate, and Potassium chloride) - 95 mg (2% DV)

AlkaLime® Blend – 179 mg
- Lemon (*Citrus limon*) fruit powder
- Lemon (*Citrus limon*) peel oil
- Lime (*Citrus aurantifolia*) peel oil

Other Ingredients - Tartaric acid, Citric acid, Stevia (*Stevia rebaudiana*) leaf extract, Magnesium phosphate

WHAT THE INGREDIENTS DO
- Calcium, Sodium, Potassium - the combined negatively and positively charged biochemical mineral cell salts work in synergy to support cellular repair, nerve function, helps muscle tissues to function correctly, strengthens bones and teeth. Together they are critical to metabolic processes and they balance the biochemistry of the blood. Sodium phosphate is an acid neutralizer.

AlkaLime® Blend
- Lemon fruit powder, Lemon peel oil, and Lime peel oil - helps minerals absorb into the body more quickly and effectively.

Other Ingredients
- Tartaric acid - increases the rate at which nutrients are absorbed into the bloodstream. Aids digestion by improving intestinal absorption.
- Magnesium phosphate - Soothes stressed nerves and muscles in the body and is effective when digestive discomfort is present.

ALKALIME®

COMMENTS FROM YOUNG LIVING®

"AlkaLime® is a precisely-balanced alkaline mineral complex formulated to neutralize acidity and maintain desirable pH levels in the body. Infused with Lemon and Lime essential oils and organic whole lemon powder, AlkaLime® also features enhanced effervescence and biochemical mineral cell salts for increased effectiveness. A balanced pH is thought to play an important role in maintaining overall health and vigor."

YOUNG LIVING STATED BENEFITS

- Absorbed easily and quickly by the body.
- Effervescent formula starts working right away to soothe the occasional upset stomach.
- Gentle on the stomach.
- Helps maintain optimal pH in the stomach.
- Free of artificial colors, flavors, or sweeteners, and formulated with nine biochemical mineral cell salts, the refreshing taste of Lemon and Lime essential oils, and organic lemon powder.
- Comes in convenient, single-serve stick packs.

DIRECTIONS FOR USE

Add 1 level tsp. (or 1 stick pack) into 4-6 oz. of distilled or purified water.
Let sit for 20–25 seconds.
Gently stir until mixed, then drink immediately.
Mix only with water.
Take 1–3 times daily, one hour before meals or bedtime as an aid in alkalizing.

ALKALIME®

The statements about the supplement and the ingredients have not been evaluated by the Food and Drug Administration. Young Living® products are not intended to diagnose, treat, cure, or prevent any disease.

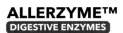

ALLERZYME™
DIGESTIVE ENZYMES

BEST WITH FOOD • NOT VEGAN • CONTAINS DAIRY • CONTAINS CORN • CONTAINS BARLEY • MINIMUM AGE 12+

Allerzyme™ is the strongest of all the digestive enzymes. Allerzyme™ is an excellent choice for bloating and gas and for those who are lactose intolerant. It is also good for people who like to eat desserts and items containing white processed sugar. It contains Plantain leaf, which is a natural anti-inflammatory and is packed with nutrients and vitamins. This enzyme contains the most essential oils out of all the Young Living® digestive enzymes.

Note on Allerzyme™: While this supplement is noted to contain Barley grass, which is a possible contaminant, the Barley grass itself does not contain any gluten. The only way to have a gluten response from Barley grass is if the production of the grass was contaminated with the Barley seed, which contains gluten. Young Living's® Allerzyme™ contains clean Barley grass, however it is up to each individual to decide if they are going to try this supplement. Allerzyme™ is specifically noted to help support the proper digestion of wheat products.

INGREDIENTS
Proprietary Allerzyme™ Blend – 193 mg
- Plantain (*Plantago major*) leaf
- Amylase
- Bromelain
- Peptidase
- Protease
- Invertase
- Phytase
- Barley (*Hordeum vulgare*) grass
- Lipase
- Lactase (as per YL, this is produced from dairy)
- Cellulase (as per YL, this is produced from dairy)
- Alpha-galactosidase
- Diastase

Proprietary Allerzyme™ Oil Blend – 12 mg
- Tarragon (*Artemisia dracunculus*) leaf oil
- Ginger (*Zingiber officinale*) root oil
- Peppermint (*Mentha piperita*) leaf oil
- Juniper (*Juniperus osteosperma*) leaf oil
- Fennel (*Foeniculum vulgare*) seed oil
- Lemongrass (*Cymbopogon flexuosus*) leaf oil
- Anise (*Pimpinella anisum*) fruit oil
- Patchouli (*Pogostemon cablin*) flower oil

Other Ingredients - Hypromellose, Water, Silica.

The statements about essential oils have not been evaluated by the Food and Drug Administration. Young Living® products and oils are not intended to diagnose, treat, cure, or prevent any disease.

WHAT THE INGREDIENTS DO

- Plantain leaf - digestive supporting herb.
- Amylase - breaks down starch, breads, and pasta.
- Bromelain - breaks down peptides and amino acids found in meats, dairy, eggs, and grains, as well as seeds, nuts, leafy greens, and many other foods. Works in the small intestine and supports blood to help ease inflammation.
- Peptidase - finishes breaking down Proteases. Helps support the immune system and ease inflammation.
- Protease 3.0 - supports blood circulation and toxicity. Higher acid content to break down animal protein.
- Protease 4.5 - helps with sinusitis and has a lower acidic content.
- Protease 6.0 - helps with edema and carries away toxins. Helps reduce pain and varicose veins. Works in the blood. Least acidic.
- Invertase - breaks down table sugar found in sweets and desserts. Breaks the connection between fructose and glucose.
- Phytase - helps with bone health and pulls needed minerals from grains making them bioavailable.
- Barley (Hordeum vulgare) grass - supports digestion and helps reduce constipation.
- Lipase - breaks down dietary fats and oils. Helps liver function.
- Lactase - breaks down dairy sugars. Helps with lactose intolerance.
- Cellulase - breaks down man-made fiber, plant fiber, fruits, and vegetables.
- Alpha-galactosidase - breaks down polysaccharides, beans, and vegetables. For gas and bloating.
- Diastase (barley grass malt - gluten) - breaks down grain sugars and starch.
- Tarragon, Ginger, Peppermint, Juniper, Fennel, Lemongrass, Anise, and Patchouli - supports digestion and bioavailability.

COMMENTS FROM YOUNG LIVING®

"Allerzyme™ is a vegetarian enzyme complex that promotes digestion. For the relief of occasional symptoms such as fullness, pressure, bloating, gas, pain, and/or minor cramping that may occur after eating."

DIRECTIONS FOR USE

Take 1 capsule three times daily just prior to meals or as needed.
Indications - For the relief of occasional symptoms such as fullness, pressure, bloating, gas, pain, and/or minor cramping that may occur after eating.

Warning - Do not give to children under 12 years of age except under the supervision of a doctor. If symptoms persist, discontinue use of this product and consult your physician. Keep in a cool dry place. Do not expose to excessive heat or direct sunlight. If pregnant or under a doctor's care, consult your physician.

The statements about essential oils have not been evaluated by the Food and Drug Administration. Young Living® products and oils are not intended to diagnose, treat, cure, or prevent any disease.

AMINOWISE®

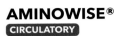

CIRCULATORY

USE ANYTIME	BEST BEFORE A WORKOUT	VEGAN	CONTAINS STEVIA	MINIMUM AGE 12+	1/2 DOSAGE IF UNDER 12

AminoWise® is one of those special necessities for those of us who love to get in a good hard workout, as well as for those who need extra amino acids to help with your circulatory system. You can drink this during your workout or directly after to help your body flush lactic acid buildup. Your body will be so happy you added this to your workout! I promise, your cells will smile!

INGREDIENTS
- Calories - 25
- Total Carbohydrates - 5 g (2% DV)
- Vitamin E (as d-alpha tocopherol acetate) - 10.8 mg (72% DV)
- Calcium (as calcium citrate) - 67 mg (5% DV)
- Magnesium (as magnesium citrate) - 2 mg (<1% DV)
- Zinc (as zinc gluconate) - 2.1 mg (19% DV)
- Potassium (as potassium citrate) - 50 mg (1% DV)
- Sodium (as sodium citrate) - 46 mg (2% DV) - *based on Mineral Blend mg breakdown*

AminoWise® Muscle Performance Blend – 5.7 g
Branched-chain amino acids (2:1:1 Leucine, Isoleucine, Valine), L-citrulline, Beta-alanine, L-glutamine, L-arginine, L-taurine

AminoWise® Recovery Blend – 1.2 g
Ningxia wolfberry (*Lycium barbarum*) fruit powder, Antioxidant blend [Red wine polyphenols, Vitamin E (D-alpha tocopherol acetate), Zinc (Zinc gluconate)], Lime (*Citrus aurantifolia*) fruit powder, Lemon (*Citrus limon*) peel oil, Lime (*Citrus latifolia*) peel oil

AminoWise® Hydration Mineral Blend – 277 mg
Sodium citrate, Potassium citrate, Calcium citrate, Magnesium citrate

Other Ingredients - Fructooligosaccharides, Tapioca maltodextrin, Citric acid, Natural flavors, Calcium silicate, Stevia (*Stevia rebaudiana*) leaf extract, Silicon dioxide.

WHAT THE INGREDIENTS DO
- Vitamin E - supports immune function and eye health; helps ease inflammation.
- Calcium citrate - helps decrease bone loss.
- Magnesium citrate - supports the normal functioning of cells, nerves, muscles, bones, and heart.
- Zinc - promotes a healthy immune system. Aids in healing of wounds.
- Potassium citrate - helps to decrease the risk of stroke, lower blood pressure, protect against loss of muscle mass, preserve bone mineral density, and reduce kidney stones.
- Sodium citrate - helps to alkalinize the urine.

AminoWise® Muscle Performance Blend
- Branched-chain amino acids (2:1:1 leucine, isoleucine, valine) - promotes healthy pathways to support weakness, supports signs of loss of brain function due to severe liver damage, reduces fatigue during exercise, promotes wound healing, and stimulates insulin production.
- L-citrulline - helps open veins and arteries to increase blood flow.
- B-alanine - improves athletic function and aids in building lean muscle mass.

The statements about essential oils have not been evaluated by the Food and Drug Administration. Young Living® products and oils are not intended to diagnose, treat, cure, or prevent any disease.

WHAT THE INGREDIENTS DO (continued)
- L-glutamine - supports immune cell activity in the gut.
- L-arginine - stimulates the release of growth hormones and insulin and promotes increased blood flow.
- L-taurine - promotes cardiovascular health and increases sports performance.

AminoWise® Recovery Blend
- Ningxia wolfberry fruit powder - Natural polysaccharide that supports the healthy function of the immune system, as well as healthy regeneration of tissues and cells
- Antioxidant blend - helps digestion, helps protect tissue against oxidative stresses.
- Lime fruit powder - promotes weight loss, improves skin quality, improves immune system, promotes consumption of water.
- Lemon peel oil - natural detoxifier, promotes weight loss, supports immune system and energy.
- Lime peel oil - supports immune system, natural detoxifier.

AminoWise® Hydration Mineral Blend – 277 mg
- Sodium citrate - helps to alkalinize the urine.
- Potassium citrate - helps to decrease the risk of stroke, lower blood pressure, protect against loss of muscle mass, preserve bone mineral density, and reduce kidney stones.
- Calcium citrate - helps decrease bone loss.
- Magnesium citrate - supports normal cell function, nerves, muscles, bones, and heart.

Other Ingredients
- Fructooligosaccharides - a prebiotic: food for gut flora.
- Tapioca maltodextrin - a carbohydrate starch base.
- Citric acid - it occurs naturally in citrus fruits and is a flavoring and preservative.
- Natural flavors - non synthetic flavors from nature.
- Calcium silicate - anti-caking agent.
- Stevia (Stevia rebaudiana) leaf extract - natural sweetener.
- Silicon dioxide - natural anti-caking agent.

AMINOWISE®

COMMENTS FROM YOUNG LIVING®
"Optimize your workout recovery with the triple-targeted formula of AminoWise®. It uses three blends for one powerful result - The Muscle Performance blend aids muscle building and repair, the Recovery blend helps reduce muscle fatigue, and the Hydration Mineral blend replenishes important minerals lost during exercise. Simply mix 1 scoop with water and drink immediately after your workout to ensure that you're getting the most out of your hard work. AminoWise® was developed and formulated to fill a need within the nutritional product line as a during and after-workout replenishing boost for the muscles. With a hydrating blend of minerals that are lost during exercise and with no added sugars, artificial sweeteners, preservatives, or artificial colors or flavors, AminoWise® is a standout in the field of workout supplementation."

DIRECTIONS FOR USE
Mix 1 scoop with 8 oz. of water and consume during or after exercise.
May also be used at anytime.

BALANCE COMPLETE™

SHAKE MIX

USE ANYTIME · NOT VEGAN · CONTAINS DAIRY · CONTAINS XYLITOL · CONTAINS BARLEY · MINIMUM AGE 1+ · DO NOT FEED TO DOGS

Balance Complete™ is the perfect meal replacement shake mix that will keep you going until your next meal. With 12 grams of protein and 180 calories, this shake packs a punch with fiber, vitamins, and minerals. Add a drop of Tangerine Vitality™ and Cinnamon Bark Vitality™ for an extra kick!

INGREDIENTS

- Calories - 180
- Total Fat - 5 g (7% DV)
  Saturated Fat 2.5 g (13% DV)
- Cholesterol - 25 mg (9% DV)
- Sodium - 75 mg (3% DV)
- Potassium - 330 mg (9% DV)
- Carbohydrates - 28 g (10% DV)
  Dietary Fiber 4 g (14%)
  Total Sugars 8 g (includes 3 g added sugars)
- Protein - 12 g (23% DV)
- D3 (Cholecalciferol) - 4 mcg (20% DV)
- A - 90 mcg (10% DV)
- C (ascorbic acid) - (25% DV)
- E - 5 mcg (35% DV)
- B1 (Thiamine HCl) - 0.4 mg (35% DV)
- B2 (Riboflavin) - 0.5 mg (40% DV)
- B3 (Niacin) - 6 mg (40% DV)
- B6 (Pyridoxine HCl) - 0.6 mg (35% DV)
- Folate - 135 mcg DFE (35% DV)
- B12 (Methylcobalamin) - 3 mcg (130% DV)
- B7 (Biotin) - 87 mcg (290% DV)
- Calcium - 454 mg (35% DV)
- Iron - 1 mg (6% DV)
- Pantothenic Acid - 3 mg (55% DV)
- Iodine (Potassium iodide) - 42 mcg (30% DV)
- Magnesium - 150 mg (35% DV)
- Zinc - 6 mg (55% DV)
- Selenium - 26 mcg (45% DV)
- Chromium - 35 mcg (100% DV)
- Molybdenum - 19 mcg (40% DV)
- Whey protein concentrate
- Natural flavors
- Nonfat dry milk
- MCT (Medium-chain triglycerides)
- Fructose
- Lecithin
- Calcium (tricalcium phosphate)

Proprietary V-Fiber™ Blend

- Larch polysaccharides, Ningxia Wolfberry fiber (*Lycium barbarum*) fruit, Rice bran, Guar gum, Glucomannan fiber (from Konjac root), Inulin fiber (from Chicory root), Sodium alginate, Whey protein concentrate, Arabinogalactan fiber (from Larch tree), Nonfat dry milk (Nonfat dry milk, lactose, Vitamin A,

BALANCE COMPLETE™

Proprietary V-Fiber™ Blend (continued)

Palmitate, Vitamin D3), Coconut creamer (Coconut oil, Maltodextrin, Sodium caseinate), Natural Flavors, Fructose, Soy lecithin, Calcium (Tricalcium phosphate)

Enzyme Complex

- Lactase, Amylase, Bromelain, Lipase, Papain

Additional Vitamins and Minerals

- Vitamin A (Mixed carotenoids), Vitamin C (Ascorbic acid), Microcrystalline cellulose, Vitamin B3 (Niacin), Zinc (Zinc oxide), Vitamin A (Beta carotene), Vitamin B5 (Pantothenic acid from Calcium pantothenate, Folic acid (from Citrus limon extracts), Biotin, Chalcone, Iodine (Potassium iodide), Vitamin B6 (Pyridoxine hydrochloride), Vitamin B2 (Riboflavin), Vitamin B1 (Thiamine hydrochloride), Chromium (Chromium polynicotinate with niacin), Vitamin D3 (Cholecalciferol), Calcium (Calcium citrate), Orange (*Citrus sinensis*) peel essential oil, Selenium (L-Selenomethionine), Molybdenum (Sodium molybdate dihydrate), Potassium (Tripotassium citrate), Vitamin B12 (methylcobalamin)

Other Ingredients

- Xylitol, Xanthan gum, Magnesium oxide, Barley (*Hordeum vulgare*) grass, Cinnamon (*Cinnamomum cassia*) bark, Lo Han Guo (*Siraitia grosvenorii*) fruit extract, Barley grass (*Hordeum vulgare*) juice, Aloe vera (*Aloe barbadensis*) leaf extract, Vitamin E (Natural mixed tocopherols)

WHAT THE INGREDIENTS DO
Proprietary V-Fiber™ Blend

- Larch polysaccharides - source of dietary fiber potent in biological immune-enhancing properties which promote healthy regeneration of tissues and cells.
- Ningxia wolfberry fruit - natural polysaccharide that supports the immune system, as well as healthy regeneration of tissues and cells.
- Rice bran - natural source of dietary fiber that promotes proper digestive function. It is nutrient-rich in bioavailable vitamins, minerals and antioxidants.
- Guar gum - stabilizes ingredients to keep fats and oils from separating. Helps promote regular bowel movements by holding water in the intestines which helps form healthy stool.
- Glucomannan fiber from Konjac root - natural source of fiber known to be low in calories and very high in fiber. Promotes a feeling of fullness along with motivating bowel movements which encourages colon health.
- Inulin fiber from Chicory root fiber - soluble plant fiber that supports digestion, curbs appetite, naturally supports cardiovascular health and improves bowel and gut health. Considered a type of prebiotic.
- Sodium alginate - brown algae source of sodium salt used as an emulsifier.
- Whey protein concentrate - high in amino acids; stimulates muscle growth.
- Arabinogalactan fiber (from Larch tree) - a complex carbohydrate that supports the immune system as a prebiotic to feed the good gut bacteria.
- Nonfat dry milk - protein source.
- Coconut creamer - MCT (Medium-chain triglycerides) - cardiovascular health.
- Natural flavors - improve taste.

Continued on next page.

These statements have not been evaluated by the Food and Drug Administration. Young Living® products are not intended to diagnose, treat, cure, or prevent any disease.

BALANCE COMPLETE™

WHAT THE INGREDIENTS DO (continued)
- Fructose - from a natural source.
- Soy Lecithin - rich in choline - beneficial to brain health.
- Calcium (Tricalcium phosphate) - helps prevent bone loss.

Proprietary Enzyme Complex - Digestive Enzymes
- Lactase - breaks down dairy sugars. Helps with lactose intolerance.
- Lipase - breaks down dietary fats and oils. Helps liver function.
- Bromelain - breaks down peptides and amino acids found in foods. Works in the small intestine and supports blood to help ease inflammation.
- Papain - digestive aid, and may help with parasites, psoriasis, shingles, diarrhea, runny nose, plus others.
- Amylase - breaks down starch, breads, and pasta.

Additional Vitamins and Minerals
- Vitamin A - phytonutrients that support cellular health and fight free radicals.
- Vitamin C - slows the effects of aging by protecting against free radical damage and oxidative stress, supports the immune system. Supports eye health and helps with absorption of iron.
- Vitamin B (Niacinamide) - a form of Vitamin B6 which is important to support the maintenance health of nerves, skin, and red blood cells.
- Zinc oxide - trace mineral that supports immune system and blood health.
- Mixed tocopherols (Vitamin E) - fat soluble with high antioxidant properties.
- Selenium (Selenomethionine) - supports normal cardiovascular function as a powerful antioxidant that defends against free radicals in the body.
- Beta-carotene - antioxidant that protects cells from free radical damage.
- Molybdenum citrate - trace mineral that is an essential nutrient that acts as a cofactor for essential enzymes which drive important chemical reactions in the body to convert, break down and remove toxic by-products of metabolism.
- Vitamin B5 - promotes healthy skin, supports the nervous system, proper digestion, creates red blood cells that carry oxygen to our cells, and is essential to hormone production within the adrenal glands.
- Vitamin B6 - supports the maintenance health of nerves, skin, and red blood cells.
- Chromium amino nicotrinate - supports metabolism and promotes improvement in blood sugar control in the body.
- Vitamin B1 - supports a healthy nervous system and promotes healthy cardiovascular function by breaking down fats and proteins. Functions by converting carbohydrates into glucose to improve energy and helps the body withstand stress while maintaining a healthy metabolism.
- Vitamin B2 - needed for overall growth. It also helps support energy levels.
- Vitamin D3 - supports bones and immune system. Helps boost weight loss, and improves moods.
- Vitamin B12 (Methylcobalamin) - the most bioavailable form of B12. Supports red blood cell production. Supports brain health, eye health, skin health, DNA production, cardiovascular health, and converts food into energy.
- Biotin B7 - helps the body convert food into energy.

These statements have not been evaluated by the Food and Drug Administration.
Young Living® products are not intended to diagnose, treat, cure, or prevent any disease.

Additional Vitamins and Minerals (continued)

- Folic acid (as folate) - required by FDA to be listed as folic acid; folic acid derived from natural sources is folate. Folate is needed for your body to make DNA. Having enough folate may prevent iron deficiency. It helps promote hair, skin and nail health through cell regeneration. Folate is an important supplement for pregnant women by helping prevent certain birth defects. It is also noted that folate supports your mood by transforming amino acids from your food into neurotransmitters such as serotonin and dopamine.
- Iodine - a trace mineral that is an essential component of the thyroid hormones; it controls metabolic rate, maintains healthy energy levels, facilitates the removal of toxins in the body, supports immune system and is critical in the prevention of an enlarged thyroid gland.

Other Ingredients

- Xanthan gum - natural emulsifier that promotes healthy stool; positively affects expediting digestion.
- Xylitol - naturally occurring plant-based sugar alcohol. 40% fewer calories than sugar.
- Magnesium oxide - supports immune system, nerves, heart, eyes, brain and muscles.
- Barley grass - supports digestion and helps reduce constipation.
- Cinnamon bark - supports blood glucose and adds flavor.
- Lo Han Guo fruit extract - monk fruit adds sweetness with no calories.
- Barley grass juice - promotes improved digestive function.
- Aloe vera leaf - rich in antioxidant properties; it soothes and aides in digestion.
- Vitamin E - high antioxidant property.

BALANCE COMPLETE™

COMMENTS FROM YOUNG LIVING®

"Balance Complete™ is a super-food-based meal replacement that is both a powerful nutritive energizer and a cleanser. Offering the benefits of Ningxia wolfberry powder, brown rice bran, barley grass, extra virgin coconut oil, aloe vera, cinnamon powder, and our premium whey protein blend, Balance Complete™ is high in fiber, high in protein, and contains the good fats, enzymes, vitamins, and minerals needed for a nutritionally dynamic meal. Balance Complete™ also features Young Living's® proprietary V-Fiber™ blend, which supplies an amazing 12 grams of fiber per serving, absorbs toxins, and satisfies the appetite while balancing the body's essential requirements."

DIRECTIONS FOR USE

Add 2 scoops of Balance Complete™ to 8 oz. of cold water. May be mixed with rice, almond, or other milk. Shake, stir or blend until smooth. For added flavor, add fruit or essential oils.

Usage: During Young Living's® 5-Day Nutritive Cleanse™, replace all three daily meals with Balance Complete™ and follow the recommended schedule.

BLM™
MOBILITY

USE ANYTIME | NOT VEGAN | CONTAINS PORK GELATIN | CONTAINS SHELLFISH | MINIMUM AGE 12+ | ½ DOSAGE IF UNDER 12

BLM™ stands for bones, ligaments, and muscles. BLM™ is an excellent addition to your mobility support regimen. It helps improve flexibility and reduces inflammation while boosting immune function. Infused with essential oils known to help support circulation and soothe muscles, this supplement may be combined with AgilEase™ and/or Sulfurzyme® or taken by itself.

INGREDIENTS
Proprietary BLM™ Blend – 715 mg
- Glucosamine Sulfate (derived from shellfish)
- Collagen type II (chicken sternum extract)
- MSM (methylsulfonylmethane)
- Balsam Canada (*Abies Balsamea*) leaf/branch oil
- Wintergreen (*Gaultheria procumbens*) leaf oil
- Manganese (Manganese citrate)
- Clove (*Syzygium aromaticum*) flower bud oil

Other Ingredients - Rice Flour, Gelatin, Magnesium stearate, Silicone dioxide

WHAT THE INGREDIENTS DO
- Glucosamine Sulfate - produces chemicals involved in building tendons, ligaments, cartilage and synovial fluid (fluid that surrounds joints). Derived from shellfish.
- Collagen type II - may improve joint flexibility, joint comfort and physical functions; supports gut integrity that helps support the immune system; helps form elastin and other compounds to help maintain healthy skin; supports healthy digestive function.
- MSM - decreases joint and muscle discomfort, significantly reduces inflammation in the body, and inhibits the breakdown of cartilage.
- Balsam Canada oil - soothes muscle discomfort and supports respiratory function.
- Wintergreen - useful to relieve discomfort and stimulate relaxation.
- Manganese - supports bone health, antioxidant activity, healthy blood sugar level management, and metabolic support.
- Clove oil - improves circulation and supports immune system.

COMMENTS FROM YOUNG LIVING®
"BLM™ supports normal bone and joint health. This formula combines powerful natural ingredients, such as type II collagen, MSM, glucosamine sulfate, and manganese citrate, enhanced with Seed to Seal® Premium essential oils. These ingredients have been shown to support healthy cell function and encourage joint health and fluid movement."

DIRECTIONS FOR USE
If you weigh less than 120 lbs., take 1 capsule three times daily. If you weigh between 120 and 200 lbs., take 1 capsule four times daily. If you weigh over 200 lbs., take 1 capsule five times daily. Allow 4-8 weeks of daily use before expecting noticeable results.

NOTE: Keep in a cool dry place. Keep out of the reach of children. Do not expose to excessive heat or direct sunlight. If pregnant or under a doctor's care, consult your physician.

The statements about the supplement and the ingredients have not been evaluated by the Food and Drug Administration. Young Living® products are not intended to diagnose, treat, cure, or prevent any disease.

CARDIOGIZE™

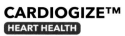

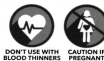

BEST WITH FOOD — **VEGAN** — **MINIMUM AGE 18+** — **DON'T USE WITH BLOOD THINNERS** — **CAUTION IF PREGNANT**

CardioGize™ was one of D. Gary Young's last formulations. The cardiovascular system is one of the most important systems in the body as it directly affects every other system. CardioGize™ is an excellent choice for all adults and will help boost antioxidant support as well as keep you moving in the right direction.

INGREDIENTS

- Carbohydrates - 1 g
- Vitamin K (as K2 menaquinone-7) - 100 mcg (83% DV)
- Folate (from Lemon peel extract) - 165 mcg DFE, 100 mcg folic acid (40% DV)
- Selenium (from yeast) 100 mcg - (182% DV)

Healthy Heart Blend – 1255 mg

- Garlic bulb extract (deodorized), Coenzyme Q10 (as ubiquinone) (90-100 mg/serving, Astragalus (*Astragalus membranaceus*) root powder, Dong Quai (*Angelica sinensis*) root powder, Motherwort (*Leonarus cardiaca*) aerial parts powder, Cat's claw (*Uncaria tomentosa*) bark powder, Hawthorn (*Crataegus oxyacantha*) berry powder, Cactus (*Opuntia ficus indica*) cladode powder, Cardamom (*Elettaria cardamomum*) seed powder

CardioGize™ Essential Oil Blend – 25 mg

- Angelica (*Angelica archangelica*) root oil, Cardamom (*Elettaria cardamomum*) seed oil, Cypress (*Cupressus sempervirens*) leaf/nut/stem oil, Lavender (*Lavendula angustifolia*) oil, Helichrysum (*Helichrysum italicum*) flower oil, Rosemary (*Rosmarinus officinalis*) leaf oil, Cinnamon (*Cinnamomum zeylanicum*) bark oil

Other Ingredients - Hypromellose, Water, Silicon dioxide

WHAT THE INGREDIENTS DO

- K2 - helps push calcium into bones preventing buildup in the coronary blood vessels.
- Folate - plant-based source of Vitamin B9. Helps cells divide.
- Selenium - supports normal cardiovascular function. Works well with CoQ10.
- Garlic bulb extract - supports healthy circulation.
- Coenzyme Q10 - helps the body produce energy, supports normal growth and repair.
- Astragalus root powder - supports immune system.
- Dong Quai root powder - nourishing to female glands, good for circulation.
- Motherwort powder - cardiovascular support. Helps to ease nervous tension.
- Cat's claw bark powder - helps the blood to flow smoother and healthier.
- Hawthorn berry powder - improves blood flow and protects blood vessels.
- Cactus cladode powder - high in beneficial fibers and antioxidants.
- Cardamom seed powder - rich in antioxidant benefits, influences healthy cholesterol levels, circulation and blood flow to protect cardiovascular health.
- Essential oil Blend - supports cardiovascular health and immune system support.

Other Ingredients - Hypromellose, Water, Silicon dioxide - capsule base and substrate.

COMMENTS FROM YOUNG LIVING®

"Formulated by D. Gary Young, CardioGize™ supports healthy heart function and blood circulation and may promote a higher quality of life. This supplement uses the proper synergistic ratio of CoQ10 and selenium, while garlic and CoQ10 provide antioxidant properties and vitamin K2 supports healthy vascular system function."

DIRECTIONS FOR USE

Take 2 capsules daily. (Best taken with food as vitamin K is fat soluble.)

NOTE: Keep out of the reach of children. Not for children under the age of 12. Not recommended while using blood thinners. Please check with personal physician if taking medication contraindicated before using CardioGize™. Dong Quai, Motherwort, and Cat's Claw are not safe during pregnancy.

The statements about the supplement and the ingredients have not been evaluated by the Food and Drug Administration. Young Living® products are not intended to diagnose, treat, cure, or prevent any disease.

CBD BY NATURE'S ULTRA
MOBILITY • EMOTIONS

Young Living® has spent a considerable amount of time researching CBD (cannabidiol) to make sure they have the best available for their loyal customers. Young Living® has partnered with Nature's Ultra as their exclusive CBD provider as a Seed to Seal® certified supplier for several reasons: purity, zero THC, synergy, and effectiveness.

The Cannabis plant is not technically hemp or marijuana. Both hemp and marijuana are from a Cannabis plant, but they differ in one main area: the THC or tetrahydrocannabinol molecule. Marijuana is a term used to describe a final plant product of cannabis that contains more than 0.3% of THC by dry weight. THC is the psychoactive molecule in the plant. Hemp is a term used when the final plant product of Cannabis has less than 0.3% THC. The Cannabis plant is often referred to as Hemp, but technically, there are many species of Cannabis. There are three main species that are recognized: Cannabis sativa, Cannabis indica, and Cannabis ruderalis. Nature's Ultra uses hemp from Cannabis sativa. The 2018 Farm Bill classified both marijuana and hemp as two different substances because they affect the endocannabinoid system differently.

Cannabinoids are plant chemicals that are secreted by cannabis flowers. When used in and on our bodies they can bind to the endocannabinoid system receptors found in our brain and body to help support various systems from cellular health, mental focus, brain health, calming, nerve support, and muscle and tissue support. There are two main cannabinoid receptors, CB-1 (nervous system, connective tissues, organs, and hormone glands) and CB-2 (immune function and blood) with a possible third CB-3 cannabinoid receptor that is a molecule known as GPR55 that is found in the brain, adrenal, spleen, and GI tract, although more research is being done on this potential CB-3 receptor. The endocannabinoid system has one main goal: to regulate your body systems. This is called homeostasis. This system wants to regulate areas such as your mood, pain, appetite, and the protection of your brain, to name a few.

Using pure CBD isolate in carrier oil such as coconut oil or olive oil, allows you to get amazing benefits without any of the psychoactive properties of marijuana or CBD laced with THC. Young Living® has raised the bar in CBD purity by creating a Smart Spectrum™ CBD which utilizes a pure isolate form of CBD that contains zero THC with Seed to Seal® Premium essential oils from Young Living® mixed into a carrier oil. THC, or tetrahydrocannabinol, is one of the 113 cannabinoids found in cannabis and is the constituent responsible for the "high" you get from marijuana. This psychoactive molecule is something that is found in many CBD oils even when they are labeled as zero percent THC.

The manufacturers of CBD know that many people want the psychoactive effects so they leave some THC in the final product labeled CBD even though it is illegal to do so. There are no regulatory agencies checking CBD companies, and it is all self-policed, meaning companies can put whatever they want into a CBD bottle and claim practically anything. The great thing about Nature's Ultra CBD from Young Living® is that it contains 0.00% THC and 99% CBD.

These statements have not been evaluated by the Food and Drug Administration.
Young Living® products are not intended to diagnose, treat, cure, or prevent any disease.

CBD PURITY

Nature's Ultra CBD by Young Living® is the purest CBD product you can purchase on the market today. Nature's Ultra is one of the very first farms to hold a USDA organic handler's certification in the United States. They do not use any pesticides; there is no need because the 1500-acre hemp farm is at a high altitude in Colorado where pests do not thrive. While many companies claim purity, Young Living's® Nature's Ultra is guaranteed synthetic and toxin free.

Something of major interest with Cannabis is that it is amazing at cleaning both the air, the soil, and groundwater. This is called phytoremediation. Simply put, Cannabis is a natural toxin vacuum cleaner. If you purchase CBD from plants that were grown in non-organic environments, or areas where a neighboring farm is not organic, you will be consuming or applying CBD that is contaminated at its core. Clean soil, zero pesticides or chemicals, and zero contaminated water from neighboring farms and even recycled rain are a must at a Cannabis farm.

SYNERGY = SMART SPECTRUM™

There are benefits from using CBD that is a full-spectrum or unmodified whole-plant extract that contains THC. This is called the entourage effect because the oil contains both CBD and THC along with the other 500+ molecules of the untouched plant. This would then be classified as a drug, aka Marijuana, and is not something that most of us are interested in using. Nature's Ultra is considered broad-spectrum and is termed "Smart Spectrum™ CBD" because it is infused with Young Living® essential oils. Infusing pure CBD isolate with the highest quality essential oils gives it back some of its entourage effect and is considered broad-spectrum. The molecules found in essential oils are extremely small (under 300 atomic mass units). They are also volatile in nature so they want to move and push. Combined with CBD, essential oils help to make the CBD more bioavailable, meaning they better absorb and are utilized by your body systems. Young Living® is the only company on the market to offer Smart Spectrum™ CBD oil.

Young Living® is also the only company in the United States to provide full-spectrum essential oils. They are unmodified, in their true botanical state. You are getting the full entourage effect when you use Young Living® essential oils. All other companies in the United States practice what is called "fractional distillation" to remove earthier smelling notes in their oils so the final product is more pleasing to the consumer. Young Living® is not concerned with their customers liking the smell of their oils, they are more concerned with the essential oil having the ability to work on and in your body for a longer amount of time and at a deeper level, to give you the greatest entourage effect. By adding these essential oils into the CBD isolate, the industry bar has been raised by Young Living® far above what any competitor has the ability to offer.

NOTE: There is a bit of controversy surrounding CBD use while pregnant or breastfeeding. All of the studies available mix up hemp or CBD with the marijuana plant that contains THC. The THC molecule is what is harmful to a growing fetus and infant during breastfeeding. Nature's Ultra™ contains zero THC, so it is the author's opinion that using this CBD during pregnancy and breastfeeding stages is safe. It is important to be your own best advocate and determine for yourself which supplements you feel comfortable using.

These statements have not been evaluated by the Food and Drug Administration.
Young Living® products are not intended to diagnose, treat, cure, or prevent any disease.

CBD BY NATURE'S ULTRA

CBD DROPPER
(NOT A SUPPLEMENT)

USE ANYTIME   KEEP REFRIGERATED   VEGAN   CONTAINS COCONUT   MINIMUM AGE 12+   ½ DOSAGE IF UNDER 12

INGREDIENTS

Strength Options:

500 mg CBD or 1000 mg CBD per 30 ml
- Coconut (*Cocos nucifera*) oil
- Cannabidiol (CBD)
- Organic Stevia (*Stevia rebaudiana*) leaf extract
- Plus one of the following:
  Cinnamon - Young Living® Cinnamon bark (*Cinnamomum zeylanicum*) oil
  Citrus - Young Living® Grapefruit (*Citrus paradisi*) oil, Orange (*Citrus sinensis*) oil
  Mint - Young Living® Peppermint (*Mentha piperita*) oil, Spearmint (*Mentha spicata*) oil

WHAT THE INGREDIENTS DO
- Coconut oil - Carrier oil base.
- Cannabidiol (CBD) - supports emotional well-being, muscle and joint tension, wake and sleep patterns, helps calm nervous tension, and helps reduce nausea.
- Organic Stevia leaf extract - natural sweetener.

CBD DROPPER CONCENTRATION CHART
Full dropper equals one single serving size.
- 500 mg CBD - 30 ml bottle - Approximately 16.66 mg of CBD per 1 ml
- 1000 mg CBD - 30 ml bottle - Approximately 33.33 mg of CBD per 1 ml

DIRECTIONS FOR USE
Shake the bottle for 10 seconds. Use a concentration of 0.5 ml - 1.0 ml and place on desired area. Use morning and night for two weeks for optimal results. Keep refrigerated.

CBD CALM ROLLER
(NOT A SUPPLEMENT)

USE ANYTIME

INGREDIENTS
Strength Options: 300 mg CBD or 600 mg CBD per 10 ml
- Cannabidiol (CBD)
- Calm - Lavender (*Lavandula angustifolia*) oil, Vetiver (*Vetiveria zizanoides*) root oil, Eucalyptus (*Eucalyptus Globulus*) leaf oil, Frankincense (*Boswellia carterii*) oil, Orange (*Citrus aurantium dulcis*) peel oil, Ylang Ylang (*Cananga odorata*) flower oil

Proprietary Carrier Oil Blend - Apricot kernel oil, Argan oil, Avocado oil, Camellia seed oil, Evening primrose oil, Hemp seed oil, Neem oil, Rosehip seed oil, Sweet almond oil

WHAT THE INGREDIENTS DO
- CBD - supports emotional well-being, muscle and joint tension, wake and sleep patterns, helps calm nervous tension, and helps reduce nausea.
- Lavender - supports focus, calming, and sleep.
- Vetiver - supports focus, calming, and sleep.
- Eucalyptus Globulus - supports calming, open air feeling, and relaxation.
- Frankincense - supports focus, calming, and sleep.
- Orange - supports emotions, focus, and calming.
- Ylang Ylang - supports balanced energies and a feeling of well-being.

DIRECTIONS FOR USE
CBD Roller - Roll on temples, wrists, or anywhere needed to soothe and calm.

These statements have not been evaluated by the Food and Drug Administration. Young Living® products are not intended to diagnose, treat, cure, or prevent any disease.

CBD JOINT & MUSCLE BALM
(NOT A SUPPLEMENT)

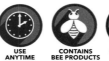

USE ANYTIME • CONTAINS BEE PRODUCTS • CAUTION IF PREGNANT

INGREDIENTS
Net weight 1.76 oz. (50 g)

Strength Options:
300 mg CBD or 600 mg CBD
- Cannabidiol (CBD)

Proprietary Young Living® Essential Oil Blend - Camphor (*Cinnamomum camphora*) leaf oil, Tea tree (M*elaleuca alternifolia*) leaf oil, Lemon (*Citrus limon*) peel oil, Peppermint (*Mentha piperita*) oil, Clove (*Eugenia caryophyllus*) bud oil, *Artemisia absinthium* leaf/stem extract (aka Wormwood), Wintergreen (*Gaultheria procumbens*) leaf oil, Helichrysum (H*elichrysum italicum*) flower oil

Proprietary Balm Blend - Camellia (*Camellia sinensis*) leaf oil (green tea), Beeswax (*Cera alba*), Shea butter (*Butyrospermum parkii*), Safflower (*Carthamus tinctorius*), Menthol, Squalane, Jojoba (*Simmondsia chinensis*) seed oil, Vitamin E (DL-alpha tocopherol), Arnica flower (*Arnica montana*)

WHAT THE INGREDIENTS DO
- Cannabidiol (CBD) - supports emotional well-being, muscle and joint tension, wake and sleep patterns, helps calm nervous tension, and helps reduce nausea.

Proprietary Young Living® Essential Oil Blend
- Camphor - supports cooling relief on muscles.
- Tea Tree - supports healthy skin.
- Lemon - supports skin brightening and skin soothing.
- Peppermint - acts as a driver or pusher to help drive and push CBD molecules in.
- Clove - supports muscle tenderness.
- *Artemisia absinthium* (Wormwood) - supports skin soothing and muscle tension.
- Wintergreen - supports joint and muscle soothing.
- Helichrysum - supports cellular tissue regeneration.

Proprietary Balm Blend - Camellia oil (green tea), Beeswax, Shea butter, Safflower, Menthol, Squalane, Jojoba seed oil, Vitamin E, Arnica flower - supports skin moisturizing, retaining, and healing benefits.

DIRECTIONS FOR USE
CBD Joint & Muscle Balm - Massage well into areas that need soothing comfort.
Note: Wormwood, Wintergreen, and Camphor are not recommended during pregnancy.

Note on CBD compliance: Even though CBD is typically a consumable supplement, and the dropper bottle contents provided by Young Living's® Nature's Ultra CBD are food grade, the FDA has excluded CBD as a dietary supplement. Young Living® abides by FDA rules and also adheres to the guidelines set forth by the Direct Selling Association (DSA). Jared O. Blum, DSA Code Administrator, stated, "Based on review of the publicly available resources, including the U.S. Food and Drug Administration (FDA), it is the determination by this office that sale of ingestible CBD products such as a foodstuff, nutritional supplement, tinctures, or for any digestible means for humans or animals is violative of the DSA Code of Ethics."

Sources:
FDA: https://www.fda.gov/media/131878/download
DSA memo: https://tinyurl.com/DSACBD

These statements have not been evaluated by the Food and Drug Administration.
Young Living® products are not intended to diagnose, treat, cure, or prevent any disease.

CBD BY NATURE'S ULTRA

COMFORTONE®

DIGESTION

USE ANYTIME

NOT VEGAN

CONTAINS BEEF GELATIN

MINIMUM AGE 12+

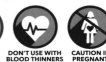
DON'T USE WITH BLOOD THINNERS

CAUTION IF PREGNANT

ComforTone® is the perfect supplement to support your stomach, digestion, liver, and gallbladder. It has herbs and roots to help with the elimination process. It is also known to help soothe discomfort from foods and will help to placate gas.

INGREDIENTS

ComforTone® Blend – 694 mg

- Cascara Sagrada bark
- Psyllium seed
- Barberry bark
- Burdock root
- Fennel seed
- Garlic bulb
- Echinacea root
- Bentonite
- Diatomaceous earth
- Ginger root
- German Chamomile flower extract
- Apple pectin
- Licorice root
- Cayenne fruit

ComforTone® Essential Oils

Tarragon, Ginger, Tangerine, Rosemary, Anise, Peppermint, Ocotea, German Chamomile

Other Ingredients - Gelatin, Water, Silicon dioxide

WHAT THE INGREDIENTS DO

- Cascara Sagrada bark - helps to support normal intestinal peristalsis (wave-like motion that moves waste out of the body). NOTE - Turns stool black and is a laxative.
- Psyllium seed - helps speed the passage of stool through the digestive tract.
- Barberry bark - helps remove morbid matter from the stomach and bowels.
- Burdock root - supports the kidneys and lymphatic system.
- Fennel seed - improves digestion and is an appetite suppressant.
- Garlic bulb - stimulates the lymphatic system to help throw off waste.
- Echinacea root - supports immune system, digestion, and lymphatic filtration.
- Bentonite - protects intestinal lining, neutralizes bacteria in the gut.
- Diatomaceous earth - soft fibers that absorb toxins to be eliminated.
- Ginger root - calms and cleanses bowels, minimizes flatulence.
- German Chamomile flower extract - helps upset stomach and gas.
- Apple pectin - natural source of dietary fiber.
- Licorice root - mild laxative. Softens, lubricates and nourishes the intestinal tract.
- Cayenne fruit - rebuilds tissue in the stomach and supports digestion.

ComforTone® Essential Oils

- Tarragon, Ginger, Tangerine, Rosemary, Anise, Peppermint, Ocotea, German Chamomile - supports proper digestion.

COMMENTS FROM YOUNG LIVING®

"ComforTone® (capsules) is an effective combination of herbs and essential oils that support the health of the digestive system by eliminating residues from the colon and enhancing its natural ability to function optimally. Because it supports normal peristalsis (the wave-like contractions that move food through the intestines), ComforTone® is ideal for strengthening the system that delivers nutrients to the rest of the body. It also contains ingredients that are beneficial to liver, gallbladder, and stomach health."

DIRECTIONS FOR USE

Take 1 capsule three times daily. Drink at least 64 oz. of distilled water throughout the day for best results. NOTE: Cascara Sagrada is not safe during pregnancy.

The statements about the supplement and the ingredients have not been evaluated by the Food and Drug Administration. Young Living® products are not intended to diagnose, treat, cure, or prevent any disease.

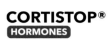

USE BEFORE BREAKFAST | NOT VEGAN | CONTAINS BEEF GELATIN | CONTAINS SOY | MINIMUM AGE 21+ | CAUTION IF PREGNANT

CortiStop® is a favorite of those who need a little help with the jitters. When life is coming at you from all sides, this is what to take first thing in the morning. Men can use it too, even though Young Living® mentions it is for women. Cortistop® contains powerful precursor hormones pregnenolone and DHEA derived from wild yams. It supports emotional fluctuations and helps improve memory and cognitive function. See each ingredient below along with the benefits of each.

INGREDIENTS
- Pregnenolone
- L-a-phosphatidylserine
- L-a-phosphatidylcholine
- Black cohosh (Actaea racemosa) root extract
- DHEA [derived from wild yam (Dioscorea Villosa) Root]
- Clary Sage (Salvia sclarea) flowering top
- Canadian Fleabane (Conyza canadensis) flowering top
- Fennel (Foeniculum vulgare) seed
- Frankincense (Boswellia carterii) gum/resin
- Peppermint (*Mentha piperita*) leaf

Other Ingredients - Rice Flour, Silica, and Gelatin (bovine)
Note: Contains Soy

WHAT THE INGREDIENTS DO
- Pregnenolone - precursor hormone that increases production of all hormones in the body such as progesterone, estrogen, and cortisol. It combats fatigue, increases energy, supports memory, supports motivation, helps increase libido, and may help improve mood swings.
- L-a-phosphatidylserine - improves mental function.
- L-a-phosphatidylcholine - improves memory function and memory loss.
- Black cohosh root - supports menopause and PMS.
- DHEA dehydroepiandrosterone - precursor hormone that helps with cognition, emotions, libido, and muscle and bone mass. May help with vaginal dryness.
- Clary Sage, Canadian Fleabane, Fennel, Frankincense, and Peppermint - all hormone supporting essential oils.

Other Ingredients - Rice Flour, Silica, and Gelatin - capsule base and substrate

COMMENTS FROM YOUNG LIVING®
"CortiStop® is a proprietary dietary supplement designed to help the body maintain its natural balance and harmony. When under stress, the body produces cortisol. When cortisol is produced too frequently, it can have negative health consequences such as feelings of fatigue, difficulty maintaining healthy weight, and difficulty maintaining optimal health of cardiovascular systems. CortiStop® supports the glandular systems of women."

DIRECTIONS FOR USE
Take 2 capsules in the morning before breakfast. If desired, for extra benefits, take another 2 capsules before retiring. Use daily for eight weeks. Discontinue use for 2-4 weeks before once more resuming. NOTE: Black Cohosh, Clary Sage, and Fennel are not recommended during pregnancy.

The statements about the supplement and the ingredients have not been evaluated by the Food and Drug Administration. Young Living® products are not intended to diagnose, treat, cure, or prevent any disease.

DETOXZYME®
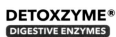

 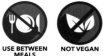

USE BETWEEN MEALS · **NOT VEGAN** · **CONTAINS DAIRY** · **MINIMUM AGE 12+**

Detoxzyme® is an enzyme powerhouse to help you cleanse your system. It is an excellent choice for bloating and gas, and for those who are lactose intolerant. Detoxzyme® helps to flush the body of dead white blood cells to allow you to function at your best. Cumin powder is added to Detoxzyme® and provides natural iron and also helps with blood sugar. It is also a good choice if you have a sweet tooth. It contains the fewest essential oils of the adult enzymes and is a vegetarian enzyme complex, but is not vegan. Below is a list of the enzymes in Detoxzyme® and their function.

INGREDIENTS
Amylase, Cumin (Cuminum cyminum) seed powder, Invertase, Protease 4.5, Glucoamylase, Bromelain, Phytase, Lipase, Cellulase (from dairy), Alpha-galactosidase, Lactase
Essential Oils - Cumin (*Cuminum cyminum*) seed oil, Anise (*Pimpinella anisum*) seed oil, Fennel (*Foeniculum vulgare*) seed oil
Other Ingredients - Hypromellose, Rice bran, Silica, Magnesium stearate, Water

WHAT THE INGREDIENTS DO
- Amylase - breaks down starches, breads, and pasta.
- Cumin - digestive supporting herb.
- Invertase - breaks down table sugar. Breaks connection between fructose and glucose.
- Protease 4.5 - helps with sinusitis and has a lower acidic content.
- Glucoamylase - breaks down starch and cereals. Flushes dead white blood cells.
- Bromelain - breaks down meats, dairy, eggs, and grains, as well as seeds, nuts, leafy greens, and other foods. Supports blood to help ease inflammation.
- Phytase - helps with bone health and pulls needed minerals from grains.
- Lipase - breaks down dietary fats and oils. Helps liver function.
- Cellulase - from dairy; breaks down man-made fiber, plant fiber, fruits, and vegetables.
- Alpha-galactosidase - breaks down beans and vegetables (for gas and bloating).
- Lactase - breaks down dairy sugars. Helps with lactose intolerance.
- Essential Oils - Cumin, Anise, and Fennel - supports digestion.
- Hypromellose - vegetable capsule
- Rice bran - natural filler for volume control
- Silica - natural substrate for anti-caking
- Magnesium stearate - natural flow agent

COMMENTS FROM YOUNG LIVING®
"Detoxzyme® combines a myriad of powerful enzymes that complete digestion, help detoxify, and promote cleansing. The ingredients in Detoxzyme® also work with the body to support normal function of the digestive system, which is essential for maintaining and building health."

DIRECTIONS FOR USE
Take 1-2 capsules three times daily between meals or as needed. This product may be used in conjunction with a cleansing or detoxifying program. For the relief of occasional symptoms such as fullness, pressure, bloating, gas, pain, and/or minor cramping that may occur after eating.
Customer Notes: Take a handful just before bed to help clean out your system.

DETOXZYME®

DIGEST & CLEANSE™
DIGESTION

JUST BEFORE MEALS

VEGAN

CONTAINS ALL OILS

CONTAINS COCONUT

MINIMUM AGE 12+

CAUTION IF PREGNANT

Digest & Cleanse® is oh so helpful for those of us who have tummy troubles. It can become your best friend! I highly recommend having this in your stash and taking it on a regular basis.

INGREDIENTS
Digest & Cleanse® Blend – 710 mg
Contains 12 drops total of Coconut carrier oil and Seed to Seal® Premium essential oils.
- Medium-chain triglycerides (from fractionated Coconut oil)
- Peppermint (*Montha piperita*) aerial parts oil
- Caraway (*Carum carvi*) fruit oil
- Coconut (*Cocus nucifera*) fruit oil
- Lemon (*Citrus limon*) peel oil
- Ginger (*Zingiber officinale*) root oil
- Fennel (*Foeniculum vulgare*) seed oil
- Anise (*Pimpinella anisum*) seed oil

Other Ingredients - Hypromellose, Water, Silica
Contains tree nuts (Coconut)

WHAT THE INGREDIENTS DO
- Medium-chain triglycerides - may help burn fat and reduce hunger.
- Peppermint oil - increases energy and improves digestion.
- Caraway oil - antioxidant that promotes digestion and increases weight loss.
- Coconut oil - supports the immune system, protects the liver from toxins, reduces inflammation, improves digestion, helps burn fat, reduces hunger.
- Lemon oil - improves digestion and stimulates lymphatic drainage.
- Ginger oil - improves digestion, reduces inflammation, and supports the liver.
- Fennel oil - improves digestion, supports blood pressure, supports weight loss.
- Anise oil - helps keep blood sugar levels stable, improves digestion.

COMMENTS FROM YOUNG LIVING®
"Digest & Cleanse® soothes gastrointestinal upset and supports healthy digestion. Stress, overeating, and toxins can irritate the gastrointestinal system and cause cramps, gas, and nausea that interfere with the body's natural digestive and detox functions. Supplementing with Digest & Cleanse® will soothe the bowel, prevent gas, and stimulate stomach secretions, thus aiding digestion. Digest & Cleanse® is formulated with clinically proven and time-tested essential oils that work synergistically to help prevent occasional indigestion and abdominal pain. Precision Delivery softgels release in the intestines for optimal absorption and targeted relief and to help prevent aftertaste."

DIRECTIONS FOR USE
Take 1 softgel one to three times daily with water 30-60 minutes prior to meals.
Caution - Keep out of the reach of children.
Note: Excessive internal use of essential oils is not considered safe during pregnancy.
Out of Stock DIY: add 2 drops each Peppermint, Caraway, Ginger, Fennel, and Lemon Vitality™ essential oils, topped off with 4 drops carrier oil to a veggie capsule.

The statements about the supplement and the ingredients have not been evaluated by the Food and Drug Administration. Young Living® products are not intended to diagnose, treat, cure, or prevent any disease.

DIGEST & CLEANSE®

ENDOGIZE™
HORMONES

USE ANYTIME   NOT VEGAN   CONTAINS BEEF GELATIN   CONTAINS SOY   MINIMUM AGE 21+   CAUTION IF PREGNANT   GOOD CHOICE FOR MEN

EndoGize™ is a strong endocrine supporting supplement for both men and women. It contains Ashwagandha root powder which is one of the most important herbs used in Ayurvedic medicine, an ancient practice that began in India 3,000 years ago and is still in use today. The root comes from India, Africa, and the Middle East and has a common name of Indian ginseng because of its energizing properties, but it is not ginseng. The plant is more like a tomato plant. "Ashwa" means horse. Ashwagandha gets its name because it smells like a horse.

Ashwagandha root has been touted to help adrenal fatigue, ease inflammation in the body, boost testosterone levels, help increase fertility in men, help to lower blood sugar levels, improve insulin sensitivity in muscle cells, improve memory and brain function, help reduce cortisol levels when chronically stressed, and also support healthy emotions, peace, and stress. Other herbs and phytonutrients in EndoGize™ are used for libido support and the overall health of the endocrine system. It contains natural DHEA found in wild yams, which is helpful for mood swings, night sweats, and general hormone support for both women and men.

There are several digestive enzymes in EndoGize™ making this supplement helpful to stressed individuals. High levels of chronic stress can cause digestive enzyme production to decrease. Using EndoGize™ will help support healthy digestion while rebuilding the strength of your endocrine system.

INGREDIENTS
- Calories - 5
- Total Carbohydrate - <1 g (1% DV)
- Protein <1 g (1% DV)
- B6 (pyridoxine HCL) - 25 mg (1470% DV)
- Zinc (zinc aspartate) - 2 mg (20% DV)
- Ashwagandha (*Withania somnifera*) root powder
- Muira puama (*Ptychopetalum olacoides*) bark
- L-arginine
- Epimedium (*Epimedium sagittatum*) aerial parts
- Tibulus (*Tribulus terrestris*) fruit extract
- Phosphatidylcholine
- Lecithin (Soy)
- DHEA (dehydroepiandrosterone)
- Black pepper (*Piper nigrum*) fruit extract
- Glucoamylase, Acid stable protease
- Longjack (*Eurycoma longifolia*) root extract
- Amylase
- Cellulase

EndoGize™ Oil Blend – 34 mg
- Ginger (*Zingiber officinale*) root oil
- Myrrh (*Commiphora myrrha*) gum/resin oil
- Cassia (*Cinnamomum aromaticum*) branch/leaf oil
- Clary sage (*Saliva sclarea*) flowering top oil
- Canadian fleabane (*Conyza canadensis*) flowering top

Other Ingredients - Rice flour, Gelatin (Bovine) (Contains Soy)

These statements have not been evaluated by the Food and Drug Administration.
Young Living® products are not intended to diagnose, treat, cure, or prevent any disease.

WHAT THE INGREDIENTS DO

- B6 - supports brain development, nervous system, and immune system.
- Zinc - supports immune system and tissue repair.
- Ashwagandha root powder - supports immune system, mental clarity, concentration, and alertness. May help boost testosterone levels, may help increase fertility in men, may help to lower blood sugar levels, may improve insulin sensitivity in muscle cells, may improve memory and brain function, may help reduce cortisol levels when chronically stressed, and may support healthy emotions, peace, and stress.
- Muira puama bark - helps improve libido and Erectile Dysfunction.
- L-arginine - an amino acid that helps support the circulatory system allowing improved blood flow.
- Epimedium aerial parts (aka "Horny Goat Weed") - used to support Erectile Dysfunction and sexual drive.
- Tribulus fruit extract - supports a healthy urinary tract, helps improve libido, and possibly increase testosterone. Supports body building.
- Phosphatidylcholine - some research suggests it may improve symptoms of ulcerative colitis. It helps with memory and also may help break down fat.
- Soy Lecithin - a fat that helps with memory. It may also help support healthy emotions, peace, eczema, the gallbladder and liver.
- DHEA dehydroepiandrosterone (from wild yams) - precursor hormone that helps with cognition, healthy emotions, libido, and muscle and bone mass. It may also help with vaginal dryness.
- Black pepper fruit extract - improves digestion, supports metabolism and energy, helps ease inflammation, and helps other supplements become more bioavailable.
- Longjack root extract - supports energy, sexual desire, and male fertility.

Digestive Enzymes
- Glucoamylase - breaks down starchy foods and cereals. Flushes the body of dead white blood cells.
- Protease 6.0 - helps with edema and carries away toxins. Helps reduce pain and varicose veins. Works in the blood. Least acidic.
- Cellulase - breaks down man-made fiber, plant fiber, fruits, and vegetables.
- Amylase - breaks down starches, breads, and pasta.

Essential Oils - Ginger, Myrrh, Cassia, Clary Sage, Canadian Fleabane

NOTE - Ashwagandha is not to be used if you are pregnant or nursing, trying to conceive, or have high cholesterol. Do not take if you are using blood glucose lowering medication as this may lower it too low. Please monitor your blood glucose closely if you choose to use this with medications and consult your doctor before you begin using it. Some drug interactions may occur. Consult your doctor prior to use. Do not use this along with Thyromin™ or Thyroid medicine due to Ashwagandha root.

COMMENTS FROM YOUNG LIVING®
"EndoGize™ is especially formulated to support a healthy and balanced endocrine system."

DIRECTIONS FOR USE
Take 1 capsule twice daily. Use daily for four weeks.
Discontinue for two weeks before resuming.
Note: Ashwagandha is not safe during pregnancy.

The statements about the supplement and the ingredients have not been evaluated by the Food and Drug Administration. Young Living® products are not intended to diagnose, treat, cure, or prevent any disease.

ENDOGIZE™

ESSENTIALZYME™
DIGESTIVE ENZYMES

USE 1 HOUR BEFORE MEAL · NOT VEGAN · CONTAINS PORK · CONTAINS SOY · MINIMUM AGE 12+

Essentialzyme™ is a good choice if you are looking for a broad-spectrum digestive enzyme that also supports hormones. It is good for those who need help absorbing B12, Calcium, Iron, and Proteins. Essentialzyme™ should be used by people who have low stomach acid. It is the only enzyme supplement from Young Living® that contains Betaine HCL, which promotes the production of hydrochloric acid which is essential for high protein diets. This enzyme contains the most herbs.

INGREDIENTS
- Carbohydrate <1g (<1% DV)
- Calcium (dicalcium phosphate) 70 mg (6% DV)

Proprietary Blend (Light) – 250 mg
- Pancrelipase, Pancreatin, Trypsin

Proprietary Blend (Dark) – 270 mg
- Betaine HCL (Betaine hydrochloride), Bromelain, Thyme (*Thymus vulgaris*) leaf powder, Carrot (*Daucus carota*) root powder, Alfalfa (*Medicago sativa*) sprout powder and leaf powder, Papain, Cumin (*Cuminum cyminum*) seed powder, Anise (*Pimpinella anisum*) seed oil, Fennel (*Foeniculum vulgare*) seed oil, Peppermint (*Mentha piperita*) leaf oil, Tarragon (*Artemisia dracunculus*) aerial parts oil, Clove (*Syzygium aromaticum*) bud oil

Other Ingredients - Microcystalline cellulose, Dicalcium phosphate, Hydroxypropylcellulose, Hydroxyproplylmethylcellulose, Stearic acid, Croscamellose sodium, Silicon dioxide, Sodium citrate, Sodium carboxymethyl cellulose, Dextrin, Lecithin, Dextrose. Contains Soy (Lecithin)

WHAT THE INGREDIENTS DO
- Pancrelipase - (pancreas from pigs) supports a poorly performing pancreas.
- Pancreatin (pancreas from pigs) - good for those with a poorly performing pancreas.
- Trypsin - breaks down proteins. For muscle growth and hormone production.
- Betaine HCL - digestive aid, helps absorb B12, Calcium, Iron, and proteins; promotes the production of hydrochloric acid.
- Bromelain - breaks down meats, dairy, eggs, and grains, as well as seeds, nuts, leafy greens, and others. Supports blood to help ease inflammation.
- Thyme leaf powder - supports digestion.
- Carrot root powder - supports digestion.
- Alfalfa sprout and leaf powder - supports digestion.
- Papain - digestive aid to help break proteins down into peptides and amino acids.
- Cumin - supports digestion.
- Anise, Fennel, Peppermint, Tarragon, and Clove essential oils - supports digestion.

Other Ingredients - substrate

COMMENTS FROM YOUNG LIVING®
"Essentialzyme™ is a bilayered, multienzyme complex caplet specially formulated to support and balance digestive health and to stimulate overall enzyme activity to combat the modern diet. Essentialzyme™ contains Tarragon, Peppermint, Anise, Fennel, and Clove essential oils to improve overall enzyme activity, and support healthy pancreatic function."

DIRECTIONS FOR USE
Take 1 caplet before meals for best results.
Customer Notes: Use many throughout the day and evening when traveling to support health.

The statements about the supplement and the ingredients have not been evaluated by the Food and Drug Administration. Young Living® products are not intended to diagnose, treat, cure, or prevent any disease.

ESSENTIALZYMES-4™

DIGESTIVE ENZYMES

BEST WITH FOOD · NOT VEGAN · CONTAINS BEEF GELATIN · CONTAINS BEE PRODUCTS · MINIMUM AGE 12+

Essentialzymes-4™ helps support proper nutrient absorption. This is the broadest reaching enzyme complex. It contains bee pollen which is rich in antioxidants, vitamins, and minerals, as well as enzymes to help build your immune system and support brain function and alertness. This digestive enzyme also contains essential oils to help it become more bioavailable. The best choice for everyone!

INGREDIENTS

WHITE CAPSULE
- Carbohydrate <1g (<1% DV)

Essentialzymes-4™ (White) Blend – 225 mg
- Bee pollen powder; Digestive Enzymes: Pancreatin, Lipase; Essential Oils: Ginger (*Zingibar officinale*) root oil, Fennel (*Foeniculum vulgare*) seed oil, Tarragon (*Artemisia dracunculus*) leaf oil, Anise (*Pimpinella anisum*) fruit oil, Lemongrass (*Cymbopogon flexuosus*) leaf oil

Other Ingredients - Rice Flour, Hypromellose, Magnesium Stearate, Silicon Dioxide

YELLOW CAPSULE
- Riboflavin (B2) 8.3 mg (638% DV)
- Sodium 10 mg (<1% DV)

Essentialzymes-4™ (Yellow) Blend – 186 mg
- Digestive Enzymes: Protease 3.0, Protease 4.5, Protease 6.0, Amylase, Cellulase, Lipase, Peptidase, Bromelain, Papain; Essential Oils: Anise (*Pimpinella anisum*) fruit oil, Ginger (*Zingibar officinale*) root oil, Rosemary (*Rosemarinus officinalis*) leaf oil, Tarragon (*Artemisia dracunculus*) leaf oil, Fennel (*Foeniculum vulgare*) seed oil

Other Ingredients - Rice Flour, Gelatin, Magnesium Stearate, Silicon Dioxide

WHAT THE INGREDIENTS DO
- Amylase - breaks down starches, breads, and pasta.
- Bromelain - breaks down meats, dairy, eggs, and grains, as well as seeds, nuts, leafy greens, and others. Supports blood to help ease inflammation.
- Cellulase - breaks down man-made fiber, plant fiber, fruits, and vegetables.
- Lipase - breaks down dietary fats and oils. Helps liver function.
- Peptidase - supports immune system and helps ease inflammation.
- Phytase - helps with bone health and pulls needed minerals from grains.
- Protease 3.0 - supports circulation and toxicity. Higher acid to break down animal protein.
- Protease 4.5 - helps with sinusitis and has a lower acidic content.
- Protease 6.0 - helps with edema and carries away toxins. Least acidic.
- Papain - digestive aid to help break proteins down into peptides and amino acids.
- Pancreatin (pancreas from pigs or cows) - helps produce other enzymes. Good for those with a poorly performing pancreas.
- Bee pollen - contains vitamins, minerals, and antioxidants.
- Digestive supporting oils - Ginger, Fennel, Tarragon, Anise, Lemongrass, Rosemary.

Other Ingredients - capsule base and substrate

COMMENTS FROM YOUNG LIVING®
"Essentialzymes-4™ is a multi-spectrum enzyme complex specially formulated to aid the critically needed digestion of dietary fats, proteins, fiber, and carbohydrates commonly found in the modern processed diet. The dual time-release technology releases the animal- and plant-based enzymes at separate times within the digestive tract, allowing for optimal nutrient absorption."

DIRECTIONS FOR USE
Take 2 capsules (one dual dose blister pack) twice daily with largest meals.

The statements about the supplement and the ingredients have not been evaluated by the Food and Drug Administration. Young Living® products are not intended to diagnose, treat, cure, or prevent any disease.

ESSENTIALZYMES-4™

FEMIGEN™
HORMONES

BEST WITH FOOD | NOT VEGAN | CONTAINS BEEF GELATIN | MINIMUM AGE 21+ | WOMEN SPECIFIC | CAUTION IF PREGNANT

FemiGen™ supports a healthy libido, stress, energy, emotions, mood swings, vaginal dryness, PMS, hot flashes, appetite, metabolism, and is a natural alternative to estrogen therapy. Other herbs found in this supplement support your immune system and help aid digestion. L-cystine is the basic building block of glutathione, which is a gem for longevity, liver detoxification, and cognitive health. FemiGen™ is a perfect supplement for hormonal changes.

INGREDIENTS
- Iron - (4% DV)
- Magnesium - (2% DV)

FemiGen™ Blend – 1.2 g
- Damiana (*Turnera diffusa*) leaf
- Epimedium (*Epimedium sagittatum*)
- Wild yam (*Dioscorea villosa*) root
- Dong quai (*Angelica sinensis*) leaf
- Muira puama (*Ptychopetalum olacoides*) bark
- American Ginseng (*Panax quinquefolius*) root and leaf
- Licorice (*Glycyrrhiza glabra*) root extract
- Black cohosh (*Cimicifuga racemosa*) root and stem
- L-carnitine L-tartrate
- Dimethylglycine
- Cramp bark (*Viburnum opulus*) bark
- L-phenylalanine
- Squaw vine (*Mitchella repens*) aerial parts
- L-cystine
- L-cysteine HCL
- Fennel (*Foeniculum vulgare*) seed oil
- Clary sage (*Salvia sclarea*) flowering top oil
- Sage (*Salvia officinalis*) leaf oil
- Ylang Ylang (*Cananga odorata*) flower oil

WHAT THE INGREDIENTS DO
- Damiana - supports libido, healthy emotions, mood swings, and helps lower stress.
- Epimedium (aka "Horny Goat Weed") - used to increase sexual drive.
- Wild Yam - natural alternative to estrogen therapy. Supports vaginal dryness, PMS, hot flashes, increased energy, and libido.
- Dong Quai - helps ease menopausal symptoms and PMS.
- Muira Puma - increases sex drive, supports PMS, and can support joint pain.
- American Ginseng - helps to lower stress; supports immune and digestive systems.
- Licorice extract - helps reduce stress and aids in digestion.
- Black Cohosh - helps ease menopause and PMS.
- L-carnitine L-tartrate - helps reduce lactic acid build up.
- Dimethylglycine - helps improve the nervous system and immune system.
- Cramp Bark - helps with fluid retention, PMS and cramps.
- Squaw Vine - supports peace, insomnia, menstruation, baby blues.
- L-phenylalanine - helps suppress appetite and help burn fat. Also helps with moods.
- L-cystine - building block of glutathione for oxidative stress, liver detox, and cognition.
- L-cysteine HCL - helps support anti-aging. Supports the immune system.
- Hormone supporting oils - Fennel, Clary Sage, Sage, Ylang Ylang

Other Ingredients - Gelatin (Bovine) capsule, Silicon dioxide - capsule and substrate.

COMMENTS FROM YOUNG LIVING®
"FemiGen™ capsules were formulated with herbs and amino acids designed to balance and support the female reproductive system from youth through menopause. FemiGen™ combines whole food herbs like wild yam, damiana, and dong quai, along with synergistic amino acids and select essential oils to supply nutrition that is supportive of the special needs of the female systems."

DIRECTIONS FOR USE
Take 2 capsules with breakfast and 2 capsules with lunch.
Customer Notes: When first starting out, use 1 capsule with breakfast and 1 capsule with lunch for 1-2 weeks. Monitor your body then increase to the recommended dose as needed.
Note: Black Cohosh, Dong Quai, Licorice Root, Clary Sage are not safe during pregnancy.

The statements about the supplement and the ingredients have not been evaluated by the Food and Drug Administration. Young Living® products are not intended to diagnose, treat, cure, or prevent any disease.

FEMIGEN™

ICP™

DIGESTION

USE ANYTIME | VEGAN | MINIMUM AGE 12+

ICP™ is a part of Young Living's® intestinal cleanse protocol. It is often said that the letters ICP stands for "I see poo." It supports healthy digestion and a healthy colon.

INGREDIENTS

- Calories - 20
  - Calories from Fat - 5
- Total Fat - 0.5 g (<1% DV)
- Total Carbohydrate - 4 g (1% DV)
  - Dietary Fiber - 2 g (10% DV)
- Iron - 1 mg (6% DV)

ICP™ Blend – 5 g

- Psyllium *(Plantago ovata)* seed powder, Oat *(Avena sativa)* bran powder , Flax *(Linum usitatissimum)* seed powder, Fennel *(Foeniculum vulgare)* seed powder, Rice *(Oryza sativa)* bran, Guar *(Cyamopsis tetragonoloba)* gum seed powder, Yucca *(Yucca filamentosa)* root, Microcrystalline cellulose, Fennel *(Foeniculum vulgare)* seed oil, Anise *(Pimpinella anisum)* seed oil, Tarragon *(Artemisia dracunuculus)* leaf oil, Aloe vera *(Aloe barbadensis)* leaf extract, Ginger *(Zingiber officinale)* root oil, Lemongrass *(Cymbopogon flexuosus)* leaf oil, Rosemary *(Rosmarinus officinalis)* leaf oil

ICP™ Enzyme Blend – 123 mg

- Lipase, Protease 4.5, 3.0, and 6.0, Phytase, Peptidase

WHAT THE INGREDIENTS DO

- Iron - may improve muscle function, increase brain function and eliminate fatigue.
- Psyllium - helps constipation, digestion, blood sugar, cholesterol, and weight loss.
- Oat bran - aids digestion, regulates blood sugar levels, can help with weight loss.
- Flax seed - rich in dietary fiber, supports cholesterol, weight loss, and blood pressure.
- Fennel seed - improves digestion, lowers blood pressure, may promote weight loss.
- Rice bran - can aid in weight loss, may lower blood pressure and cholesterol levels.
- Guar gum seed - natural bonding agent.
- Yucca root - may relieve pain and supports the immune system.
- Microcrystalline cellulose - an important source of fiber.
- Fennel seed oil - improves digestion, lowers blood pressure, may promote weight loss.
- Anise seed oil - helps keep blood sugar levels stable, improves digestion.
- Tarragon leaf oil - improves digestion, fights bacteria.
- Aloe vera leaf extract - antioxidant and antimicrobial properties, can aid in digestion.
- Ginger root oil - improves digestion, reduces inflammation, improves liver function.
- Lemongrass leaf oil - supports the immune system, digestion, and cholesterol levels.
- Rosemary leaf oil - helps cleanse the liver, aids in digestion.

ICP™ Enzyme Blend 123 mg

- Lipase, Protease (4.5, 3.0, 6.0), Phytase, Peptidase - breaks down food for digestion and absorption.

COMMENTS FROM YOUNG LIVING®

"ICP™ helps keep your colon clean with an advanced mix of fibers that scour out residues. A healthy digestive system is important for the proper functioning of all other systems because it absorbs nutrients that are used throughout the body. Enhanced with a special blend of essential oils, the fibers work to decrease the buildup of wastes, improve nutrient absorption, and help maintain a healthy heart."

DIRECTIONS FOR USE

Mix 2 rounded teaspoons with at least 8 oz. of juice or water. If cleansing or eating a high-protein diet, use three times daily. If eating a low-protein diet, use once daily. Drink immediately as this product tends to thicken quickly when added to liquid. Tastes best in juice or smoothies.

The statements about the supplement and the ingredients have not been evaluated by the Food and Drug Administration. Young Living® products are not intended to diagnose, treat, cure, or prevent any disease.

ICP™

ILLUMINEYES™
VISION

BEST WITH FOOD — VEGAN — MINIMUM AGE 12+ — ½ DOSAGE IF UNDER 12

IlluminEyes™ is a natural combination of Acerola Cherry, Marigold Flower, and Goji berry (Wolfberry) that supports eye and skin health. The high amounts of Beta-carotene are derived from Lyceum barbarum (Wolfberry) fruit powder as well as the Acerola Cherry, and Marigold Flower.

These three powerhouse ingredients have some incredible benefits. IlluminEyes™ helps to protect your eyes from damaging blue light found in our computers, mobile devices, and from the sun. It helps to protect and maintain our eye health and helps to increase macular pigment optical density (MPOD). This means it helps lower the risk of age-related macular degeneration, it helps to absorb harmful blue light which in turn protects the photo-receptors in your eyes from further damage, and it helps to improve visual acuity (such as low light reading or small type reading on the back of labels).

Your MPOD can also determine your ability to see contrast in lower contrast situations such as seeing a white airplane in a light blue sky, your glare recovery in situations when you go from dark to light, as well as light sensitivity and visual discomfort when exposed to bright light or sunlight. IlluminEyes™ will help reduce eye fatigue and eye strain.

The Marigold Flower found in IlluminEyes™ is high in zeaxanthin which has been studied for its remarkable ability to absorb blue light, and its high antioxidant behavior helps to protect tissue from oxidative stress. Marigolds also contain Lutein. Vitamin A, Zeaxanthin, and Lutein are carotenoids that help reduce oxidation for better cellular and tissue health to help support healthy looking skin by strengthening your skin and increasing its durability.

Vitamin A can be obtained from three sources: as preformed retinol found in animal sources such as dairy, certain meats, and fish; as provitamin A, called Beta-carotene, found in plant pigments; or as synthetic vitamin A. There are some concerns in the medical community surrounding smokers taking supplements with vitamin A, that it can cause an increase in lung cancer for a small percentage of the participants. The studies that are sited were based on previous data pooling of other studies where people took a multivitamin containing synthetic vitamin A. Other studies were conducted using retinoids, a form of vitamin A derived from animals, that showed an increase in lung cancer in patients who were smokers. Beta-carotene is vitamin A found naturally in fruits and vegetables. Studies have shown protective activity when using this form of vitamin A. Not all vitamin A is equal. It is important to know your source.

IlluminEyes™ uses Beta-carotene sourced from Wolfberries, Acerola Cherries, and Marigold Flowers. If you are a smoker, and are concerned, you are welcome to make your own choice when it comes to IlluminEyes™, however the vitamin A is derived from natural plant sources, and if there was a valid medical caution, Young Living® would have put that caution on the label.

These statements have not been evaluated by the Food and Drug Administration.
Young Living® products are not intended to diagnose, treat, cure, or prevent any disease.

INGREDIENTS
- A (Beta-carotene from Acerola Cherry, Marigold, and Wolfberry) - 1300 mg (144% DV)
- C (from Acerola Cherry) - 10 mg (11% DV)
- E (D-alpha tocopherol) - 10 mg (67% DV)
- Lutein (from Marigold flower) - 20 mg
- Zeaxanthin (from Marigold flower and Wolfberry) - 4 mg

IlluminEyes™ Blend – 273 mg
- Wolfberry (*Lycium barbarum*) fruit powder
- Marigold (*Tagetes erecta*) flower extract
- Acerola cherry (*Malpighia glabra*) extract

Other Ingredients - Microcrystalline cellulose, Capsule (Hypromellose), Water, Purple carrot concentrate, Magnesium stearate, Silicon dioxide

WHAT THE INGREDIENTS DO
- A - supports immune function, decreases oxidative stress, supports eye and skin health.
- C - supports immune function and decreases oxidative stress.
- E - antioxidant to support eye health and free radicals.
- Lutein - supports eye health and decreases oxidative stress. Helps prevent eye diseases, supports tissue health, heart health, and blood health.
- Zeaxanthin - supports eye health and decreases oxidative stress. Helps protect eyes from harmful blue light.

IlluminEyes™ Blend – 273 mg
- Wolfberry fruit powder - supports immune function, and decreases oxidative stress.
- Marigold flower extract - high in lutein and zeaxanthin for eye health.
- Acerola cherry extract - high in antioxidants and supports immune function.

Other Ingredients - Microcrystalline cellulose, Capsule (Hypromellose, Water, Purple carrot concentrate), Magnesium stearate, Silicon dioxide - for capsule and substrate.

COMMENTS FROM YOUNG LIVING®
"Support your eyes and skin with the powerful ingredients in IlluminEyes™! Featuring lutein and zeaxanthin, this proprietary formula helps reduce eye strain, protects eyes from damaging blue light, and maintains vibrant skin. IlluminEyes™ can also help support your eye health in the long-term – vitamins A and C both have properties that may help reduce eye health deterioration commonly related to age."

BENEFITS
- Protects eyes from damaging blue light.
- Improves visual performance.
- Helps protect and maintain proper eye health.
- Helps support vision in low light settings.
- Helps reduce eye fatigue and eye strain.
- Increases macular pigment optical density.
- May help reduce eye health deterioration common with age.
- Maintains healthy looking skin.
- Helps support skin strength and durability.

DIRECTIONS FOR USE
Take 1 capsule daily with food.

Customer Notes: For children under 12, you may use one capsule every other day, or mix half a capsule into a shake mix or in applesauce.

The statements about the supplement and the ingredients have not been evaluated by the Food and Drug Administration. Young Living® products are not intended to diagnose, treat, cure, or prevent any disease.

ILLUMINEYES™

IMMUPRO™

SLEEP • IMMUNE SUPPORT

USE JUST
BEFORE BED

MELATONIN
SLEEP AID

VEGAN

CONTAINS
STEVIA

MINIMUM
AGE 14+

ImmuPro™ helps strengthen the immune system and helps you fall asleep faster. Take one chewable tablet of ImmuPro™ about 30 minutes before bedtime. It has just the right amount of non-habit forming melatonin, because it is from a natural source, to help you drift off to dreamland and then it gets to work with its amazing ability to fight all that oxidative stress that you built up during the day.

INGREDIENTS
- Calories - 5
- Total Carbohydrate - 1 g
- Total Sugars (includes added sugars) - <1 g
- Calcium (calcium carbonate) - 84 mg (6% DV)
- Zinc (zinc bisglycinate chelate) - 5 mg (45% DV)
- Selenium (elenium glycinate chelate) - 68 mcg (124% DV)
- Copper (copper bisglycinate chelate) - 0.16 mg (18% DV)

ImmuPro™ Blend – 940 mg
- Strawberry (*Fragaria chiloensis*) fruit powder
- Wolfberry (*Lycium barbarum*) fruit polysaccharide
- Raspberry (*Rubus idaeus*) fruit powder
- Reishi (*Ganoderma lucidum*) whole mushroom powder
- Maitake Mushroom (*Grifola frondosa*) mycelia powder
- Arabinogalactan [from larch tree (*Larix laricina*) wood extract]
- Mushroom (*Agaricus blazei*) mycelia powder
- Orange (*Citrus sinensis*) peel oil

Melatonin – 4.2 mg
Other Ingredients - Dextrose (non-GMO), Hydroxylproply cellulose, Stevia (*Stevia rebaudiana*). Silicon dioxide, Magnesium stearate, Maltodextin (non-GMO) - capsule and substrate

WHAT THE INGREDIENTS DO
- Zinc - highly absorbable form of zinc. Supports immune function.
- Selenium - a powerful antioxidant that defends against free radicals in the body.
- Copper - supports red blood cell production, immune system, bones, vessels, and nerves.
- Strawberry fruit powder - antioxidant and source of soluble and insoluble fiber.
- Wolfberry polysaccharides - Supports immune system.
- Reishi mushroom - supports anti-aging and immune system.
- Maitake mushroom - contains beta-glucan which supports the immune system.
- Agaricus blazei mushroom - supports immune function and helps fight weight gain.
- Wolfberry and Larch Tree extracts - supports immune function and regeneration of cells.

COMMENTS FROM YOUNG LIVING®
"ImmuPro™ has been specially formulated to provide exceptional immune system support when combined with a healthy lifestyle and adequate sleep to support the body's needs. This power-packed formula combines naturally-derived immune-supporting Ningxia wolfberry polysaccharides with a unique blend of reishi, maitake, and agaricus blazei mushroom powders to deliver powerful antioxidant activity to help reduce the damaging effects of oxidative stress from free radicals."

DIRECTIONS FOR USE
Take 1-2 chewable tablets at bedtime. Do not exceed 2 tablets per day.
Caution: contains Melatonin which may cause drowsiness. Do not drive or operate machinery while taking products containing Melatonin. Keep out of the reach of children.

The statements about the supplement and the ingredients have not been evaluated by the Food and Drug Administration. Young Living® products are not intended to diagnose, treat, cure, or prevent any disease.

INNER DEFENSE®
IMMUNE SYSTEM

USE ANYTIME · BEST WITH FOOD · CONTAINS ALL OILS · NOT VEGAN · CONTAINS FISH GELATIN · CONTAINS COCONUT · MINIMUM AGE 14+ · CAUTION IF PREGNANT

Inner Defense® is an immune system supporting essential oil supplement. It is safe to consume daily, but can also be taken on days you are not feeling your best. Contrary to popular assumption, taking this daily will not upset your good gut flora. The oils in this capsule work in harmony with your gut, helping to strengthen your terrain, rather than beat it up. It is best to take Inner Defense® as needed rather than on a daily basis. If you choose to take it at night before bed, do not take Life 9® that night. Monitor your daily wellness and if you feel a little dip in your wellness, use Inner Defense® as a one-time "bomb". This means you would take 1-2 capsules right at the very first signs of a wellness dip.

INGREDIENTS
Inner Defense® 03 Super Blend – 405 mg
- Virgin Coconut (*Cocos nucifera*) fruit oil
- Oregano (*Origanum vulgare*) leaf/stem oil
- Thyme (*Thymus vulgaris*) leaf oil
- Lemongrass (*Cymbopogon flexuosus*) leaf oil

Thieves® Essential Oil Blend – 225 mg
Contains 13 drops total of Coconut carrier oil and Seed to Seal® Premium essential oils.
- Clove (*Syzygium aromaticum*) bud oil
- Lemon (*Citrus Limon*) peel oil
- Eucalyptus radiata (*Eucalyptus radiata*) leaf oil
- Rosemary (*Rosmarinus officinalis*) leaf oil
- Cinnamon (*Cinnamomum verum*) bark oil

Other Ingredients - Fish gelatin, Glycerin, Water.
Note: Contains fish (tilapia, carp) and tree nuts (Coconut)

WHAT THE INGREDIENTS DO
- Virgin Coconut Oil - contains vitamins and minerals that support overall health.
- Oregano - rich in antioxidants and supports the immune system.
- Thyme - supports respiratory, digestive, immune and nervous systems, and mood.
- Lemongrass - supports immune and circulatory systems.
- Clove - supports healthy microbial balance.
- Lemon - helps improve mental clarity and supports the immune system.
- Eucalyptus - supports immune and respiratory systems; helps ease inflammation.
- Rosemary - supports cognition and the immune system.
- Cinnamon Bark - supports immune and respiratory systems.

COMMENTS FROM YOUNG LIVING®
"Young Living's® Inner Defense® reinforces systemic defenses, creates unfriendly terrain for yeast/fungus, promotes healthy respiratory function, and contains potent essential oils like Oregano, Thyme, and Thieves® which are rich in thymol, carvacrol, and eugenol for immune support. The liquid softgels dissolve quickly for maximum results. Softgel capsule has been reformulated with fish gelatin to remove the need for carrageenan and beeswax used in the porcine gelatin based softgel."

DIRECTIONS FOR USE
Take 1 softgel daily (a.m.) or take 1 softgel 3-5 times daily when needed.
For best results use Life 9® eight hours later. NOTE: Excessive internal use of essential oils is not considered safe during pregnancy.

The statements about the supplement and the ingredients have not been evaluated by the Food and Drug Administration. Young Living® products are not intended to diagnose, treat, cure, or prevent any disease.

INNER DEFENSE®

JUVAPOWER®

LIVER & INTESTINE SUPPORT

 BEST WITH FOOD **VEGAN** **CONTAINS BARLEY** **MINIMUM AGE 12+** **CAUTION IF PREGNANT**

JuvaPower® is the supplement to take when you need extra help with alkalizing your body. It is a source of antioxidants and it supports your liver and helps to bind acids. JuvaPower® is an easy way to get added nutrients to support immune and digestive systems, as well as helps support cardiovascular health.

INGREDIENTS

- Calories - 30
- Total Fat - 0.5 g
- Total Carbohydrates - 5 g (2% DV)
    Dietary Fiber - 2 g (6% DV)
    Total Sugars - 1 g
- Protein - 1 g
- Iron - 1.7 mg (10% DV)
- Sodium - 25 mg (1% DV)

JuvaPower® Blend – 7.5 g

- Rice (*Oryza sativa*) seed bran
- Spinach (*Spinacia oleracea*) leaf powder
- Tomato (*Lycopersicon esculentum*) fruit flakes
- Beet (*Beta vulgaris*) root powder
- Flaxseed (*Linum usitatissumum*) bran
- Oat seed (*Avena sativa*) bran
- Broccoli (*Brassica oleracea*) floret/stalk powder
- Cucumber (*Cucumis sativus*) fruit powder
- Dill (*Anethum graveolens*) seed
- Barley (*Hordeum vulgare*) sprouted seed
- Ginger (*Zingiber officinale*) root/rhizome powder
- Slippery elm (*Ulmus fulva*) bark
- Psyllium (*Plantago ovata*) seed husk
- Anise (*Pimpinella anisum*) seed
- Fennel (*Foeniculum vulgare*) seed
- Aloe vera (*Aloe barbadensis*) leaf extract
- Peppermint (*Mentha piperita*) leaf
- Anise (*Pimpinella anisum*) seed oil
- Fennel (*Foeniculum vulgare*) seed oil

WHAT THE INGREDIENTS DO

- Rice bran - can aid in weight loss, may lower blood pressure and cholesterol levels.
- Spinach leaf powder - has beta-carotene, iron, and fiber providing benefits to support aging, immune system, digestion, and blood.
- Tomato fruit flakes - a good source of antioxidants and nutrients to support proper immune system functioning.
- Beet root powder - a health-promoting food that aids in increasing nitric oxide availability and can support hypertension and endothelial function.
- Flaxseed bran - rich in alpha-linolenic acid (ALA, omega-3 fatty acids), lignans, and fiber that can support the cardiovascular and immune systems.

WHAT THE INGREDIENTS DO (continued)

- Oat seed bran - a good source of B complex vitamins, vitamin E, protein, fat, minerals, and is rich in beta-glucan which is heart-healthy soluble fiber.
- Broccoli floret/stalk powder - an excellent source of vitamins K, E, C, B6, and A, phosphorus, potassium, magnesium, as well as folate and fiber.
- Cucumber fruit powder - antioxidant and skin-conditioning properties.
- Dill seed - assists with relief of abdominal discomfort, colic, and digestion. It can also assist with ulcers, eye diseases, and uterine pains.
- Barley sprouted seed - contains a variety of vitamins, minerals, and polyphenolic compounds that may improve cholesterol metabolism.
- Ginger root/rhizome powder - improves digestion, reduces inflammation, reduces cholesterol levels, and improves liver function.
- Slippery elm bark - supports common cold symptoms, supports digestion, urinary tract, and bowel.
- Psyllium seed husk - stimulates the intestines to contract and helps speed the passage of stool through the digestive tract.
- Anise seed and seed oil - helps keep blood sugar levels stable and improves digestion.
- Fennel seed and seed oil - improves digestion, helps move waste material out of the body, and is a mild appetite suppressant.
- Aloe vera leaf extract - has antioxidant properties and can aid in digestion.
- Peppermint leaf - increases energy and improves bowel movements.

COMMENTS FROM YOUNG LIVING®

"JuvaPower® is a high antioxidant vegetable powder complex and is one of the richest sources of acid-binding foods. JuvaPower® is rich in liver-supporting nutrients and has intestinal cleansing benefits."

DIRECTIONS FOR USE

Sprinkle 7.5 grams (1 Tbsp.) on food (i.e., baked potato, salad, rice, eggs, etc.) or add to 4-8 oz. purified water or rice/almond milk and drink.
Use JuvaPower® three times daily for maximum benefits.

NOTE: Anise and Slippery Elm is likely safe during pregnancy when used in food use but does have estrogenic effects.

JUVAPOWER®

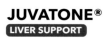

BEST BETWEEN MEALS

NOT VEGAN

CONTAINS BEE PRODUCTS

MINIMUM AGE 12+

¼-½ DOSAGE IF UNDER 12

CAUTION IF PREGNANT

JuvaTone® is a liver-supporting supplement and is helpful for those who tend to eat more animal protein. This supplement should be used when desiring to have optimal liver function. Whether you have had a bit too much to drink or you indulged in a meal high in animal protein, JuvaTone® is your go-to source! It is a powerful herbal supplement to support healthy liver function.

INGREDIENTS
- Calcium (dicalcium phosphate) - 344 mg (35% DV)
- Copper (Copper citrate) - 1.6 mg (80% DV)
- Sodium - 16 mg

Proprietary JuvaTone® Blend – 3.3 g
- Choline (C. bitarate)
- Dl-methionine
- Inositol
- Beet (*Beta vulgaris*) root
- Dandelion (*Taraxacum officinale*) root
- L-cysteine HCl
- Alfalfa (*Medicago sativa*) sprout
- Oregon grape (*Berberis aquifolium*) root
- Parsley (*Petroselinum crispum*) leaf powder
- Bee propolis
- Echinacea purpurea root

Proprietary Essential Blend – 11 mg
- Lemon (*Citrus limon*) peel oil
- German chamomile (*Matricaria recutita*) flower oil
- Geranium (*Pelargonium graveolens*) aerial parts oil
- Rosemary (*Rosmarinus officinalis*) leaf oil
- Myrtle (*Myrtus communis*) leaf oil
- Blue tansy (*Tanacetum annuum*) flowering top oil

Other Ingredients - Cellulose, Silicon dioxide, Magnesium stearate, Cellulose film-coating

WHAT THE INGREDIENTS DO
- Calcium - helps prevent bone loss and repairs joints.
- Copper - important in growth and development.
- Sodium - supports nerve impulses and maintains the balance of water and minerals.
- Choline - supports metabolism, liver, and brain function.
- Dl-methionine - supports the liver, skin, hair, and strengthens nails, plus detoxes cells.
- Inositol - helps turn food into energy. Supports the immune system, hair and nails.
- Beet root - a health-promoting and disease-preventing functional food. Supports hypertension and endothelial function.
- Dandelion root - a rich source of vitamin A. Supports the liver, gallbladder, bile ducts, and for minor digestive problems.
- L-cysteine HCl - supports glutathione for lung and brain function. Supports the liver.
- Alfalfa sprout - a source of Vitamins A, C, E, and K4 and minerals calcium, potassium, phosphorous, and iron. Supports urinary system and cholesterol.

The statements about the supplement and the ingredients have not been evaluated by the Food and Drug Administration. Young Living® products are not intended to diagnose, treat, cure, or prevent any disease.

WHAT THE INGREDIENTS DO (continued)

- Oregon grape root - supports immune and digestive systems.
- Parsley leaf powder - improves digestion.
- Bee propolis - supports the immune system.
- Echinacea purpurea root - supports the immune system.
- Lemon peel oil - supports the immune, digestive, and lymphatic systems.
- German chamomile flower oil - supports digestion and gas.
- Geranium aerial parts oil - anti-inflammatory properties.
- Rosemary leaf oil - supports the liver and immune system.
- Myrtle leaf oil - supports the immune system.
- Blue tansy flowering top oil - supports the immune system and the liver.

COMMENTS FROM YOUNG LIVING®

"JuvaTone® is a powerful herbal complex designed to promote healthy liver function. It is an excellent source of choline, a nutrient that is vital for proper liver function and necessary for those with high protein diets. JuvaTone® also contains inositol and dl-methionine, which helps with the body's normal excretion functions. Methionine also helps recycle glutathione, a natural antioxidant crucial for normal liver function. Other ingredients include Oregon grape root, a source of the liver-supporting compound berberine, and Seed to Seal® Premium essential oils to enhance overall effectiveness."

DIRECTIONS FOR USE

Take 2 tablets twice daily. Increase as needed up to 4 tablets four times daily. Best when taken between meals.
Note: Oregon Grape root contains Berberine, and is not advised for pregnancy.

JUVA PRODUCT LINE

Young Living's® Juva product line assists the body's natural cleansing functions. The word "Juva" comes from the idea of re-JUVA-nate. Using the Juva product line helps to rejuvenate your liver. The liver, one of the main filtration organs in your body, cleanses your blood that comes from your digestive tract. It has a wonderful ability to detoxify chemicals and metabolize alcohol, drugs, and synthetics. Keeping your liver clean can help correct several issues according to Functional Diagnostic Nutrition[1] such as poor digestion, hormone imbalances, weight gain, skin problems, fatigue, bad breath, the white coating on your tongue, chemical sensitivities, and food cravings to name a few.

- JuvaCleanse® essential oil blend helps support the body's digestive system.
- JuvaFlex® essential oil blend helps support the body's digestive system.
- JuvaPower® adds extra fiber and nutrients to your digestive system.
- JuvaTone® tablets provide vital nutrients to support a healthy digestive system.

Source:
1. https://www.functionaldiagnosticnutrition.com/10-signs-congested-liver/

JUVATONE®

K & B™

RENAL SUPPORT

USE ANYTIME | NOT VEGAN | CONTAINS BEE PRODUCTS | MINIMUM AGE 12+ | ½ DOSAGE IF UNDER 12

K & B™ is a liquid tincture that is a must for renal system support. The K and B stand for Kidney and Bladder. It supports the renal system to help increase urination and the liver to help support detoxification. It contains natural antioxidants and natural anti-inflammatory properties. K & B™ may be taken by adding to distilled water or added directly to veggie capsules.

INGREDIENTS

Proprietary K & B™ Blend – 3 ml
- Juniper (*Juniperus communis*) berry extract
- Parsley (*Petroselinum crispum*) leaf extract
- Uva-ursi (*Arctostaphylos uva-ursi*) leaf extract
- Dandelion (*Taraxacum officinale*) root extract
- German chamomile (*Matricaria recutita*) flower extract
- Royal Jelly (from bees)
- Geranium (*Pelargonium graveolens*) aerial parts oil
- Fennel (*Foeniculum vulgare*) seed oil
- Clove (*Syzygium aromaticum*) flower bud oil
- Roman chamomile (*Chamaemelum nobile*) aerial parts oil
- Sage (*Salvia officinalis*) leaf oil
- Juniper (*Juniperus communis*) branch/leaf/fruit oil

Other Ingredients - Water, Ethyl alcohol

WHAT THE INGREDIENTS DO
- Juniper berry extract - supports digestion, intestinal gas, heartburn, bloating, and loss of appetite. Also supports the urinary tract, kidneys and bladder.
- Parsley leaf extract - supports the urinary tract, and gastrointestinal tract.
- Uva-ursi leaf extract - supports the urinary tract and painful urination.
- Dandelion root extract - supports digestion. Used to increase urine production and as a laxative to increase bowel movements. Rich in antioxidants. Supports liver health.
- German chamomile flower extract - supports digestion and gas.
- Royal Jelly - produced by honey bees. Source of B vitamin complex and 50+ minerals and vitamins. Supports the cardiovascular, kidneys, lungs, and immune systems.
- Essential oils - Geranium, Fennel, Clove, Roman chamomile, Sage, Juniper - supports digestion.

COMMENTS FROM YOUNG LIVING®

"K & B™ is formulated to nutritionally support normal kidney and bladder health. It contains extracts of juniper berries, which enhance the body's efforts to maintain proper fluid balance; parsley, which supports kidney and bladder function and aids overall urinary health; and uva-ursi, which supports both urinary and digestive system health. K & B™ is enhanced with Seed to Seal® Premium essential oils."

DIRECTIONS FOR USE

Take 3 half droppers (3 ml) three times daily in distilled water, or as needed. Shake well before using.

The statements about the supplement and the ingredients have not been evaluated by the Food and Drug Administration. Young Living® products are not intended to diagnose, treat, cure, or prevent any disease.

K & B™

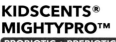
KIDSCENTS®
MIGHTYPRO™
PROBIOTIC + PREBIOTIC

USE ANYTIME | BEST WITH FOOD | VEGAN | CONTAINS NO OILS | CONTAINS XYLITOL | MINIMUM AGE 2+ | 1-2X ADULT DOSAGE | DO NOT FEED TO DOGS

KidScents® MightyPro™ is the perfect way to introduce prebiotics and probiotics to your little ones or even your big ones. The convenient single-serving packets make them the perfect travel companion. The over eight billion active cultures in MightyPro™ work to support your gut for a healthier immune system. They taste just like a Pixie Stix® so everyone in your family is sure to become an instant fan. Just be sure not to let your fur babies have any. MightyPro™ contains xylitol, which can be toxic to dogs.

INGREDIENTS

Prebiotic Blend
- Fructooligosaccharides (FOS), Ningxia wolfberry (*Lycium barbarum*) fruit fiber

Probiotic Strains
- *Lactobacillus paracasei* Lpc-37
- *Lactobacillus acidophilus* LA-14
- Ningxia wolfberry (*Lycium barbarum*) fruit powder
- *Lactobacillus plantarum* LP-115
- *Lactobacillus rhamnosus* GG AF
- *Streptococcus thermophilus*
- *Lactobacillus rhamnosus* 6594
- *Bifidobacterium infantis* Bl-26

Other Ingredients - Xylitol, Erythritol, Natural fruit punch flavor, Citric acid

WHAT THE INGREDIENTS DO
- Fructooligosaccharides - a prebiotic: food for gut flora.
- Ningxia Wolfberry fiber from fruit - food for gut flora.
- *Lactobacillus paracasei* Lpc-37 - supports the digestive and immune system.
- *Lactobacillus acidophilus* LA-14 - has anti-inflammatory effects.
- Ningxia wolfberry fruit powder - supports good bacteria in the gut.
- *Lactobacillus plantarum* LP-115 - inhibits the growth of pathogenic microorganisms.
- *Lactobacillus rhamnosus* GG AF - supports gastrointestinal infections and immune system.
- *Streptococcus thermophilus* - breaks down lactose, supports digestion and immune system.
- *Lactobacillus rhamnosus* 6594 - supports a healthy gut and the immune system.
- *Bifidobacterium infantis* Bl-26 - improves digestion and supports the immune system.
- Xylitol - a natural sugar substitute from food.
- Erythritol - a natural zero-calorie sweetener for food.
- Natural fruit punch flavor - provides a sweet taste.
- Citric acid - it occurs naturally in citrus fruits and is a flavoring and preservative.

COMMENTS FROM YOUNG LIVING®

"MightyPro™ is a unique, synergistic blend of prebiotics and probiotics in a supplement specially formulated for children. Packaged in easy, one-dose packets that can be taken almost anywhere you go, this supplement features over eight billion active, live cultures to support digestive and immune health."

DIRECTIONS FOR USE

For children 2 years and older, empty contents of 1 packet into mouth and allow to dissolve. Take 1 packet daily with food to provide optimal conditions for healthy gut bacteria. Can be combined with cold food or drinks. Do not add to warm or hot food or beverages. May be used anytime, but best with food.

The statements about the supplement and the ingredients have not been evaluated by the Food and Drug Administration. Young Living® products are not intended to diagnose, treat, cure, or prevent any disease.

KIDSCENTS® **MIGHTYPRO™**

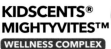
KIDSCENTS®
MIGHTYVITES™
WELLNESS COMPLEX

USE ANYTIME

BEST WITH FOOD

VEGAN

CONTAINS NO OILS

CONTAINS STEVIA

CONTAINS BARLEY

MINIMUM AGE 4+

2X ADULT DOSAGE

KidScents® MightyVites™ are a chewable multi-vitamin that is perfect for your little

ones. They contain vitamins, minerals, plant nutrients, and antioxidants to help support your child's healthy active lifestyle. MightyVites™ are also a great option for adults who have a hard time swallowing pills.

INGREDIENTS

- Calories - 15
- Total Carbohydrates - 5 g
- Total Sugars - 3 g (Includes 2 g Added Sugars)
- Vitamin A (Beta-carotene from organic food blend) - 60 mg (18% DV)
- Vitamin C (from organic food blend) - 27 mg (30% DV)
- Vitamin D (Cholecalciferol) - 5 mcg (25% DV)
- Vitamin E (from organic food blend) - 30 mg (201% DV)
- B1 Thiamin (from organic food blend) - 0.8 mg (67% DV)
- B2 Riboflavin (from organic food blend) - 0.9 mg (69% DV)
- B3 Niacin (from organic food blend) - 9 mg (56% DV)
- B6 (from organic food blend) - 2.2 mg (129% DV)
- B9 Folate (from organic food blend) - 200 mcg DFE (120 mcg folic acid) (50% DV)
- B12 (Methylcobalamin) - 3.2 mcg (133% DV)
- B7 Biotin (from organic food blend) - 40 mcg (133% DV)
- B5 Pantothenic acid (from organic food blend) - 1.8 mg (36% DV)
- Zinc (from organic food blend) - 1.1 mg (10% DV)
- Selenium (from organic food blend) - 8 mcg (15% DV)

MightyVites™ Wild Berry Blend – 973 mg
- Orgen-Kid® Blend:
  - Curry (*Murraya koenigii*) leaf extract
  - Guava (*Psidium Guajava*) fruit extract
  - Lemon (*Citrus limon*) peel extract
  - Sesbania (*Sesbania grandiflora*) leaf extract
  - Amala (P*hyllanthus emblica*) fruit extract
  - Holy Basil (*Ocimum sanctum*) aerial parts extract
  - Annatto (*Bixa orellana*) seed extract
- Beet (*Beta vulgaris*) root juice powder
- Orange (*Citrus sinensis*) fruit juice powder
- Strawberry (*Fragaria ananassa*) fruit juice powder
- Wolfberry (*Lycium barbarum*) fruit powder
- Citrus flavonoids [from Tangerine (*Citrus tangeria*) peel]
- Barley grass (*Hordeum vulgare*) leaf powder
- Broccoli (*Brassica oleracea*) sprout powder

Other Ingredients - Sorbitol, Fructose, Natural Flavors, Natural Sweetener (erythritol, oligaosaccharide), Malic Acid, Stevia (*Stevia rebaudiana*) leaf extract, Silicon dioxide, Magnesium stearate

Orgen-Kid® contains the following natural food-based key ingredients - Natural mixed carotenoids, Natural vitamin B1 (Thiamin), Natural vitamin B2 (Riboflavin), Natural vitamin B3 (Niacin), Natural vitamin B5 (Pantothenate), Natural vitamin B6 (Pyridoxine), Natural vitamin B9 (Folate), Natural vitamin C, Natural vitamin E, Natural biotin, Natural magnesium, Natural zinc, Natural copper, Natural manganese, Natural potassium, Natural selenium, Wolfberry powder, Barley grass, Broccoli sprouts, Kosher vitamin D3, and Vitamin B12.

WHAT THE INGREDIENTS DO

- A - protects the eyes and supports a healthy immune system.
- C - supports cartilage, ligaments, tendons and skin. Helps healing.
- D - helps maintain healthy bones, and supports a healthy immune system.
- E - helps to prevent damage to cells.
- B1 Thiamin - beneficial to a healthy nervous system.
- B2 Riboflavin - needed for overall growth and supports energy levels.
- B3 Niacin - supports circulation and cholesterol.
- B6 - supports the immune system and supports moods.
- B9 Folate - supports the heart.
- B12 - is essential in red blood cell production and DNA synthesis.
- B7 Biotin - is important for healthy skin and nails.
- B5 Pantothenic acid - supports regeneration of the skin during wound healing.
- Zinc - helps growth and repair, supports immune function, hormones and digestion.
- Selenium - a powerful antioxidant that defends against free radicals in the body.

MightyVites™ Wild Berry Blend
- Curry - helps with digestion and liver detoxification.
- Guava - supports the immune system and healthy digestion.
- Lemon - supports the body when cold symptoms occur.
- Sesbania - supports blood vessels to stay flexible.
- Amala - helps fend off free radicals which can cause aging.
- Holy Basil - helps to lower stress.
- Annatto - supports wound healing and healthy bones.
- Beet root juice - supports blood flow and may increase energy.
- Orange - has antioxidants that defend against free radicals.
- Strawberry - improves the skin and supports a healthy immune system.
- Wolfberry - supports eye health and overall health.
- Tangerine - supports eye health and reduces stress.
- Barley grass - is a detoxifier and natural antioxidant.
- Broccoli - is disease protection, supports a healthy immune system.

Other Ingredients - Sorbitol, Fructose, Natural Flavors, Natural Sweetener (erythritol, oligaosaccharide), Malic Acid, Stevia (*Stevia rebaudiana*) leaf extract, Silicon dioxide, Magnesium stearate - sweeteners and substrate

KIDSCENTS® MIGHTYVITES™

COMMENTS FROM YOUNG LIVING®

"KidScents® MightyVites™ include a full range of vitamins, minerals, antioxidants, and phytonutrients that deliver whole-food multinutrient support to your child's general health and well-being. Following in the footsteps of the recent Master Formula™ reformulation, MightyVites™ benefit from Orgen-kids®, a nutrient-dense, food-based superfruit, plant, and vegetable complex. Free of preservatives and artificial colors and flavors, these delicious, berry-flavored chewables give your children full nutritional support. Orgen-kids® is formulated with Orgen-FA®, which is the best source for natural folate available. Orgen-FA® is 100 percent USDA Certified Organic and does not contain synthetic folic acid or additives. It is extracted using hot water and is no different than the folic acid that is produced when boiling broccoli."

DIRECTIONS FOR USE

Children ages 4–12, take 4 chewable tablets daily. Best with breakfast.
Can be taken separately or in a single daily dose.

The statements about the supplement and the ingredients have not been evaluated by the Food and Drug Administration. Young Living® products are not intended to diagnose, treat, cure, or prevent any disease.

KIDSCENTS® MIGHTYZYME™

DIGESTIVE ENZYMES

BEST WITH FOOD · VEGAN · CONTAINS STEVIA · MINIMUM AGE 2+ · 2X ADULT DOSAGE

KidScents® MightyZyme™ chewables contain enzymes that naturally occur in the body that support and assist the digestive needs of growing bodies and the normal digestion of food.

INGREDIENTS
- Calcium (from calcium carbonate) - 50 mg (DV Kids <4yo 6%, >4yo 5%)

MightyZyme™ Blend – 79.3 mg
- Lipase
- Alfalfa (Medicago sativa) leaf powder
- Amylase
- Protease 4.5
- Bromelain
- Carrot (Daucus carota sativa) root powder
- Peptidase
- Phytase
- Protease 6.0
- Protease 3.0
- Peppermint (Mentha Piperita) aerial parts oil
- Cellulase

Other Ingredients - Sorbitol, Dextrates, Natural mixed berry flavor, Microcrystalline cellulose, Magnesium stearate, Steric acid, Silica, Apple juice powder, Stevia (Stevia rebaudiana) leaf extract

WHAT THE INGREDIENTS DO
- Calcium - supports bone, muscle, heart, and blood health.
- Lipase - breaks down dietary fats and oils. Helps liver function.
- Alfalfa leaf powder - for vitamins A, C, E, and K4, as well as minerals, calcium, potassium, phosphorus and iron.
- Amylase - breaks down starches, breads, and pasta.
- Protease 4.5 - helps with sinusitis and has a lower acidic content.
- Bromelain - breaks down meats, dairy, eggs, grains, seeds, and nuts.
- Carrot root powder - natural source of vitamin A, B, K, and potassium.
- Peptidase - breaks down Proteases. Supports immune function.
- Phytase - helps with bone health and pulls needed minerals from grains.
- Protease 6.0 - helps with edema and carries away toxins. Least acidic.
- Protease 3.0 - supports circulation and toxicity. Higher acid breaks down animal protein.
- Peppermint oil - supports the healthy functioning of the digestive system.
- Cellulase - breaks down man-made fiber, plant fiber, fruits, and vegetables.

Other Ingredients - Sorbitol, Dextrates, Natural mixed berry flavor, Microcrystalline cellulose, Magnesium stearate, Steric acid, Silica, Apple juice powder, Stevia leaf extract - for flavor and formation.

COMMENTS FROM YOUNG LIVING®
"MightyZyme™ chewables contain enzymes that naturally occur in the body that support and assist the digestive needs of growing bodies and the normal digestion of foods."

DIRECTIONS FOR USE
For children ages 6 or older: Chew 1 tablet 3 times daily prior to or with meals. For children 2-6 years of age: Chew 1/2 to 1 tablet (crushed if needed and mixed with yogurt or applesauce). For relief of occasional symptoms including fullness, pressure, bloating, stuffed feeling (commonly referred to as gas), pain and/or minor cramping that may occur after eating.

The statements about the supplement and the ingredients have not been evaluated by the Food and Drug Administration. Young Living® products are not intended to diagnose, treat, cure, or prevent any disease.

KIDSCENTS®
UNWIND™
AM: FOCUS • PM: SLEEP

USE ANYTIME | VEGAN | CONTAINS STEVIA | CONTAINS XYLITOL | MINIMUM AGE 4+ | DO NOT FEED TO DOGS

KidScents® Unwind™ helps to calm and relax the mind. When used during the day, it helps those both young and old to have better daytime focus. When used just before bed, with low light, it helps the body naturally fall asleep faster by producing the precursor hormone called serotonin. When your body produces serotonin, it can naturally produce the right amount of melatonin. This supplement will not make you sleepy during the day, unless you create a low light nap time environment. So if you need extra focus during the day, something to calm your nerves, or the ability to fall asleep naturally at night, this is the perfect supplement for both young and old alike. It tastes best when mixed into four ounces of cold water.

INGREDIENTS AND WHAT THEY DO
- Magnesium 42mg 10% DV

KidScents® Unwind™ Blend – 337 mg
- L-theanine - an amino acid that promotes calmness without the side effects of drowsiness.
- Marine mineral magnesium complex - helps to increase GABA which helps your mind to relax. Plays a role in regulating the stress-response in the body.
- 5-HTP (*Griffonia simplicifolia* seed extract) - helps the body naturally produce melatonin by producing the precursor hormone called serotonin. It is best experienced with low light situations. 5-HTP also helps to improve mood by calming the mind and easing emotional stress.
- Lavender (*Lavandula angustifolia*) flower essential oil - known to help calm the mind and support hormone and mood balance.
- Roman Chamomile (*Chamaemelum nobile*) flower essential oil - known to promote relaxation and helps decrease the time it takes to fall asleep.

Other Ingredients
- Erythritol - a type of sugar alcohol that works as a low-calorie sweetener.
- Xylitol - a type of sugar alcohol that works as a low-calorie sweetener. NOTE: Toxic to dogs!
- Magnesium citrate - a flow agent that helps guarantee the consistency of the ingredients.
- Natural watermelon flavor - naturally sourced flavor.
- Stevia (*Stevia rebaudiana*) leaf extract - natural sweetener.

COMMENTS FROM YOUNG LIVING®
"The world is a big, exciting place for kids, with plenty to learn and do every day. From school and piano lessons to playdates and finger painting new masterpieces, it's no surprise kids' minds and bodies don't always want to settle down at the end of the day. Help ease overstimulation with KidScents® Unwind™! This simple supplement features calming superstars like L-theanine, 5-HTP, and magnesium that are must-haves for bringing a sense of chill when energy is high."

DIRECTIONS FOR USE
Label: For children 4 years and older, empty contents of 1 packet into mouth to dissolve. For best taste: Empty contents into 4 ounces of cold water, stir, and drink.

Customer Notes: Unwind™ is used by adults with great success to help with stress and multitasking during the day and also at night to get better sleep.

KIDSCENTS® UNWIND™

The statements about the supplement and the ingredients have not been evaluated by the Food and Drug Administration. Young Living® products are not intended to diagnose, treat, cure, or prevent any disease.

LIFE 9®

DIGESTIVE ENZYMES

USE 1-4 HRS AFTER DINNER · KEEP REFRIGERATED · VEGAN · CONTAINS NO OILS · MINIMUM AGE 12+

Young Living® offers a synergy of nine different strains with 17 billion live active cultures in a delayed-release capsule to deliver the cultures directly to your intestines. Life 9® is designed to give you the greatest possible benefits. It has nine strains to give you full-spectrum support, but what is interesting is that the best time to take it is at night just before bed or a few hours after dinner on an empty stomach. You should take this without any other supplement. Once you swallow it, it goes to work. All those beautiful healthy bacteria helping support your beautiful gut! It is said that 85% of all our issues stem from the gut. You may take these every day or at least 3-4 times a week. This may also be used as a way to rapidly support your gut when you are feeling a dip in your immune system by consuming 5-6 at once right before bed. This is only to be done as needed and no more than once a month. Life 9® will help to regulate your bowel movements. If you take too many for too long you may experience diarrhea. When you are having one bowel movement per full meal per day that is the right consistency, not too soft and not too hard, this means your gut is working correctly. There are no essential oils in Life 9®.

INGREDIENTS

- *Lactobacillus acidophilus, Bifidobacterium lactis, Lactobacillus plantarum, Lactobacillus rhamnosus, Lactobacillus salivarius, Streptococcus thermophilus, Bifidobacterium breve, Bifidobacterium bifidum, Bifidobacterium longum*

WHAT THE INGREDIENTS DO

- *Lactobacillus acidophilus* - antagonizes pathogens and has anti-inflammatory effects.
- *Bifidobacterium lactis* - aids in absorption of vitamins and minerals.
- *Lactobacillus plantarum* - improves immune response, and helps ease IBS.
- *Lactobacillus rhamnosus* - promotes a healthy gut and supports the immune system.
- *Lactobacillus salivarius* - targets pathogenic bacteria; produces lactic acid that helps fight bad bacteria. Improves digestive health, immune function, and dental health.
- *Streptococcus thermophilus* - breaks down lactose; supports immune and digestive systems.
- *Bifidobacterium breve* - competes with other bacteria, breaks down foods that are considered non-digestible; ferments sugars, produces lactic and acetic acids.
- *Bifidobacterium bifidum* - produces natural antibiotics that kill bad bacteria. Supports immune function and digestion.
- *Bifidobacterium longum* - Aids in normal digestion and balance of the intestinal tract.

COMMENTS FROM YOUNG LIVING®

"Life 9® is a proprietary, high-potency probiotic that combines 17 billion live cultures from nine beneficial bacteria strains that promotes healthy digestion, supports gut health, and helps maintain normal intestinal function for overall support of a healthy immune system. Life 9® is specially designed with special delayed-release capsules, a dual-sorbent desiccant, and a special bottle and cap that ensure your Life 9® stays fresh and effective. Each bottle contains 30 capsules, making it easy to use this helpful supplement daily."

DIRECTIONS FOR USE

Take 1 capsule 1-4 hours after dinner, on an empty stomach, or as needed. Refrigerate after opening.

The statements about the supplement and the ingredients have not been evaluated by the Food and Drug Administration. Young Living® products are not intended to diagnose, treat, cure, or prevent any disease.

LONGEVITY™
ANTIOXIDANT

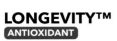

USE ANYTIME · BEST WITH FOOD · VEGAN · CONTAINS COCONUT · CONTAINS ALL OILS · MINIMUM AGE 12+

Longevity™ softgels are a pre-mixed essential oil synergy, high in antioxidant power, that is ready to consume. The best part is they come in thick-walled capsules that are designed to dissolve in your intestines rather than your stomach. This is important because getting oils into your intestines promotes better health than allowing your stomach acids to come in contact with the oils. While stomach acid is not a huge offense to oils, there are some added benefits to getting them into your intestines rather than your digestive system. Supporting your gut goes a long way toward longevity!

INGREDIENTS
Longevity™ Blend – 720 mg
- Medium-chain triglycerides (from fractionated Coconut oil)
- Coconut (*Cocos nucifera*) fruit oil
- Thyme (*Thymus vulgaris*) leaf oil
- Orange (*Citrus sinensis*) peel oil
- Clove (*Syzygium aromaticum*) flower bud oil
- Frankincense (*Boswellia carterii*) gum/resin oil

Contains 14 drops total of Coconut carrier oil and essential oils.
Other Ingredients - Hypromellose, Water, Silica, Mixed tocopherols (vitamin E)
Note: Contains tree nuts (Coconut)

WHAT THE INGREDIENTS DO
- Medium-chain triglycerides - beneficial for cognitive function, mood balance and weight management; assists in digestion and nutrient absorption; heart protective with antioxidant properties.
- Coconut fruit oil - supports immune function and digestion; beneficial for brain, heart and oral health; protective for kidneys, liver and urinary tract; supports energy.
- Thyme leaf oil - beneficial for immune, respiratory, digestive and nervous systems; assists in cognitive function, hormone balance and relaxation; supports oral, eye and skin health.
- Orange peel oil - supports immune function, improves blood flow and assists a healthy blood pressure; promotes the production of collagen for healthy skin.
- Clove flower bud oil - high in antioxidants; supports the immune system, supports oral, digestive and cardiovascular health and is protective for the liver.
- Frankincense gum/resin oil - immune enhancing and stress reducing; beneficial for skin health and to fight signs of aging; supports hormone balance, cognitive function, digestion and sleep.

COMMENTS FROM YOUNG LIVING®
"Longevity™ softgels are a potent, proprietary blend of fat-soluble antioxidants. Longevity™ blend should be taken daily to strengthen the body's systems to prevent the damaging effects of aging, diet, and the environment. Enriched with the Seed to Seal® Premium essential oils Thyme, Orange, and Frankincense. Longevity™ protects DHA levels, a nutrient that supports brain function and cardiovascular health, promotes healthy cell regeneration, and supports liver and immune function. Longevity™ also contains clove oil, nature's strongest antioxidant, for ultra antioxidant support."

DIRECTIONS FOR USE
Take 1 softgel capsule once daily with food or as needed.
Out of stock: add 4-9 drops of Longevity Vitality™ to a capsule with 4 drops carrier oil.

The statements about the supplement and the ingredients have not been evaluated by the Food and Drug Administration. Young Living® products are not intended to diagnose, treat, cure, or prevent any disease.

LONGEVITY™

MASTER FORMULA™
WELLNESS COMPLEX

USE ANYTIME · BEST WITH FOOD · VEGAN · CONTAINS BARLEY · CONTAINS CAFFEINE · MINIMUM AGE 12+

If you want to choose an "All Star" for daily supplementation, Master Formula™ would be the way to go. It is designed to support full-spectrum health. It contains a complete B vitamin complex, vegan D3, and gut supporting pre-biotics. It contains the coveted Turmeric Root Essential Oil, which is loaded with antioxidants and amazing for glowing skin and hair. Master Formula™ also contains 60% of your daily iron needs and the vitamin K2 for bone and heart health. This supplement is packed full of herbs and vegetables that have been juiced and dried to deliver pure phytonutrients from plants that have been picked at the peak of harvest.

LIQUID VITAMIN CAPSULE INGREDIENTS & WHAT THEY DO

The Liquid Vitamin Capsule contains powerful essential oils including Turmeric root oil, a powerfully oxygenating oil that supports overall health. This capsule contains fat soluble vitamins E, K, and a vegan sourced vitamin D3. These all provide excellent antioxidant support.

- D3 (Cholecalciferol) - 10 mcg (400 IU) (50% DV) - helps your body absorb calcium and phosphorus, strong bones.
- E (D-alpha tocopherol) - 33.5 mg (223% DV) - antioxidant, helps to protect cells from the damage caused by free radicals.
- K2 (Menaquinone-7) - 50 mcg (42% DV) - metabolizes calcium, the main mineral found in your bones and teeth.

Proprietary Master Formula™ Essential Oil Blend – 7.5 mg
- Turmeric (*Curcuma longa*) root oil - supports mobility, liver function, and brain health.
- Cardamom (*Elettaria cardamomum*) fruit/seed oil - supports respiratory and immune systems, as well as the bioavailability of herbs.
- Clove (*Syzygium aromaticum*) flower bud oil - supports immune system.
- Fennel (*Foeniculum vulgare*) seed oil - supports the immune and digestive systems.
- Ginger (*Zingiber officinale*) root oil - supports immune function and bioavailability.

Other Ingredients - Sunflower lecithin (non-GMO), Hypromellose, beta-carotene.

MICRONIZED NUTRIENT CAPSULE INGREDIENTS & WHAT THEY DO

This capsule supports the body naturally through lycopene, wolfberry powder, and citrus bioflavonoids. The capsule also contains Orgen-B®, which is a blend of certified organic guava, mango, and lemon extracts for a perfect synergy of B vitamins and chelated minerals. It contains 100% natural vitamin B1, B2, B3, B5, B6, and B9. Orgen Family® states, "B-vitamins help critically with a range of normal body functions, from cellular growth to metabolism. Vitamin B3, also known as Niacin, helps in the metabolism of glucose and fat. Vitamin B6, also known as pyridoxine, dominates the metabolism of amino acids and lipids. Vitamin B9 acts as a coenzyme in the form of folates that aids the production of red blood cells."

- A (Beta-carotene) - 675 mcg RAE (75% DV) - supports health and immune function.
- B1 (Thiamin) - 11 mg (917% DV) - enables the body to use carbohydrates as energy.
- B2 (Riboflavin) - 10 mg (769% DV) - helps break down proteins, fats, and carbohydrates into energy.
- B3 (Niacin) - 17 mg (106% DV) - supports blood and brain function; eases joint stiffness.
- B5 (Pantothenic acid) - 19 mg (380% DV) - supports blood; converts food into energy.
- B6 (Pyridoxine) - 11 mg (647% DV) - creates red blood cells.
- B7 (Biotin or Vitamin H) - 300 mcg (1000% DV) - supports metabolism and enzymes.
- B9 (Folate) - 583.3 mcg DFE (350 mcg Folic Acid) (146% DV) - Folic Acid from organic food blend; plays a crucial role in cell growth.

The statements about the supplement and the ingredients have not been evaluated by the Food and Drug Administration. Young Living® products are not intended to diagnose, treat, cure, or prevent any disease.

MASTER FORMULA™

MICRONIZED NUTRIENT CAPSULE INGREDIENTS & WHAT THEY DO (continued)

- B12 (Methylcobalamin) - 12 mcg (500% DV) - supports production of red blood cells.
- Iron (Ferrous bisglycinate chelate) 10 mg (56% DV) - supports healthy blood and immune function; may support fatigue.
- Magnesium (Magnesium glycinate chelate) - 60 mg (14% DV) - regulates muscle and nerve function, blood sugar levels, and blood pressure.
- Zinc (Zinc glycinate chelate) - 15 mg (136% DV) - helps the immune system fight off invading bacteria and viruses.
- Selenium (Selenium glycinate chelate) - 75 mcg (136% DV) - is a powerful antioxidant that defends against free radicals in the body.
- Copper (Copper glycinate chelate) - 350 mcg (39% DV) - enables red blood cell production, supports immune system, bones, vessels, and nerves.
- Manganese (Manganese glycinate chelate) - 2 mg (87% DV) - helps activate enzymes.
- Chromium (Chromium nicotinate glycinate chelate) - 120 mcg (343% DV) - improves insulin sensitivity, enhances protein, carbohydrate, and lipid metabolism.
- Molybdenum (Molybdenum glycinate chelate) - 75 mcg (167% DV) - removes toxins from the metabolism of sulfur containing amino acids.

Proprietary Master Formula Capsule Blend – 42 mg
- Atlantic kelp - rich source of iodine.
- Inositol - helps turn food into energy. Supports the immune system, hair, and nails.
- PABA (Para amino benzoic acid) - supports skin elasticity, joints, and hair health.
- Spirulina algae - supports blood lipids, blood sugar, and blood pressure.
- Barley grass - supports digestion and helps reduce constipation.
- Citrus bioflavonoids (whole fruit powders) - supports immune system and oxidative stress.
- Olive (Olea europaea) leaf extract - supports the brain and heart.
- Boron citrate - supports bones, muscles, testosterone levels, and mental clarity.
- Lycopene - fights oxidative stress and supports heart health.

Other Ingredients - Hypromellose, Magnesium stearate (vegetable source), Silicon dioxide, Microcrystallinec ellulose - capsule and substrate content.

PHYTO-CAPLET INGREDIENTS & WHAT THEY DO

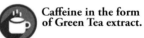

Caffeine in the form of Green Tea extract.

Contains trace minerals and gut flora-supporting prebiotics. Phyto-caplet also contains Spectra™, a powerful antioxidant that contains fruit, veggie, and herb extracts with Vitamin C. FutureCeuticals, Inc. states, "Spectra™ represents the latest evolution in the fight against potentially-damaging free radicals. For the first time anywhere, the biological effects of a natural supplement on the changes of oxidative and Nitrosative stress markers, as well as cellular metabolic activity, have been clinically observed in the human body. Exclusively available from FutureCeuticals, Spectra™ has been reported to decrease ROS, increase cellular oxygen consumption in blood and mitochondria, decrease extracellular H2O2, and reduce TNFa-induced inflammatory response in humans."

- C (calcium ascorbate and acerola cherry) - 61 mg (68% DV) - supports immune system.
- Calcium carbonate - 200 mg (5% DV) - for healthy bones, muscles, nervous system, and heart.
- Potassium chloride - 50 mg (<2% DV) - helps regulate muscle contractions, supports nerve function and fluid balance.

Proprietary Master Formula Tablet Blend – 208 mg
- Choline bitartrate (this is not B4 as some assume) - supports brain memory.
- Prebiotics (Wolfberry Fiber and Fructooligosaccharides) - food for good gut flora.

Continued on next page.

MASTER FORMULA™

PHYTO-CAPLET INGREDIENTS & WHAT THEY DO (continued)

Spectra™ Fruit, Vegetable, and Herb Blend – 100 mg

- Coffea arabica fruit extract - antioxidants known to protect brain cells.
- Broccoli seed concentrate - detoxification to support brain and increases glutathione.
- Camellia sinensis leaf extract - aka Green Tea - supports oxidative stress.
- Onion bulb extract - high in vitamins, minerals, and antioxidants.
- Apple fruit skin extract - supports digestion and cardiovascular health.
- Acerola fruit extract - high in vitamin C, supports immune health.
- Camu-camu fruit concentrate - high in vitamin C and antioxidants.
- Japanese sophora flower extract - has anti-oxidative and anti-inflammatory activities.
- Tomato fruit concentrate - source of vitamin C, potassium, folate, and vitamin K.
- Broccoli floret and stem concentrate - vitamins K, A, C, calcium, phosphorus, and zinc.
- Cabbage palm fruit concentrate - high in vitamin C and K.
- Turmeric root concentrate - antioxidants that support heart health, memory, and mood.
- Garlic clove concentrate - antioxidants that support the brain, blood, and cells.
- Basil leaf concentrate - reduces stress and has anti-inflammatory and antioxidant properties.
- Oregano leaf concentrate - antioxidant and antibacterial.
- Cassia branch/stem concentrate - supports renal, circulatory, and immune systems.
- European elder fruit concentrate - supports heart health, immune function, and stress.
- Carrot root concentrate - good source of vitamin A and antioxidants to support blood.
- Mangosteen fruit concentrate - supports skin, immune function, and blood sugar.
- Black currant fruit extract - high in vitamin C, antioxidants for skin and anti-aging.
- Blueberry fruit extract - high in nutrients and antioxidants to support blood and cells.
- Sweet cherry fruit concentrate - supports joints, muscles, brain, sleep, and immune function.
- Blackberry fruit concentrate - high in antioxidants, vitamins C, K, and A.
- Chokeberry fruit concentrate - high in phenols, supports immune function.
- Raspberry fruit concentrate - antioxidants that support heart health and circulation.
- Spinach leaf concentrate - supports blood; high in calcium, folic acid, and vitamins A and C.
- Collards leaf concentrate - high in folate, calcium, and vitamins E, A, K, and C.
- Bilberry fruit extract - supports blood vessels, cellular health, and circulation.
- Brussels sprout head concentrate - antioxidants that support cells; high in vitamin K.

MASTER FORMULA™

COMMENTS FROM YOUNG LIVING®

"Master Formula™ is a full-spectrum, multinutrient complex, providing premium vitamins, minerals, and food-based nutriment to support general health and well-being. By utilizing a Synergistic Suspension Isolation process – SSI Technology – ingredients are delivered in three distinct delivery forms. Collectively, these ingredients provide a premium, synergistic complex to support your body."

BENEFITS

- Naturally supports general health and well-being for the body
- Gut flora supporting prebiotics
- Ingredients help neutralize free radicals in the body
- Includes antioxidants, vitamins, minerals, and food-based nutriment
- Pre-packaged sachets are convenient to take your vitamins on the go
- SSI Technology delivers ingredients in three forms chosen for their complementary properties

DIRECTIONS FOR USE

Take 1 packet (1 liquid capsule, 1 caplet, 2 capsules) daily with water.

The statements about the supplement and the ingredients have not been evaluated by the Food and Drug Administration. Young Living® products are not intended to diagnose, treat, cure, or prevent any disease.

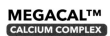

MEGACAL™
CALCIUM COMPLEX

USE 1 HOUR AFTER MEAL

VEGAN

CONTAINS XYLITOL

MINIMUM AGE 12+

¼-½ DOSAGE IF UNDER 12

DO NOT FEED TO DOGS

MegaCal™ was formulated to help support the body's calcium needs. It contains a synergistic blend of multiple calciums, along with magnesium, manganese, and vitamin C to support cell health and proper bone formation and maintenance. MegaCal™ is a powdered formula to be mixed with water or juice for proper calcium absorption.

INGREDIENTS
- Calories 15
- Total Carbohydrate - 3 g
- Vitamin C (Calcium ascorbate) - 8.2 mg (9% DV)
- Calcium (Calcium carbonate, Calcium lactate pentahydrate, Calcium glycerophosphate, and Calcium ascorbate) - 206 mg (16% DV)
- Magnesium (Magnesium citrate, Magnesium sulfate, and Magnesium carbonate) - 191 mg (46% DV)
- Zinc (Zinc gluconate) - 320 mcg (3% DV)
- Manganese (Manganese sulfate) - 320 mcg (14% DV)

MegaCal ™ Blend
- Xylitol
- Lemon (*Citrus limon*) peel oil

Other Ingredients - Caprylic/capric glycerides, Copper gluconate

WHAT THE INGREDIENTS DO
- Vitamin C - antioxidant that supports cartilage, ligaments, tendons and skin.
- Calcium carbonate - for healthy bones, muscles, heart, and nervous system.
- Calcium lactate pentahydrate - supports calcium deficiencies.
- Calcium glycerophosphate - supports calcium and phosphorus levels.
- Calcium ascorbate - a form of vitamin C that contains 10% absorbable calcium.
- Magnesium (as citrate, sulfate, and carbonate) - important for bone formation, calcium absorption, and carbohydrate and glucose metabolism; helps maintain muscle health and heart health; helps reduce muscle tension.
- Zinc gluconate - important for growth and healthy development of body tissues.
- Manganese sulfate - essential for bone development and maintenance; promotes normal functioning of the brain, nervous system and enzyme systems; protects against free radicals; promotes healthy blood sugar levels.

MegaCal ™ Blend
- Xylitol - sugar substitute.
- Lemon rind oil - promotes skin health, aids in weight loss efforts, improves bone density.

Other Ingredients
- Caprylic/capric glycerides - used as a dispersing agent.
- Copper gluconate - supports red blood cells; supports cardiovascular and bone health.

COMMENTS FROM YOUNG LIVING®
"MegaCal™ is a wonderful source of calcium, magnesium, manganese, and vitamin C. MegaCal™ supports normal bone and vascular health as well as normal nerve function and contains 207 mg of calcium and 188 mg of magnesium per serving."

DIRECTIONS FOR USE
Take 1 scoop (1 tsp.) (5g) with 1 cup (240 ml) of water or juice daily, one hour after a meal or taking medication or one hour before bedtime.
Do not exceed three servings daily. DO NOT FEED TO DOGS.

MEGACAL™

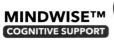

MINDWISE™
COGNITIVE SUPPORT

MindWise™ is formulated to help healthy brain function. It supports cardiovascular health for better cognition. Antioxidants support immune function and proper cell function. Taken on a regular basis, MindWise™ is a smart choice for a healthy heart and mind. It comes in two packages: as a serum to be taken by the spoonful, and in single-serving sachets for easy storing and use.

INGREDIENTS
- Vitamin D3 (Cholecalciferol)

Proprietary Memory Blend – 378.4 mg
- Pomegranate fruit extract
- Rhododendron leaf extract
- L-alpha glycerylphosphorylcholine (GPC)
- Acetyl-L-Carnitine (ALCAR)
- Coenzyme Q10 (31.8 mg per serving)
- Turmeric root powder

Proprietary Oil Blend – 397.4 mg
- Sacha inchi seed oil, Medium-chain triglycerides, Essential Oils - Lemon, Peppermint, Fennel, Anise, Lime

Other Ingredients - Water, Pomegranate juice concentrate, Acai puree, Glycerin, Sunflower lecithin, Natural flavors, Malic acid, Citric acid, Luo Han Guo fruit extract, No preservatives

WHAT THE INGREDIENTS DO
- Vitamin D3 - supports mood, healthy bones, and immune function.
- Pomegranate fruit extract - high antioxidant benefits.
- Rhododendron leaf extract - beneficial polyphenols and flavonoids.
- L-alpha glycerylphosphorylcholine (GPC) - builds cell membranes and contributes to the production of neurotransmitters.
- Acetyl-L-Carnitine (ALCAR) - antioxidant that supports normal brain function.
- Coenzyme Q10 - helps produce energy, normal growth, maintenance and repair.
- Turmeric root powder - helps ease inflammation in the body.

Proprietary Oil Blend
- Sacha inchi seed oil - vegetarian oil supports healthy brain and cardiovascular health.
- Medium-chain triglycerides - supports cardiovascular health and cognitive function.
- Lemon, Peppermint, Fennel, Anise, Lime - supports absorption of other ingredients; high in antioxidants and supports immune function.

Other Ingredients
- Pomegranate juice - adds flavor and high in antioxidants.
- Acai puree - adds flavor and high in antioxidants.
- Glycerin - adds base and sweet taste.
- Sunflower lecithin - rich in choline - beneficial to brain health.
- Malic acid - found in apples and pears; supports energy.
- Citric acid - it occurs naturally in citrus fruits and is a flavoring and preservative.
- Luo Han Guo - adds sweetness with no calories (Monk fruit).

These statements have not been evaluated by the Food and Drug Administration. Young Living® products are not intended to diagnose, treat, cure, or prevent any disease.

COMMENTS FROM YOUNG LIVING®
"Support normal cardiovascular health and cognitive health with the fruity, nutty flavor of MindWise™! With a vegetarian oil made from cold-pressed sacha inchi seeds harvested from the Peruvian Amazon and other medium-chain triglyceride oils, MindWise™ has a high proportion of unsaturated fatty acids and omega-3 fatty acids. Plus, it uses a combination of fruit juices and extracts, turmeric, and Seed to Seal® Premium essential oils to create a heart and brain function supplement with a taste you'll love! MindWise™ also includes our proprietary memory function blend made with bioidentical CoQ10, ALCAR, and GPC—ingredients that have been studied for their unique benefits. With generous amounts of vitamin D3, this premium supplement is equipped to support normal brain function and overall cognitive and cardiovascular health."

BENEFITS
- Supports normal brain and heart function
- Contains a high proportion of unsaturated fatty acids and omega-3 fatty acids
- Includes beneficial GPC, ALCAR, and bioidentical CoQ10
- Supports heart health by replenishing the body with CoQ10
- Features an improved, smoother texture
- Includes no added preservatives
- Formulated with turmeric

DIRECTIONS FOR USE
16 oz. Bottle
Take 1 Tbsp. (3 teaspoons) once daily.
Children (4-12 years) should take 1–2 tsp. once daily.
Should be taken with a meal.
Shake well before each use.
Consume within 30 days of opening.
Refrigerate after opening.

Original packaging usage:
- For optimal results follow this schedule when using the bottled version:
  Adult Initial Dose: 2 Tbsp. once daily for 7-10 days followed by maintenance schedule. Adult Maintenance Dose: 1 Tbsp. once daily.
- Children (4-12) should follow children's schedule (see above under 16 oz. Bottle).
- If you are pregnant, nursing, taking medication, or have a medical condition, consult a health care professional prior to use.

Single-Serve Packet
Drink 1 sachet daily.
Consume promptly after opening.
Should be taken with a meal.
Shake well before use.
Packets do not need to be refrigerated, but they taste better cold.

MINDWISE™

The statements about the supplement and the ingredients have not been evaluated by the Food and Drug Administration. Young Living® products are not intended to diagnose, treat, cure, or prevent any disease.

MINERAL ESSENCE™
MINERAL COMPLEX

USE ANYTIME — KEEP REFRIGERATED — NOT VEGAN — CONTAINS BEE PRODUCTS — MINIMUM AGE 12+ — ¼-½ DOSAGE IF UNDER 12

We often find ourselves depleted of the vital minerals we need every day. This powerful, fully balanced mineral tincture is the perfect way to supplement our growing mineral needs. Shake this well before using. You can add the 5 ml needed to five 00 capsules or simply add it to 4-8 oz. of water.

INGREDIENTS
- Calories per serving - 10
- Carbohydrates - 3 g (<1% DV)
- Sugars - 2 g
- Includes 2 g Added Sugars (3% DV)
- Magnesium - 350 mg (80% DV)
- Chloride - 1,000 mg (45% DV)
- Sodium - 10 g (<1% DV)

Mineral Essence™ Blend – 5 ml
- Salt (trace mineral complex)
- Honey
- Royal Jelly (from bees)
- Lemon (*Citrus limon*) peel oil
- Cinnamon (*Cinnamomum verum*) Bark oil
- Peppermint (*Mentha piperita*) aerial parts oil

WHAT THE INGREDIENTS DO
- Magnesium - supports bone formation, calcium absorption, carbohydrate and glucose metabolism, muscle health, and heart health.
- Chloride - supports blood volume and pressure. Supports fluid balance in cells.
- Sodium - supports nerve impulses and maintains the balance of water and minerals.

Mineral Essence™ Blend
- Salt - supports nerve impulses and maintains the balance of water and minerals.
- Honey - antioxidant that supports immune, digestive, heart, and gut health.
- Royal Jelly - produced by honey bees. Source of B vitamin complex and 50+ minerals and vitamins. Supports the cardiovascular, kidneys, lungs, and immune systems.
- Lemon peel oil - natural detoxifier, supports immune system, moods and energy.
- Cinnamon Bark oil - supports the immune, digestive, and circulatory systems.
- Peppermint oil - supports energy, brain health, and immune and digestive systems.

COMMENTS FROM YOUNG LIVING®
"Mineral Essence™ is a balanced, full-spectrum ionic mineral complex enhanced with essential oils. According to two time Nobel Prize winner Linus Pauling PhD. "You can trace every sickness, every disease, and every ailment to a mineral deficiency." Ionic minerals are the most fully and quickly absorbed form of minerals available."

DIRECTIONS FOR USE
Take 5 half-droppers (1ml each) morning and evening or as needed as a mineral supplement. May be added to 4-8 oz. of water or juice before drinking.

Customer Notes: Many find it beneficial to add several droppers directly to a warm bath.

NOTE: This product contains Royal Jelly, which may cause allergic reactions. Shake well before using and refrigerate after opening. Mineral Essence™ contains many minerals such as zinc, iron, and 50 other minerals not listed in the ingredients. These are called ionic trace minerals and are found in Royal Jelly.

The statements about the supplement and the ingredients have not been evaluated by the Food and Drug Administration. Young Living® products are not intended to diagnose, treat, cure, or prevent any disease.

MINERAL ESSENCE™

MULTIGREENS™
PHYTONUTRIENTS

 USE ANYTIME   **NOT VEGAN**   **CONTAINS BEEF GELATIN** 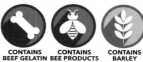 **CONTAINS BEE PRODUCTS** **CONTAINS BARLEY**   **MINIMUM AGE 12+**   **½ DOSAGE IF UNDER 12**

MultiGreens™ is the perfect daily pairing to NingXia Red® for general health support. It is rich in antioxidants to support proper cell function. MultiGreens™ supports healthy memory, mood, and other nervous system functions. It contains sea kelp, which is a great source of minerals, most notably, iodine. It also contains spirulina, which is an excellent source of bioavailable calcium, niacin, potassium, magnesium, iron, and B vitamins.

INGREDIENTS
- Calories - 5
- Total Carbohydrate - <1 g
- Protein <1 g
- Iron 0.8 mg (4% DV)
- Sodium 8 mg (<1 % DV)

Proprietary MultiGreens™ Blend – 1.5 g
- Bee pollen, Barley (*Hordeum vulgare*) grass juice concentrate, Spirulina (*Spirulina platensis*), Choline (as choline bitartrate), Eleuthero (*Eleutherococcus senticosus*) root, Alfalfa (*Medicago sativa*) stem/leaf extract, Kelp (*Laminaria digitata*) whole thallus
- MultiGreens™ Oil Blend - Rosemary (*Rosmarinus officinalis*) leaf oil, Lemon (*Citrus limon*) peel oil, Lemongrass (*Cymbopogon flexuosus*) leaf oil, Melissa (*Melissa officinalis*) leaf/flower oil
- Amino Acid Complex (L-Arginine, L-Cysteine, L-Tyrosine)

Other Ingredients - Gelatin, Silica

WHAT THE INGREDIENTS DO
- Bee pollen - antioxidants that protect against free radicals in the body.
- Barley grass juice concentrate - source of minerals; improves digestive function.
- Spirulina - contains calcium, niacin, potassium, magnesium, B vitamins and iron.
- Choline - supports brain memory, mood, muscle control, and nervous system functions.
- Eleuthero root - helps the body better adapt to stress; supports nervous system function.
- Alfalfa stem/leaf extract - supports healthy cholesterol and glucose levels.
- Kelp - supports metabolism. Sea kelp is the richest natural source of iodine.

MultiGreens™ Oil Blend
- Rosemary leaf oil - supports hair growth, mental acuity, and respiratory function.
- Lemon peel oil - cleanses toxins from the body and stimulates lymphatic drainage.
- Lemongrass leaf oil - supports immune and circulatory systems.
- Melissa leaf/flower oil - is used as a digestive aid.

Amino Acid Complex
- L-arginine - supports blood and circulation.
- L-cysteine - supports metabolism and energy.
- L-tyrosine - supports nerve cell communication and may support moods.

Other Ingredients - Gelatin (vegetable), Silica - capsule and substrate.

COMMENTS FROM YOUNG LIVING®
"MultiGreens™ is a nutritious chlorophyll formula designed to boost vitality by working with the glandular, nervous, and circulatory systems. MultiGreens™ is made with spirulina, alfalfa sprouts, barley grass, bee pollen, eleuthero, Pacific kelp, and Seed to Seal® Premium essential oils."

DIRECTIONS FOR USE
Take three capsules twice daily.
Customer Notes: You may break open the capsules and mix in with applesauce for those who cannot swallow pills.

The statements about the supplement and the ingredients have not been evaluated by the Food and Drug Administration. Young Living® products are not intended to diagnose, treat, cure, or prevent any disease.

MULTIGREENS™

NINGXIA RED®
ANTIOXIDANTS • IMMUNE

USE ANYTIME | KEEP REFRIGERATED | VEGAN | CONTAINS STEVIA | MINIMUM AGE 1+

NingXia Red® is a powerhouse of antioxidants and nutrients that the whole family will benefit from using. It is a whole body supplement for a more healthful life experience. The wolfberry, also known as the goji berry, is touted for having high antioxidant properties. A daily shot helps support better energy and normal cellular function, as well as whole-body health and wellness. Four ounces of NingXia Red® equals one serving of fruit; however, one ounce has the antioxidant equivalent to eating four pounds of carrots or eight whole oranges! NingXia Red® is safe for all people from solid-food eating children to adults. Pregnant and nursing women should also consider using NingXia Red® as part of their healthy daily regimen. The Orange, Yuzu, Lemon, and Tangerine essential oils in NingXia Red® contain d-limonene, which is a powerful wellness-promoting constituent. NingXia Red® is free of high fructose sweeteners. Wolfberries and exotic fruits such as blueberry, cherry, aronia, pomegranate, and plum give NingXia Red® its delicious flavor.

INGREDIENTS
- Calories - 25
- Carbohydrates - 6 g (2% DV)
- Sugars - 5 g
- Protein - <1 g
- Calcium - 40 mg (4% DV)
- Iron - 0.4 mg (2% DV)
- Sodium - 35 mg (2% DV)
- Potassium - 414 mg (9% DV)

Proprietary NingXia Red® Blend – 58 g
Ningxia Wolfberry (*Lycium barbarum*) whole fruit puree, Aronia fruit juice concentrate (*Aronia melanocarpa*), Sweet Cherry fruit juice concentrate (*Prunus avium*), Plum juice concentrate (*Prunus domestica*), Blueberry fruit juice concentrate (*Vaccinium corymbosum*), Pomegranate fruit juice concentrate (*Punica granatum*)

Proprietary Essential Oil Blend – 100 mg
Grape (*Vitis vinifera*) seed extract, Orange (*Citrus sinensis*) peel oil, Yuzu (*Citrus junos*) rind oil, Lemon (*Citrus limon*) peel oil, Tangerine (*Citrus reticulata*) rind oil

Other Ingredients - Water, Tartaric acid, Natural blueberry flavor, Pure vanilla extract, Malic acid, Sodium benzoate (to maintain freshness), Pectin, Stevia rebaudiana extract.

WHAT THE INGREDIENTS DO
- Calcium - for healthy bones, muscles, nervous system, and heart.
- Iron - supports healthy blood and immune function; helps combat fatigue.
- Sodium - supports nerve impulses and maintains the balance of water and minerals.
- Potassium - maintains fluid and electrolyte balance.

Proprietary NingXia Red® Blend
- Ningxia Wolfberry puree - rich in vitamins and minerals including vitamin A, C, zinc, and iron. High in complex carbohydrates and antioxidants. Supports the immune system and liver and eye health.
- Blueberry juice concentrate, Plum juice concentrate, Cherry juice concentrate, Aronia juice concentrate, Pomegranate juice concentrate - a unique collection of all extremely high antioxidant rich fruit juices that are known to support immune function and protect against oxidative stress.

These statements have not been evaluated by the Food and Drug Administration.
Young Living® products are not intended to diagnose, treat, cure, or prevent any disease.

NINGXIA RED®

WHAT THE INGREDIENTS DO (continued)
Proprietary Essential Oil Blend
- Grape seed extract - rich in antioxidants including flavonoids and phytonutrients; protects against oxidative stress and supports healthy whole-body wellness.
- Essential Oils - Orange, Yuzu, Lemon, Tangerine - high in limonene, these antioxidant rich citrus oils support immune function, cleanse toxins from the body, support circulation and digestive health and stimulate lymphatic drainage. Tangerine is particularly beneficial for respiratory health while Yuzu has beneficial properties that support nerve and brain health.

Other Ingredients
- Water - drink base
- Tartaric acid - antioxidant.
- Natural blueberry flavor - to enhance flavor.
- Pure vanilla extract - to enhance flavor.
- Malic acid - found in apples and pears; supports energy.
- Sodium benzoate (natural source) - natural preservative.
- Pectin - supports digestion and blood.
- Stevia extract - adds no-calorie sweetness.

COMMENTS FROM YOUNG LIVING®
"Young Living® NingXia Red® benefits include support for energy levels, normal cellular function, and whole-body and normal eye health. A daily shot of 2–4 oz. helps support overall wellness with powerful antioxidants. The wolfberries sourced for NingXia Red® hail from the Ningxia province in northern China. This superfruit has one of the highest percentages of fiber of any whole food and contains zeaxanthin—a carotenoid important to maintaining healthy vision. It also contains polysaccharides, amino acids, and symbiotic vitamin mineral pairs that when present together promote optimum internal absorption. By using whole wolfberry puree—juice, peel, seeds, and fruit—Young Living® is able to maintain more of the desired health-supporting benefits in every bottle of NingXia Red®."

DIRECTIONS FOR USE
- Drink 1-2 oz. twice daily. Best served chilled. Shake well before use. Refrigerate after opening and consume within 30 days. Do not drink directly from the bottle. Do not use if the seal is broken.

- Blend NingXia Red® into a shake mix, acai bowl, or morning juice as part of a quick, convenient breakfast.

- Chill and serve NingXia Red® to family and guests at gatherings and celebrations when you're looking for a healthy alternative to sparkling drinks.

- Treat children to this tasty drink instead of sugary sodas or juice cocktails.

- Combine with NingXia Nitro® for a nourishing drink that also supports cognitive wellness.

- Add a drop or two of your favorite dietary essential oil for an extra flavor boost! Try Peppermint Vitality™, Thieves® Vitality™, Cinnamon Bark Vitality™, or Grapefruit Vitality™.

NINGXIA RED®

The statements about the supplement and the ingredients have not been evaluated by the Food and Drug Administration. Young Living® products are not intended to diagnose, treat, cure, or prevent any disease.

NINGXIA NITRO®
ENERGY • COGNITION

USE BEFORE 3PM — NOT VEGAN — CONTAINS DAIRY — CONTAINS CAFFEINE — CONTAINS COCONUT — MINIMUM AGE 14+

NingXia Nitro® is a non-habit forming energy shot that contains natural sources of energy from green tea extract, ginseng, and choline to help support mental clarity. It should be used anytime there is a need for heightened cognition and energy. Consider using Nitro® for the afternoon lull, to help ease head tension, for added clarity before a test or presentation, for an energy boost before a workout, or anytime extra energy is needed.

INGREDIENTS
- Contains 40 mg of naturally occurring caffeine.
- Calories - 20
- Carbohydrates - 5 g (2% DV)
- Sugars - 4 g
- B3 - Niacin (as niacinamide) - 10 mg (50% DV)
- B6 (pyridoxine HCI) - 1 mg (50% DV)
- B12 (methylcobalamin) - 6 μg (100% DV)
- Iodine - 75 μg (50% DV)

Proprietary Nitro® Energy Blend – 476 mg
- D-Ribose
- Green tea (*Camellia sinsnis*) leaf extract
- Choline (as Choline bitartrate)
- Mulberry leaf extract
- Korean ginseng root extract

Proprietary Nitro® Alert Oil Blend – 5 mg
- Vanilla (*Vanilla planifolia*) fruit oil (absolute)
- Chocolate (*Theobroma Cacao*) bean oil
- Yerba mate (*Ilex paraguariensis*) leaf oil
- Spearmint (*Mentha spicata*) leaf oil
- Peppermint (*Menta piperita*) leaf oil
- Nutmeg (*Myristica fragrans*) fruit oil
- Black Pepper (*Piper nigrum*) fruit oil
- Wolfberry (*Lycium barbarum*) seed oil

Nitro® Fruit Juice Blend Concentrate - Sweet Cherry, Kiwi, Blueberry, Acerola, Bilberry, Black currant, Raspberry, Strawberry, Cranberry, Coconut nectar, Natural flavors, Pectin, Xanthan gum

Other Ingredients - Purified water. Contains dairy and tree nut (coconut)

WHAT THE INGREDIENTS DO
- B3 - converts food into usable energy.
- B6 - supports healthy nerves, skin, and red blood cells.
- B12 - supports red blood cells, brain health, eye health, skin health, DNA production, cardiovascular support, and converts the food you eat into energy.
- Iodine - supports the thyroid, metabolic rate, energy levels, helps remove toxins, supports immune system, and is critical in the prevention of an enlarged thyroid gland.

Proprietary Nitro® Energy Blend
- D-Ribose - supports energy, metabolism, and improved muscle function.
- Green tea extract - antioxidants that support energy, heart, liver and brain health.
- Choline (as Choline bitartrate) - cognitive enhancer that supports brain health.
- Mulberry leaf extract - antioxidant to support cholesterol, triglycerides, and glucose.
- Korean ginseng extract - improves antioxidant activity in cells and mental fatigue.

WHAT THE INGREDIENTS DO (continued)
Proprietary Nitro® Alert Oil Blend
- Vanilla absolute oil - flavor enhancer and may reduce stress and support feelings of peace.
- Chocolate oil - (absolute) may relax muscles and help balance the body and the mind.
- Yerba mate oil - antioxidants support energy, immune function, and clarity.
- Spearmint oil - soothes digestion, cools and promotes energy and emotionally uplifting.
- Peppermint oil - supports digestive and immune systems, brain function, energy, and focus.
- Nutmeg oil - supports lymphatic, immune, and digestive health. Supports adrenals.
- Black Pepper oil - supports the liver; helps promote bioavailability of other supplements.
- Wolfberry seed oil - exceptionally high in essential fatty acids; stimulates intracellular oxygenation and blood circulation.

Nitro® Juice Blend Concentrate
- Sweet Cherry - antioxidants to support immune function and protect against oxidative stress.
- Kiwi - antioxidants with vitamin C, vitamin K, vitamin E, folate, and potassium.
- Blueberry - supports blood vessels, cellular health, and circulation.
- Acerola - high in vitamin C, supports immune health.
- Bilberry - strengthens blood vessels, improves circulation.
- Black currant - antioxidants with vitamin C for immune system support.
- Raspberry - antioxidants with vitamins and minerals.
- Strawberry - improves the skin and supports a healthy immune system.
- Cranberry - supports renal system, immune system, and blood.
- Coconut nectar - contains a wide range of vitamins, minerals, and amino acids.
- Natural flavors - extracted from fruit or fruit juice to enhance flavor.
- Pectin - supports digestion and blood.
- Xanthan gum - adds sweet taste.

COMMENTS FROM YOUNG LIVING®
"When you need a midday boost, it's easy to reach for things like soda and energy drinks. Skip the sugary solution and reboot with an option from Young Living®. With NingXia Nitro®, you'll get a quick pick-me-up without the sugar or caffeine overload. Infused with essential oils, botanical extracts, D-ribose, Korean ginseng, and green tea extract, NingXia Nitro® supports alertness, as well as cognitive and physical fitness. A great support for body and mind wellness, use NingXia Nitro® for running, weight-lifting, or getting through your afternoon slump. The naturally occurring caffeine in Young Living's® NingXia Nitro® supports normal energy levels and alertness to help you with a busy day or a tough workout. Stash Nitro® wherever you need it! The small, convenient packaging makes it a great addition to your office desk, gym bag, or purse. Each box contains fourteen 20 ml tubes."

DIRECTIONS FOR USE
Consume NingXia Nitro® directly from the tube or mix with 2-4 oz. of NingXia Red®, 1 can of NingXia Zyng®, or 4 oz. of water anytime you need a pick-me-up. Best served chilled. Shake well before use.

Not recommended for children under 14.

NINGXIA NITRO®

NINGXIA ZYNG®

ENERGY DRINK

USE BEFORE 3PM   VEGAN   CONTAINS STEVIA   CONTAINS CAFFEINE   MINIMUM AGE 18+

NingXia Zyng® is the healthy alternative to the dangerously unhealthy energy drinks. Drink NingXia Zyng® when you need a quick pick-me-up, or enjoy a NingXia "cocktail" by combining a can of NingXia Zyng®, 2 ounces of NingXia Red®, and one tube of NingXia Nitro® with a few drops of your favorite Vitality™ essential oils.

INGREDIENTS

- Calories per serving - 35
- Total Carbohydrates - 9 g
- Sugars (organic cane sugar) - 8 g (7 g added)
- A (Retinyl palmitate) - 150 mcg (15% DV)
- E (D-alpha tocopherol acetate) - 2 mg (15% DV)
- B3 (Niacin / Niacinamide) - 10 mg (60% DV)
- B5 (Pantothenic acid) - 5 mg (100% DV)
- B6 (Pyridoxine hydrochloride) - 1.5 mg (90% DV)
- Carbonated water, Organic cane sugar, Pear juice concentrate, Wolfberry (*Lycium barbarum*) puree, Citric acid, Blackberry juice concentrate, Natural flavors, White tea leaf extract - 35 mg, Stevia rebaudiana leaf extract, Black Pepper (*Piper nigrum*) fruit oil, Lime (*Citrus latifolia*) peel oil

WHAT THE INGREDIENTS DO

- A as Retinyl palmitate - used as an antioxidant, a source of A in a more stable form.
- E - the form of vitamin E that exhibits the greatest bioavailability in the body.
- B3 Niacin - converts consumed food into usable energy.
- B5 - antioxidants to reduce the amount of water lost through the skin.
- B6 - supports the health of nerves, skin, and red blood cells.
- Carbonated water - makes the drink bubbly.
- Evaporated cane sugar - less-processed, more nutritious form of cane sugar.
- Pear juice concentrate - antioxidants with vitamin C, K, B, potassium, copper, phosphorus, magnesium, calcium, and iron, as well as others.
- Wolfberry puree - supports immune system and healthy regeneration of cells.
- Citric acid - preservative and flavor enhancer; antioxidant and alkalizing properties.
- Blackberry juice - antioxidant with manganese, copper, Vitamins A, C, E, and K.
- Natural flavor - extracted from fruit or fruit juice to enhance flavor.
- White tea leaf extract - high in antioxidants; natural source of caffeine.
- Stevia rebaudiana leaf extract - healthy, no calorie natural sweetener.
- Black Pepper fruit oil - supports liver and energy; helps bioavailability.
- Lime peel oil - supports digestion and is a natural detoxifier.

COMMENTS FROM YOUNG LIVING®

"A hydrating splash of essential oil-infused goodness, NingXia Zyng® uses the same whole-fruit wolfberry puree found in our popular superfruit supplement, NingXia Red®. We add sparkling water, pear and blackberry juices, and a hint of Lime and Black Pepper essential oils for a dynamic, unique taste. You'll enjoy a refreshing boost that's full of flavor without artificial flavors and preservatives."

DIRECTIONS FOR USE

Drink 1 can as desired. Best served chilled. Lightly invert can once before opening.

CAUTIONS: Contains naturally occurring caffeine from white tea extract (35 mg); use in moderation if consuming after 3 p.m. Not intended for young children or those who may be sensitive to caffeine.

The statements about the supplement and the ingredients have not been evaluated by the Food and Drug Administration. Young Living® products are not intended to diagnose, treat, cure, or prevent any disease.

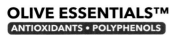

USE ANYTIME   VEGAN   MINIMUM AGE 12+   ½ DOSAGE IF UNDER 12

Olive Essentials™ is a game-changer for optimal health. It gives you the same amount of the polyphenol called hydroxytyrosol in one capsule as if you consumed a full liter of olive oil. Polyphenols are medically recognized to support heart health, immune system, and help to decrease oxidative stress. Studies on hydroxytyrosol have shown cardiovascular benefits as well as reductions in LDL cholesterol. Hydroxytyrosol is considered to be one of the most powerful antioxidant compounds available from nature, and has two times more antioxidant power than the well-known powerhouse, green tea. It is known to benefit the cells, skin, and eyes, as well as help ease inflammation, and support overall body health.

INGREDIENTS
- Hydroxytyrosol (from Olive fruit) - 20 mg

Olive Essentials™ Blend – 231 mg
- Olive fruit extract
- Olive leaf extract
- Parsley (*Petroselinum crispum*) essential oil
- Rosemary (*Rosmarinus officinalis*) essential oil

Other Ingredients
- Microcrystalline cellulose
- Capsule (Hypromellose, Water)
- Magnesium stearate

WHAT THE INGREDIENTS DO
- Hydroxytyrosol - supports cardiovascular health and may reduce LDL cholesterol.

Olive Essentials™ Blend
- Olive fruit extract - antioxidant that supports blood, heart, and immune function.
- Olive leaf extract - reduces inflammation, supports immune function.
- Parsley essential oil - supports internal cleansing, digestion, and immune function.
- Rosemary essential oil - supports immune function and respiratory health.

Other Ingredients
- Microcrystalline cellulose - anti-caking agent for powder.
- Hypromellose and Water - for capsule.
- Magnesium stearate - substrate.

COMMENTS FROM YOUNG LIVING®
"Discover a keystone of the Mediterranean lifestyle with Olive Essentials™. Featuring ingredients handpicked to support your overall well-being and healthy heart, it's sure to become a staple in your home. Olive Essentials™ features hydroxytyrosol from Spanish olives, a naturally occurring compound that contributes to the fruit's healthy reputation. Each capsule of Olive Essentials™ has as much hydroxytyrosol as a liter of extra virgin olive oil, delivering a concentrated amount of this invaluable compound. Hydroxytyrosol is a phenolic compound obtained from olive fruit and leaves. It is considered a powerful antioxidant compound with beneficial properties that support overall health. The formula also features Rosemary Vitality™ essential oil to help keep your healthy immune system in top shape, while Parsley Vitality™ essential oil goes to work promoting internal cleansing."

DIRECTIONS FOR USE
Take 1 capsule daily.

The statements about the supplement and the ingredients have not been evaluated by the Food and Drug Administration. Young Living® products are not intended to diagnose, treat, cure, or prevent any disease.

OLIVE ESSENTIALS™

OMEGAGIZE3®
OMEGA-3 FATTY ACIDS

USE ANYTIME | NOT VEGAN | CONTAINS FISH | MINIMUM AGE 12+ | ¼-½ DOSAGE IF UNDER 12 | DON'T USE WITH BLOOD THINNERS

There are so many fish oil omega-3 fatty acid supplements from which to choose, but Young Living® has far exceeded all the others with OmegaGize3®! OmegaGize3® is a core omega-3 supplement infused with an essential oil blend. Many of the Young Living® supplements are infused with essential oils. Essential oils, when taken internally, can support health in a myriad of ways. Studies have shown that when infused with essential oils, the nutrients in the supplements become more bioavailable.

INGREDIENTS
- Calories per serving - 10
- Total fat - 1 g (1% DV)
- Vitamin D3 (Cholecalciferol) - 24 mcg (120% DV)

Proprietary OmegaGize3® Blend – 1.1 g
- Omega-3 fatty acids (from Basa fish oil) - 445 mg
- Eicosapentaenoic acid (EPA) - 135 mg
- Docosahexaenoic acid (DHA) - 310 mg
- Coenzyme Q10 (as ubiquinone)

Omega Enhancement Blend – 156 mg
- Clove (*Syzygium aromaticum*) flower bud oil
- German Chamomile (*Matricaria recutita*) flower oil
- Spearmint (*Mentha spicata*) leaf oil

Other Ingredients - Gelatin (from fish), Rice bran oil, Silicon dioxide, Purified water, Mixed carotenoids. Contains fish (Basa)

WHAT THE INGREDIENTS DO
- Vitamin D (D3) - supports healthy bones and helps support immune function. Helps boost weight loss, and improves moods.

Proprietary OmegaGize3® Blend
- Omega-3 fatty acids - supports healthy brain function and cardiovascular health.
- Eicosapentaenoic acid (EPA) - supports the heart and reduces menopause symptoms.
- Docosahexaenoic acid (DHA) - supports the brain and fetal development.
- Coenzyme Q10 - helps produce energy, normal growth, maintenance and repair.

Omega Enhancement Blend
- Clove flower bud oil - supports a healthy microbial balance in the body.
- German Chamomile flower oil - for stomach upset, and helps minimize flatulence.
- Spearmint leaf oil - Soothes digestion and promotes energy.

Other Ingredients - Gelatin, Rice bran oil, Silicon dioxide, Purified water, Mixed carotenoids - capsule and substrates.

COMMENTS FROM YOUNG LIVING®
"OmegaGize3® combines the power of three core daily supplements - omega-3 fatty acids, vitamin D-3, and CoQ10 (ubiquinone). These supplements combine with our proprietary enhancement essential oil blend to create an omega-3, DHA-rich fish oil supplement that may support general wellness. Used daily these ingredients work synergistically to support normal brain, heart, eye, and joint health."

DIRECTIONS FOR USE
Take 2-4 capsules twice daily. Do not exceed 8 capsules per day.

The statements about the supplement and the ingredients have not been evaluated by the Food and Drug Administration. Young Living® products are not intended to diagnose, treat, cure, or prevent any disease.

OMEGAGIZE3®

PD 80/20™
HORMONES

USE ANYTIME | BEST WITH FOOD | CONTAINS NO OILS | NOT VEGAN | CONTAINS BEEF GELATIN | MINIMUM AGE 21+

PD 80/20™ is the most basic of all the hormone supplements but has a perfect balance of pregnenolone to natural DHEA from wild yams. This supplement contains 400 mg of pregnenolone and 100 mg of DHEA which is where its name is derived from - 80% Pregnenolone to 20% DHEA.

INGREDIENTS
- Pregnenolone - 400 mg
- DHEA (dehydroepiandrosterone derived from wild yams) - 100 mg

Other Ingredients - Rice flour, Gelatin (bovine)

WHAT THE INGREDIENTS DO
- Pregnenolone - a precursor hormone that increases the production of all hormones in the body such as progesterone, estrogen, and cortisol. It helps combat fatigue, increases energy, supports memory, supports motivation, helps increase libido, and may help improve mood swings. According to a study published in 2009 by Marx, Keefe, and Buchanan, in Neuropsychopharmacology titled "Proof-of-concept trial with the neurosteroid pregnenolone targeting cognitive and negative symptoms in schizophrenia," they found that patients with schizophrenia saw improvements with their symptoms when they used pregnenolone for eight weeks.
- DHEA (dehydroepiandrosterone) - a precursor hormone that helps with cognition, healthy emotions, libido, vaginal dryness, and helps improve muscle and bone mass.

Other Ingredients - Rice flour (substrate powder), Gelatin (capsule).

NOTE: there are no essential oils in this supplement.

COMMENTS FROM YOUNG LIVING®
"PD 80/20™ is a dietary supplement formulated to help maximize internal health and support the endocrine system. It contains pregnenolone and DHEA, two substances produced naturally by the body that decline with age. Pregnenolone is the key precursor for the body's production of estrogen, DHEA, and progesterone, and it also has an impact on mental acuity and memory. DHEA is involved in maintaining the health of the cardiovascular and immune systems."

DIRECTIONS FOR USE
1 capsule per day as needed. Best absorbed with food.
Do not take if under the age of 21.

PD 80/20™

These statements have not been evaluated by the Food and Drug Administration.
Young Living® products are not intended to diagnose, treat, cure, or prevent any disease.

PARAFREE™

CLEANSING

| USE ANYTIME | BEST WITH FOOD | CONTAINS ALL OILS | NOT VEGAN | CONTAINS FISH | MINIMUM AGE 18+ | CAUTION IF PREGNANT |

ParaFree™ supports digestion, circulation, respiratory, and immune function by helping your body rid itself of unwanted hitch-hikers. This essential oil capsule combines powerful essential oils that cleanse the body and fight oxidative stress.

INGREDIENTS

ParaFree™ Blend – 2250 mg

- Sesame (*Sesamum indicum*) seed oil
- Cumin (*Cuminum cyminum*) seed oil
- Olive (*Olea europaea*) fruit oil
- Anise (*Pimpinella anisum*) fruit oil
- Fennel (*Foeniculum vulgare*) seed oil
- Vetiver (*Vetiveria zizanioides*) root oil
- Bay Laurel (*Laurus nobilis*) leaf oil
- Nutmeg (*Myristica fragrans*) seed oil
- Tea tree (*Melaleuca alternifolia*) leaf oil
- Thyme (*Thymus vulgaris*) leaf oil
- Clove (*Syzygium aromaticum*) flower bud oil
- Ocotea (*Ocotea quixos*) leaf oil
- Dorado Azul (*Hyptis suaveolens*) aerial parts oil
- Tarragon (*Artemisia dracunculus*) leaf oil
- Ginger (*Zingiber officinale*) root oil
- Peppermint (*Mentha piperita*) aerial parts oil
- Juniper (*Juniperus osteosperma*) aerial parts oil
- Lemongrass (*Cymbopogon flexuosus*) leaf oil
- Patchouli (*Pogostemon cablin*) leaf oil

Other Ingredients - Fish Gelatin (tilapia or carp for capsule), Glycerin, Water

WHAT THE INGREDIENTS DO

ParaFree™ Blend

- Sesame seed oil - carrier oil rich in vitamin B with high antioxidant properties.
- Cumin seed oil - aids in digestion and promotes a reduction of potential flatulence.
- Olive fruit oil - antioxidants protect cells and promote cardiovascular health.
- Anise fruit oil - helps keep blood sugar levels stable, improves digestion.
- Fennel seed oil - improves digestion, and is a mild appetite suppressant.
- Vetiver root oil - known for its soothing, grounding abilities.
- Bay Laurel leaf oil - is renewing and purifying.
- Nutmeg seed oil - supports lymphatic, digestive, and immune health; helps energy.
- Tea tree leaf oil - supports respiratory and intestinal tract. Research: may help prevent antibiotic resistance; positive synergistic effect when combined with antibiotics.
- Thyme leaf oil - supports digestive cleansing, urinary, immune, and respiratory systems.
- Clove flower bud oil - antioxidants support a healthy microbial balance in the body.
- Ocotea leaf oil - stimulates digestion and supports the liver; supports blood sugar, cardiovascular, and blood flow; helps curb cravings and promote feelings of fullness.
- Dorado Azul oil - supports the respiratory system.
- Tarragon leaf oil - improves digestion, fights bacteria.
- Ginger root oil - supports digestion, cleanses bowels, minimizes flatulence.
- Peppermint oil - supports digestive and immune function; supports energy, and focus.
- Juniper oil - is a powerful cleanser and detoxifier.
- Lemongrass leaf oil - supports immune and digestive functions; supports healthy blood.
- Patchouli leaf oil - is soothing and releasing to the body.

COMMENTS FROM YOUNG LIVING®

"ParaFree™ is formulated with an advanced blend of some of the strongest essential oils studied for their cleansing abilities."

DIRECTIONS FOR USE

Take 3 softgels twice daily or as needed. For best results, take for 21 days and rest for seven days. Cycle may be repeated three times. Take on an empty stomach for maximum results. NOTE: Excessive internal use of essential oils is not considered safe during pregnancy.

The statements about the supplement and the ingredients have not been evaluated by the Food and Drug Administration. Young Living® products are not intended to diagnose, treat, cure, or prevent any disease.

POWERGIZE™
STAMINA • STRENGTH

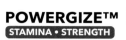

USE ANYTIME · BEST BEFORE A WORKOUT · NOT VEGAN · CONTAINS DAIRY · MINIMUM AGE 18+ · CAUTION IF PREGNANT · GOOD CHOICE FOR MEN

A favorite among athletes, PowerGize™ can be utilized by any adult wishing to boost their physical game. Formulated with Ashwagandha root (also found in EndoGize™), PowerGize™ helps support male testosterone, physical performance, and sexual drive. Both men and women may use this supplement.

INGREDIENTS
- B6 (pyridoxine HCL) - 12 mg
- Magnesium (magnesium bisglycinate) - 20 mg
- Zinc (zinc glycinate chelate) - 5 mg

PowerGize™ Energy Blend – 995.25 mg
- Ashwagandha (*Withania somnifera*) root extract
- Longjack (*Eurycoma longifolia*) root powder
- Fenugreek (Trigonella foenum-graecum) (50% saponin) seed extract
- Epimedium (*Epimedium brevicornum*) leaf powder
- Desert hyacinth (*Cistanche tubulosa*) root extract
- Tribulus (*Tribulus terrestris*) (45% saponin) fruit/leaf extract
- Muira puama (*Ptychopetalum olacoides*) bark powder

Essential Oils - Idaho Blue spruce (*Picea pungens*) aerial parts oil, Goldenrod (*Solidago canadensis*) flowering top oil, Cassia (*Cinnamomum aromaticum*) branch/leaf oil
Other Ingredients - Hypromellose, Rice flour, Silicon dioxide
Note: Contains milk

WHAT THE INGREDIENTS DO
- B6 - supports brain development, nervous system, and immune system.
- Magnesium - aids in normal function of the cells, nerves, muscles, bones, and heart.
- Zinc - supports immune function, tissue growth, and skin, eye and heart health.

PowerGize™ Energy Blend
- Ashwagandha root extract - supports immune function, mental clarity, concentration, and alertness. May improve memory and brain function, reduce cortisol levels when chronically stressed, and support healthy emotions, peace, and stress.
- Longjack root powder - may boost testosterone, increase energy, and physical endurance.
- Fenugreek seed extract - supports digestion and blood; improves exercise performance.
- Epimedium leaf powder - boosts stamina, focus, and energy.
- Desert hyacinth root powder - supports cardiovascular and renal health; muscle building.
- Tribulus fruit/leaf extract - enhances libido, natural diuretic properties, supports heart.
- Muira puama bark powder - promotes nerve function and cognitive health.
- Idaho Blue spruce aerial parts oil - supports respiratory, endocrine, and immune health.
- Goldenrod flowering top oil - supports respiratory, lymphatic, circulatory and heart health.
- Cassia branch/leaf oil - supports nervous, digestive, circulatory and immune systems.

Other Ingredients - Hypromellose, Rice flour, Silicon dioxide - capsule and substrate.

COMMENTS FROM YOUNG LIVING®
"Inspire your inner athlete with PowerGize™! This supplement is specially formulated to help individuals of all ages boost stamina and performance. PowerGize™ helps sustain energy levels, strength, mental and physical vibrancy, and vitality when used in addition to physical activity. PowerGize™ is also formulated with KSM-66, a premium ashwagandha root extract, which is touted for its properties that support immunity, mental clarity, concentration, and alertness."

DIRECTIONS FOR USE
Take 2 capsules daily. NOTE: Ashwagandha is not advised during pregnancy.

The statements about the supplement and the ingredients have not been evaluated by the Food and Drug Administration. Young Living® products are not intended to diagnose, treat, cure, or prevent any disease.

POWERGIZE™

PROSTATE HEALTH™
HORMONES

USE ANYTIME | BEST WITH FOOD | NOT VEGAN | CONTAINS PORK | CONTAINS BEEF GELATIN | MINIMUM AGE 21+ | DON'T USE WITH BLOOD THINNERS | MEN SPECIFIC

Specifically formulated for men, Prostate Health™ targets key elements to support the prostate. It helps elevate moods, balances testosterone levels, supports the body's inflammatory response, and provides antioxidant support. The essential oils in Prostate Health™ are known to help support healthy digestion.

INGREDIENTS
- Saw palmetto (*Serenoa Replens/serrulata*) fruit extract - 235 mg
- Pumpkin (*Cucurbita pepo*) seed oil - 175 mg

Essential Oil Blend – 100 mg
- Geranium (*Pelargonium graveolens*) flower/leaf oil
- Fennel (*Foeniculum vulare*) seed oil
- Lavender (*Lavandula angustifolia*) flowering top oil
- Myrtle (*Myrtus communis*) leaf oil
- Peppermint (*Mentha piperita*) aerial parts oil

Other Ingredients - Porcine gelatin, Water, Silica

WHAT THE INGREDIENTS DO
- Saw palmetto fruit extract - balances testosterone and improves prostate health.
- Pumpkin seed oil - reduces inflammation, supports a healthy prostate; supports mental health, combats stress, and supports healthy emotions.
- Geranium flower/leaf oil - promotes urination, reduces inflammation, balances hormones.
- Fennel seed oil - improves digestion, and is a mild appetite suppressant.
- Lavender flowering top oil - supports moods, immune and respiratory systems.
- Myrtle leaf oil - supports urinary tract, bladder, digestion, and respiratory health.
- Peppermint oil - supports digestive and immune function; supports energy, and focus.

Other Ingredients - Porcine gelatin, Water, and Silica - capsule and substrate.

COMMENTS FROM YOUNG LIVING®
"Prostate Health™ is uniquely formulated for men concerned with supporting the male glandular system and maintaining healthy, normal prostate function. Prostate Health™ is an essential oil supplement featuring powerful saw palmetto and pumpkin seed oil—ingredients known for their support of a healthy prostate gland. A proprietary blend of pure Geranium, Fennel, Myrtle, Lavender, and Peppermint essential oils provides the body with key components. The benefits of liquid capsules include a targeted release for ideal absorption and minimal aftertaste. For maximum benefit, Prostate Health™ should be taken consistently over time."

DIRECTIONS FOR USE
Take 1 liquid capsule twice daily. Best with food.
Note: Saw palmetto could interfere with Coumadin® or blood thinners.
This supplement contains carrier oil in the form of Pumpkin seed oil, which helps with the fat-solubility of Saw Palmetto. You do not need to take with food, but it will better absorb if you take it with a little fat-containing food.

PURE PROTEIN™ COMPLETE

SHAKE MIX

USE ANYTIME · NOT VEGAN · CONTAINS DAIRY · CONTAINS EGG · CONTAINS STEVIA · MINIMUM AGE 1+

Pure Protein™ Complete shake mix comes in both vanilla and chocolate. It contains five different proteins that your body processes at different rates to keep you full longer. It is gluten free and helps you have sustained energy and contains digestive enzymes and amino acids that are crucial for energy production and healthy immune function.

INGREDIENTS

- Calories - 170
- Total Fat - 2.5 g (3% DV)
    - Saturated Fat - 1 g (5% DV)
    - Trans Fat - 0 g
- Cholesterol - 50 mg (15% DV)
- Total Carbohydrate - 14 g (5% DV)
    - Dietary Fiber - 2 g (7% DV)
    - Sugars - 9 g
        - Added Sugars 6 g (13%)
- Protein - 25 g (50% DV)
- Calcium - 135 mg (10% DV)
- Iron 7 mg (41%)
- Sodium - 200 mg (9% DV)
- Potassium 375.4 mg (8% DV)
- B1 Thiamin (as thiamin hydrochloride) - 0.75 mg (63% DV)
- B2 Riboflavin - 0.85 mg (65% DV)
- B3 Niacin - 10 mg (63% DV)
- B6 (Pyridoxine hydrochloride) - 1 mg (59% DV)
- B12 (Methylcobalamin) - 3 mcg (125% DV)
- B7 (Biotin) - 150 mcg (500% DV)
- B5 (Pantothenic Acid as d-calcium pantothenate) - 5 mg (100% DV)
- Zinc (Zinc picolinate) - 15 mg (136% DV)

Pure Protein™ Proprietary Blend – 31.75 gm
rBGH-free whey protein concentrate, Pea protein isolate, Goat whey protein concentrate, Egg albumin, Organic hemp seed protein, elevATP® (Ancient peat, Apple extract)
Enzyme Proprietary Complex – 55 gm
Alpha and Beta Amylase, Protease, Lipase, Cellulase, L. acidophilus, Papain, Bromelain
Amino Acid Blend - L-glutamine, L-methionine, L-lysine, L-leucine, L-isoleucine, L-valine
Other Ingredients - Organic evaporated cane juice, Cocoa powder, Xanthan gum, Natural flavors, Sodium chloride, Stevia (*Stevia rebaudiana*) leaf extract, Orange (*Citrus sinensis*) peel oil, Luo han guo (*Siraitia grosvenorii*) fruit extract

WHAT THE INGREDIENTS DO

- Protein - to repair cells and make new ones.
- Calcium - specific calcium to reduce the amount of water lost through the skin.
- Iron - may improve muscle function, increase brain function and eliminate fatigue.
- Sodium - supports fluid balance and electrolytes.
- Potassium - maintains fluid and electrolyte balance.
- B1 - beneficial to a healthy nervous system.
- B2 - needed for overall growth. It also helps support energy levels.
- B3 - helps lower cholesterol, ease arthritis and boost brain function.
- B6 - supports the health of nerves, skin, and red blood cells.
- B12 - supports the body to make red blood cells.
- B7 - supports a healthy metabolism and creates enzymes.
- B5 - reduces the amount of water lost through the skin.
- Zinc - helps ease inflammation; supports the blood and heart.

Continued on next page.

PURE PROTEIN™

WHAT THE INGREDIENTS DO (continued)

Pure Protein™ Proprietary Blend
- rBGH-free whey protein concentrate - stimulates muscle growth.
- Pea protein isolate - easily digested protein.
- Goat whey protein concentrate - promotes a healthy immune and digestive system.
- Egg albumin - excellent source of protein.
- Organic hemp seed protein - easily digestible, plant-based complete protein.
- Ancient peat and Apple extract (as elevATP) - supports ATP production for energy.

Enzyme Proprietary Complex
- Alpha and Beta amylase - breaks down starch, breads, and pasta.
- Protease - digests proteins to allow absorption of amino acids; converts food to energy.
- Lipase - breaks down dietary fats and oils. Helps liver function.
- Cellulase - breaks down man-made fiber, plant fiber, fruits, and vegetables.
- L. acidophilus - breaks down dairy sugars and helps minimize lactose intolerance.
- Papain - digestive aid to help break proteins down into peptides and amino acids.
- Bromelain - breaks down peptides and amino acids; helps ease inflammation.

Amino Acid Blend
- L-leucine, L-isoleucine, and L-valine - supports the brain and lessens exercise fatigue.
- L-methionine - supports growth of new blood vessels; supports the immune system.
- L-lysine - converts fatty acids into energy and supports absorption of calcium.
- L-glutamine - supports immune cell activity in the gut.

Other Ingredients
- Organic evaporated cane juice - natural sweetener.
- Cocoa Powder - natural flavor (chocolate flavor only).
- Xanthan gum - adds sweet taste.
- Natural flavors - extracted from fruit or fruit juice to enhance flavor.
- Sodium chloride - supports fluid balance and electrolytes.
- Stevia - no calorie natural sweetener.
- Orange rind oil - supports immune function and improves blood flow.
- Luo han guo fruit extract - adds sweetness with no calories (Monk fruit).

Allergens: Contains dairy and egg.

COMMENTS FROM YOUNG LIVING®

"Pure Protein™ Complete is a comprehensive protein supplement that combines a proprietary 5-Protein Blend, amino acids, and ancient peat and apple extract to deliver 25 grams of protein per serving in two delicious flavors, Vanilla Spice and Chocolate Deluxe. Its foundation of cow and goat whey, pea protein, egg white protein, and organic hemp seed protein provide a full range of amino acids including - D-aspartic acid, Threonine, L-serine, Glutamic acid, Glycine, Alanine, Valine, Methionine, Isoleucine, Leucine, Tyrosine, Phenylalanine, Lysine, Histidine, Arginine, Proline, Hydroxyproline, Cystine, Tryptophan, and Cysteine. Along with a proprietary enzyme blend, these amino acids support overall protein utilization in the body. Ancient peat and apple extract, along with a powerful B-vitamin blend, complete the formula. Together they support ATP production, the energy currency of the body. This innovative formula makes Pure Protein™ Complete the perfect option for those looking for a high protein supplement that features a full range of amino acids."

DIRECTIONS FOR USE

Add 2 scoops of Pure Protein™ Complete to 8 oz. of cold water. May also be mixed with rice, almond, or other milk. Shake or stir until smooth. For added flavor, add fruit or essential oils. Blend with ice for a nice shake.

REHEMOGEN™

CLEANSING

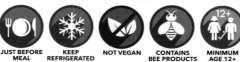

JUST BEFORE MEAL • KEEP REFRIGERATED • NOT VEGAN • CONTAINS BEE PRODUCTS • MINIMUM AGE 12+ • ¼-½ DOSAGE IF UNDER 12 • CAUTION IF PREGNANT

Rehemogen™ helps cleanse your intestinal tract as a mild laxative and supports healthy blood and detoxification. It helps to calm nervous energy and supports the digestive, nervous, renal, respiratory, lymphatic, endocrine, and immune systems. Rehemogen™ is a tincture, which means it is in liquid form that you may add from the dropper bottle directly to water or juice. You may also put each half dropper into a veggie capsule. Three veggie capsules will hold one serving.

INGREDIENTS

- Red clover (*Trifolium pratense*) blossom
- Licorice (*Glycyrrhiza glabra*) root
- Poke (*Phytolacca americana*) root
- Peach (*Prunus persica*) bark
- Oregon grape (*Berberis aquifolium*) root
- Stillingia (*S. sylvatica*) root
- Sarsaparilla (*Smilax medica*) root
- Cascara sagrada (*Frangula purshiana*) bark
- Prickly ash (*Zanthoxylum americanum*) bark
- Burdock (*Arctium lappa*) root
- Buckthorn (*Rhamnus frangula*) bark
- Royal jelly (from bees)
- Roman chamomile (*Chamaemelum nobile*) flower oil
- Rosemary (*Rosmarinus officinalis*) leaf oil
- Thyme (*Thymus vulgaris*) leaf oil
- Tea tree (*Melaleuca alternifolia*) leaf oil

Other Ingredients - Distilled water, Ethanol

WHAT THE INGREDIENTS DO

- Red clover blossom - source of vitamin A, B-complex, C, F and P, and trace minerals.
- Licorice root - mild laxative; softens, lubricates, and nourishes the intestinal tract.
- Poke root - stimulates congested and sluggish glandular system.
- Peach bark - strengthens the nervous system and stimulates the flow of urine.
- Oregon grape root - supports immune function, diarrhea, and digestion.
- Stillingia root - effective glandular stimulant as well as an activator for the liver.
- Sarsaparilla root - hormone balancing; supports metabolism.
- Cascara sagrada bark - moves waste out of the body. NOTE - Turns stool black.
- Prickly ash bark - supports circulation; improves blood purification.
- Burdock root - supports kidneys, lymphatics, and increases the flow of urine.
- Buckthorn bark - supports the gastrointestinal tract; eases constipation.
- Royal Jelly - produced by honey bees. Source of B vitamin complex and 50+ minerals and vitamins. Supports the cardiovascular, kidneys, lungs, and immune systems.
- Roman chamomile flower oil - antioxidant; supports GI tract by reducing digestive discomfort.
- Rosemary leaf oil - aids in digestion and supports liver cleansing.
- Thyme leaf oil - supports digestive cleansing, promotes healthy renal and urinary systems.
- Tea tree leaf oil - supports respiratory and intestinal tract.

Other Ingredients - Distilled water and Ethanol - tincture base.

COMMENTS FROM YOUNG LIVING®

"Rehemogen™ contains Cascara sagrada, red clover, poke root, prickly ash bark, and burdock root, which have been historically used for their cleansing and building properties. Rehemogen™ is also formulated with essential oils to enhance digestion."

DIRECTIONS FOR USE

Shake well. Take 3 half droppers (3ml) three times daily in distilled water just prior to or with meals containing protein. Refrigerate after opening.

NOTE: Oregon Grape root contains Berberine, which is not recommended during pregnancy, and Cascara Sagrada is also not recommended during pregnancy.

Do not exceed recommended dosage. Not for long term use.

SLEEPESSENCE™
SLEEP • IMMUNE SUPPORT

USE JUST BEFORE BED | MELATONIN SLEEP AID | CONTAINS ALL OILS | VEGAN | CONTAINS CORN | CONTAINS COCONUT | MINIMUM AGE 18+ | CAUTION IF PREGNANT

SleepEssence™ is an essential oil filled capsule used to support natural sleep patterns to help calm your mind so you can fall asleep faster. It contains a small amount of melatonin to help you drift off to sleep and the oils, when taken consistently over time, help you stay asleep longer. You may take 1 capsule for light support or 2 if you need more help getting a restful night's sleep.

INGREDIENTS
SleepEssence™ Blend – 637 mg
Contains 12.8 drops total of Coconut carrier oil and Seed to Seal® Premium essential oils.
- Lavender (*Lavandula officinalis*) flowering top oil
- Vetiver (*Vetiveria zizanioides*) root oil
- Valerian (*Valeriana officinalis*) root oil
- Tangerine (*Citrus reticulata*) rind oil
- Rue (*Ruta graveolens*) flower oil
- Melatonin - 3.2 mg per serving (2 capsules)

Other Ingredients - Lecithin, Coconut (Cocos nucifera) fruit oil, Carrageenan, Glycerin, Modified cornstarch, Sorbitol, Water
NOTE: Contains tree nuts (Coconut)

WHAT THE INGREDIENTS DO
- Lavender oil - provides antioxidant protection; supports moods and sleep.
- Vetiver oil - antioxidant; helps ease sleeplessnes and stress.
- Valerian oil - supports sleep, calms moods, reduces brain activity, improves sleep quality, and relaxes muscles.
- Tangerine oil - relaxes nerves and muscles, reduces tension, promotes healthy sleep.
- Rue oil - antioxidant; relaxing benefits.
- Melatonin - improves sleep quality. Helps people with disrupted circadian rhythm. Leads to the recovery of pituitary and thyroid functions. Has anti-inflammatory and antioxidant effects. Strengthens the immune system. Helps to relieve stress.

Other Ingredients
- Lecithin - supports positive moods and peace.
- Coconut fruit oil - carrier base.
- Carrageenan - supports immune function, and is an antioxidant and prebiotic.
- Glycerin - adds base and sweet taste.
- Modified cornstarch - stabilizer and emulsifier for ingredients.
- Sorbitol - sweetener and mild laxative.
- Water - supplement base.

COMMENTS FROM YOUNG LIVING®
"SleepEssence™ contains four powerful Young Living® Seed to Seal® Premium essential oils that have unique sleep-enhancing properties in a softgel vegetarian capsule for easy ingestion. Combining Lavender, Vetiver, Valerian, and Ruta Graveolens essential oils with the hormone melatonin — a well-known sleep aid — SleepEssence™ is a natural way to enable a full night's rest."

DIRECTIONS FOR USE
Take 1–2 softgels 30–60 minutes before bedtime.
CAUTION: Do not operate heavy machinery for 8-10 hours after using. Not recommended for long-term use or with products containing echinacea. Adult use only.
NOTE: Rue is not advised during pregnancy.

The statements about the supplement and the ingredients have not been evaluated by the Food and Drug Administration. Young Living® products are not intended to diagnose, treat, cure, or prevent any disease.

SLIQUE® SHAKE
SHAKE MIX • WEIGHTLOSS

USE ANYTIME

VEGAN

CONTAINS STEVIA

CONTAINS CORN

CONTAINS CAFFEINE

MINIMUM AGE 12+

½ DOSAGE IF UNDER 12

INGREDIENTS

- Calories - 190
- Total Fat - 6g (9% DV)
  - Saturated Fat 4 g (21% DV)
- Sodium - 410 mg (17% DV)
- Total Carbohydrate - 23 g (8% DV)
  - Dietary Fiber - 5 g (20% DV)
  - Sugars 11 g
- Protein - 16 g (32% DV)

A (Retinyl acetate)	8% DV	B7 Biotin	8% DV
C	20% DV	B5 Pantothenic acid	10% DV
Calcium	6% DV	Phosphorus	25% DV
Iron	20% DV	Iodine	6% DV
B1 Thiamin	20% DV	Magnesium	15% DV
B2 Riboflavin	25% DV	Zinc	20% DV
B3 Niacin	30% DV	Selenium	50% DV
B6 Pyridoxine HCl	20% DV	Copper	25% DV
B9 Folate	15% DV	Chromium	15% DV
B12	6% DV	Molybdenum	60% DV

Ingredients List - Pea protein isolate, Isomalto-oligosaccharide, Medium-chain triglycerides, Tapioca dextrose, Organic Coconut palm sugar, Natural flavor, Organic quinoa powder, Organic pumpkin seed protein, Xanthan gum, Strawberry fruit powder, Sodium citrate, Malic acid, **Fruit and vegetable extract blend** (Green tea leaf extract, Guarana seed extract, Red and white grape extracts, Grapefruit extract, Black carrot extract, Vitamin B3), Alfalfa grass juice powder, Organic wolfberry fruit powder, Stevia, **Slique® essential oil** (Grapefruit rind oil, Tangerine rind oil, Spearmint leaf oil, Lemon rind oil, Ocotea leaf oil, Stevia leaf extract), **Vitamins and Minerals** - Dipotassium phosphate, Monosodium phosphate, Magnesium oxide, Zinc gluconate, **Organic B vitamin blend** (Guava extract, Holy basil extract, Citrus limon extract), Ascorbic acid, Molybdenum glycinate, Niacin, Copper gluconate, Biotin, Vitamin A acetate, Sodium selenite, d-Calcium pantothenate, Chromium nicotinate glycinate chelate, Riboflavin, Pyridoxine HCl, Potassium iodide, Methylcobalamin

WHAT THE INGREDIENTS DO

- A as retinyl acetate - a natural form of A that supports immune function and oxidation.
- C - supports immune function and overall health.
- Calcium - supports healthy bones, heart, muscles, and nerves.
- Iron - supports healthy blood and immune function; helps reduce fatigue.
- Pea protein isolate - is easily digested, rich in iron, arginine and branched-chain amino acids known to support muscle growth, feelings of fullness and cardiovascular health.
- Isomalto-oligosaccharide - (IMO) is a moderately sweet carbohydrate that occurs naturally in honey. It is also found in fermented foods and made up of carbohydrate chains that are resistant to digestion and low in calories.
- Medium-chain triglycerides - (MCT) are fats found in foods like coconut oil. They are metabolized faster than long-chain triglycerides (LCT). They are less likely to be stored as fat.
- Tapioca dextrose - is a very quickly digested, simple sugar that offers immediate energy and is easily digested.
- Organic Coconut palm sugar - is the dehydrated sap of the coconut palm. It retains nutrient minerals like iron, zinc, calcium and potassium, along with some short-chain fatty acids like polyphenols and antioxidants.
- Natural flavor - is the flavorful constituents derived from a spice, fruit, vegetable, herb, bark, bud, root, leaf or similar plant material.

Continued on next page.

SLIQUE® SHAKE

WHAT THE INGREDIENTS DO (continued)

- Organic quinoa powder - provides a complete plant-based protein whose benefits include improved solubility and stability. It contains all nine essential amino acids, is rich in omega 3, 6, and 9, potassium, iron, magnesium, and antioxidants. Naturally gluten-free, organic quinoa powder is easily digested and optimally absorbed because of its unique breakdown of starch bonds.
- Organic pumpkin seed protein - is a great source of tryptophan, manganese, magnesium, phosphorus, copper, protein, zinc and iron. Organic pumpkin seed protein can support normal blood pressure and sugar levels, as well as a healthy heart, bones, muscle and nerve function. Pumpkin seeds are full of antioxidants that may help reduce inflammation and support the immune system.
- Xanthan gum - is a complex exopolysaccharide, a polymer composed of sugar residues, secreted by a microorganism into the environment. Produced by plant-pathogenic bacterium – xanthan gum is often used as a thickening and stabilizing agent.
- Strawberry fruit powder - rich in fiber and helps the body to absorb key nutrients. Can help stabilize blood sugar levels and is high in vitamin C while low in calories.
- Sodium citrate - used as a food preservative, flavoring agent, and stabilizer.
- Malic acid - is a component of most fruits and can promote energy production, increase endurance and help prevent muscle fatigue while exercising; natural preservative.

Fruit and Vegetable Extract Blend

- Green tea leaf extract - is rich in antioxidants called catechins, which have been shown to increase antioxidant capacity and protect against oxidative stress.
- Guarana seed extract - contains the stimulants caffeine, theophylline and theobromine. It is also rich in antioxidants, including tannins, saponins and catechins, which can neutralize free radicals in the body.
- Red and white grape extracts - contain beneficial plant compounds, resveratrol, quercetin, anthocyanins and catechins - combat oxidative stress that can lead to illness.
- Grapefruit extract - contains many powerful antioxidants that can protect your body from oxidative stress and free radicals.
- Black carrot extract - is rich in anthocyanins which are powerful antioxidants.
- B3 (Niacin) - helps the body convert food into glucose used for energy. Niacin supports the healthy function of the nervous system and normal psychological processes. It may also help ward off undue tiredness.

Slique® Essential Oil Blend

- Grapefruit rind oil - is naturally high in antioxidants and phytochemicals that reduce oxidative stress and inflammation. Limonene protects cells from damage.
- Tangerine rind oil - promotes good digestion while supporting the immune system.
- Spearmint leaf oil - promotes healthy digestion and acid secretion. Can also support the breakdown of food.
- Lemon rind oil - cleanses toxins from the body and stimulates lymphatic drainage.
- Ocotea leaf oil - has the highest levels of alpha-humulene in the world, known for its ability to minimize inflammation and irritation.
- Stevia leaf extract - is used as a natural sweetener, that has no accumulation in the body, which can promote healthy insulin production.

Vitamins and Minerals

- Dipotassium phosphate - is commonly used as an emulsifier and is a great source of potassium and phosphorus.
- Monosodium phosphate - is used as an emulsifying agent and protein modifier. It is a good source of phosphorus, which is necessary for healthy bones.
- Magnesium oxide - is beneficial for the proper functioning of the immune system, nerves, heart, eyes, brain and muscles.
- Zinc gluconate - is important for growth and healthy development of body tissues.

WHAT THE INGREDIENTS DO (continued)
Organic B Vitamin Blend
- Guava extract - is rich in antioxidants, vitamin C, potassium and fiber and is used to make collagen, a protein required to help wounds heal.
- Holy basil extract - is an adaptogen with anti-inflammatory and antioxidant properties.
- Citrus limon extract - helps in the absorption of iron.

Other Ingredients
- Alfalfa grass juice powder - has a high concentration of antioxidants, vitamins C and K, copper, folate and magnesium. It is also very low in calories.
- Organic wolfberry fruit powder - supports healthy vision thanks to high levels of an antioxidant called zeaxanthin. High amounts of Vitamins A and C help support a healthy immune system and fight oxidative stressors.
- Stevia - a natural sweetener that is low in calories, derived from the Stevia leaf.
- Ascorbic acid - acts as an antioxidant, protecting cells from free radicals.
- Molybdenum glycinate - acts as a cofactor for the enzymes involved in processing sulfites and breaking down toxins in the body.
- B3 (Niacin) - helps the body convert food into glucose, used for energy. Niacin supports the healthy function of the nervous system and normal psychological processes. It may also help ward off undue tiredness.
- Copper gluconate - helps the body form collagen, absorb iron and supports energy.
- B7 (Biotin) - a water-soluble vitamin that helps your body convert food into energy.
- Vitamin A acetate - is a powerful antioxidant necessary for eye health, immune function, cell growth and fetal development.
- Sodium selenite - is an essential trace mineral that plays an important role in reducing oxidative stress on the body.
- B5 (D-calcium pantothenate) - protects cells against damage by increasing levels of glutathione in the body.
- Chromium nicotinate glycinate chelate - is a high-quality, chelated form of the mineral chromium, an amino acid that binds to minerals and assists in their bioavailability through the intestinal walls.
- B2 (Riboflavin) - is also known as Vitamin B2. It helps the break down of proteins, fats and carbohydrates. Riboflavin maintains the body's energy supply and converts carbohydrates into adenosine triphosphate (ATP), while absorbing and activating iron, folic acid, and vitamins B1, B3 and B6.
- B6 (Pyridoxine HCl) - helps the body convert food into fuel, metabolize fats and proteins, maintain proper nerve functions and produce red blood cells.
- Potassium iodide - is stored in the thyroid gland and is necessary for normal function.
- B12 (Methylcobalamin) - acts as a cofactor for enzymes, providing functional support of neurons. B12 can also reduce the neurotoxicity of cells.

SLIQUE® SHAKE

COMMENTS FROM YOUNG LIVING®
"Slique® Shake is a complete meal replacement that provides quick, satisfying, and delicious nutrition. Formulated with Slique® Essence essential oil blend, this shake may support healthy weight management when combined with regular exercise and a sensible diet. In a convenient single-serving size packet, it's easy to slip into a purse or pocket for healthy eating on the go."

DIRECTIONS FOR USE
Add 1 Slique® Shake packet to 8 oz. of water or the milk of your choice.
Shake, stir, or blend until smooth.

SLIQUE® BARS
WEIGHTLOSS

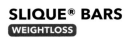

USE ANYTIME | NOT VEGAN | CONTAINS EGG | CONTAINS BEE PRODUCTS | CONTAINS NUTS | CONTAINS COCONUT | MINIMUM AGE 2+

Simply put, Slique® Bars are delicious. Both the regular and chocolate coated are incredible! They are the perfect mix of chewy, crunchy, and sweet. Eat a Slique® bar for breakfast or take with you as a midday snack. You will want to hide these from your kids!

INGREDIENTS

- Baru nuts
- Almonds
- Honey
- Chicory root inulin
- Dates
- Coconut
- Cacao nibs
- Goldenberries
- Bing cherries
- Wolfberries (*Lycium barbarum*)
- Quinoa crisps
- Chia seeds
- Potato skin extract
- Sea salt
- Vanilla (*Vanilla planifolia*) oil
- Sunflower lecithin
- Orange (*Citrus aurantium dulcis*) peel oil
- Cinnamon (*Cinnamomum verum*) bark oil.

Allergens - Contains baru nuts, almonds, and Coconut.
Manufactured in a facility that also processes tree nuts, peanuts, soy, milk, and eggs.

WHAT THE INGREDIENTS DO

- Baru nuts - high in fiber, protein, essential fatty acids and antioxidants.
- Almonds - high in protein, fiber, vitamin E, copper and magnesium.
- Honey - good source of antioxidants; beneficial to the cardiovascular system.
- Chicory root inulin - good source of prebiotic fiber; supports digestion and blood sugar.
- Dates - high in polyphenols, fiber, protein, B6, iron, and potassium.
- Coconut - may boost fat-burning and provide quick energy.
- Cacao nibs - high in antioxidants, fiber, magnesium and iron; supports mood.
- Goldenberries - high in antioxidants; supports immunity.
- Bing cherries - high in antioxidants; supports cardiovascular and blood pressure.
- Wolfberries - high in antioxidants, vitamins and minerals; beneficial for eye, brain, skin and heart health; may assist with healthy blood sugar and cholesterol levels.
- Quinoa crisps - high in amino acids, fiber, Bs, calcium, iron, magnesium and phosphorus.
- Chia seeds - high in antioxidants, fiber, protein, iron, calcium and omega-3 fatty acids.
- Potato skin extract - natural antioxidant; increases the duration of satiety.
- Sea salt - trace minerals; supports cardiovascular and electrolyte balance.
- Vanilla oil - high in antioxidants; curbs cravings.
- Sunflower lecithin - an emulsifier that supports brain, skin and digestive health.
- Orange peel oil - supports circulation, immune function, skin, and moods.
- Cinnamon Bark oil - high in antioxidants; supports circulatory and immune systems.

COMMENTS FROM YOUNG LIVING®

"Members have always enjoyed Slique® Bars as a safe, delicious weight-management tool that utilizes a dual-target approach to help manage satiety. Now this innovative bar is coated in delicious dark chocolate! To support any weight-management plan, Slique® Bars are loaded with exotic baru nuts and wholesome almonds, which promote satiety when combined with protein and fiber. We also use a potato skin extract that, when ingested, triggers the release of cholecystokinin in the body, increasing the duration of feelings of fullness."

DIRECTIONS FOR USE

Consume before or between meals with 12 oz. of water to help control hunger.

The statements about the supplement and the ingredients have not been evaluated by the Food and Drug Administration. Young Living® products are not intended to diagnose, treat, cure, or prevent any disease.

SLIQUE® CITRASLIM™

WEIGHTLOSS

DUAL TIMING   NOT VEGAN   CONTAINS BEEF GELATIN   CONTAINS COCONUT   MINIMUM AGE 14+   CAUTION IF PREGNANT

Slique® CitraSlim™ is a great way to help support your metabolism and healthy weight. The ingredients help break down excess fat and help support a healthy appetite. This is recommended when using the full Slique® protocol or it may be used by itself for healthy weight maintenance.

INGREDIENTS

1 Liquid Capsule Ingredients
Proprietary Liquid Blend – 460 mg

USE BEFORE BREAKFAST   CONTAINS ALL OILS   NOT VEGAN   CONTAINS BEEF GELATIN

- Lemongrass (*Cymbopogon flexuosus*) leaf oil
- Caprylic/capric glycerides
- Pomegranate (*Punica granatum*) seed oil
- Lemon myrtle (*Backhousia citriodora*) leaf oil
- Idaho Balsam Fir (*Abies balsamea*) branch/leaf oil

Other Ingredients - Silicon dioxide, Gelatin (from bovine), Water
Contains nut (coconut)

3 Powder Capsule Ingredients
Proprietary Powder Blend – 2088 mg

USE BEFORE 3PM   CONTAINS CAFFEINE

- Cassia (*Cinnamomum cassia*) dried bark powder
- Citrus based fruit blend - Orange (*Citrus sinesis*) whole fruit extract, Grapefruit (*Citrus Paradisi*) whole fruit extract, Guarana (*Paulinia cupana*) whole fruit extract
- Pterostilbene
- Bitter Orange (*Citrus aurantium*) unripened fruit extract
- Ocotea (*Ocotea quixos*) leaf powder
- Fenugreek (*Trigonella foenum-graecum*) seed extract
- Digestive Enzymes - Amylase, Cellulase, Lipase, Protease
- Spearmint (*Mentha spicata*) leaf oil
- Ocotea (*Ocotea quixos*) leaf oil
- Cassia (*Cinnamomum aromaticum*) leaf oil
- Fennel (*Foeniculum vulgare*) seed oil

Other Ingredients - Hypromellose, Rice Flour, Silicon dioxide.

WHAT THE INGREDIENTS DO

Liquid Capsule Ingredients
- Lemongrass leaf oil - supports immune function and digestion.
- Caprylic/capric glycerides - from Coconut oil as a carrier base.
- Pomegranate seed oil - supports immune and circulatory systems, as well as blood pressure.
- Lemon Myrtle leaf oil - supports immune function and digestion.
- Idaho Balsam Fir branch/leaf oil - soothes muscles and supports respiratory function.

3 Powder Capsule Ingredients
- Cassia dried bark powder - helps support metabolism and immune function.
- Orange whole fruit extract - helps metabolize fat, supports immune and circulatory systems.
- Grapefruit whole fruit extract - helps metabolize fat cells.
- Guarana whole fruit extract - helps boost energy.
- Pterostilbene - supports healthy weight.
- Bitter orange unripened fruit extract - helps metabolize fat cells.
- Ocotea leaf powder - helps reduce blood sugars and supports sugar cravings.
- Fenugreek seed extract - supports digestion and improves exercise performance.

Continued on next page.

WHAT THE INGREDIENTS DO (continued)
3 Powder Capsule Ingredients (continued)

Digestive Enzymes
- Amylase - breaks down starch.
- Cellulase - breaks down cellulose (plant fiber).
- Lipase - breaks down dietary fats and oils, helps liver function.
- Protease - digests proteins and helps carry away toxins.

Essential Oils
- Spearmint leaf oil - soothes digestion and promotes energy.
- Ocotea leaf oil - stimulates and optimizes digestion, helps lower blood sugar level, benefits cardiovascular health and promotes blood flow in the arteries and blood vessels, helps curb cravings and promote feelings of fullness, and stimulates the body to remove toxins through the liver.
- Cassia leaf oil - assists with nervous, digestive, circulatory and immune system health, and may assist with blood sugar balance.
- Fennel seed oil - supports digestion, metabolism, and fights free radical damage.

Other Ingredients - Hypromellose, Rice Flour, Silicon dioxide - anti-caking ingredient.

COMMENTS FROM YOUNG LIVING®
"Slique® CitraSlim™ is formulated with naturally derived ingredients to promote healthy weight management when combined with a balanced diet and regular exercise. Slique® CitraSlim™ also includes a proprietary citrus extract blend, which some studies suggest may help support the body in burning excess fat when used in conjunction with a healthy weight-management plan. This polyphenolic mixture of flavonoids offers powerful antioxidants that are touted for their health benefits. This blend may also support the release of free fatty acids, which help break down fat."

Once-Daily Liquid Capsule - The liquid capsule delivers pomegranate seed oil, Lemongrass, Lemon Myrtle, and Idaho Balsam Fir Essential Oils. This blend is high in citral, which is a constituent that may increase metabolic activity.

Powder Capsules - Three power-packed powder capsules contain a proprietary citrus extract blend, cinnamon powder, bitter orange extract, fenugreek seed, ocotea leaf extract, and a customized blend of enzymes and four Essential Oils - Ocotea, Cassia, Spearmint, and Fennel.

DIRECTIONS FOR USE
Consume 2 powder capsules in the morning with 8 oz. of water. Consume 1 powder and 1 liquid capsule with 8 oz. of water in the afternoon, before 3 p.m. If you miss taking your capsules in the morning, you may take all 4 capsules together in the afternoon, before 3 p.m.

Note: Fenugreek, natural stimulants and excessive internal use of essential oils while pregnant is not advised.

SLIQUE® CITRASLIM™

SLIQUE® ESSENCE ESSENTIAL OIL

WEIGHTLOSS • HYDRATION

USE ANYTIME — CONTAINS ALL OILS — VEGAN — CONTAINS STEVIA — MINIMUM AGE 6+

Slique® Essence essential oil blend is the perfect addition to your healthy weight loss goals. A few drops per day is all that is needed. Simply add 1-2 drops to a glass or stainless steel water bottle and fill with cold water. Sip throughout the day to get the cleansing benefits of this blend. Slique® Essence adds a refreshing citrus flavor to your water, which helps you drink more water without all the added sugar and chemicals found in store brand flavored waters.

INGREDIENTS

- Grapefruit (*Citrus paradisi*) rind oil
- Tangerine (*Citrus reticulata*) rind oil
- Spearmint (*Mentha spicata*) leaf oil
- Lemon (*Citrus limon*) rind oil
- Ocotea (*Ocotea quixos*) leaf oil
- Stevia (*Stevia Rebaudiana*) leaf extract

WHAT THE INGREDIENTS DO

- Grapefruit rind oil - boosts metabolism, stimulates the lymphatic system, supports detoxification and digestion, helps reduce sugar cravings, balances blood sugar levels, and reduces your appetite.
- Tangerine rind oil - relaxes nerves and muscles, and reduces tension, helps the body remove toxins, supports the digestive system and speeds up the metabolism.
- Spearmint leaf oil - relieves gas and indigestion and improves digestion.
- Lemon rind oil - improves digestion, supports metabolism, and cleanses the lymphatic glands. Stimulates lymphatic drainage for toxin removal. Promotes detoxification through the blood and liver. Helps support the immune system.
- Ocotea leaf oil - stimulates and optimizes digestion, helps lower blood sugar levels, supports cardiovascular health, and promotes blood flow in the arteries and blood vessels. Helps promote feelings of fullness and helps curb sugar cravings.
- Stevia leaf extract - provides sweetness with zero calories.

COMMENTS FROM YOUNG LIVING®

"Slique® Essence combines Grapefruit, Tangerine, Lemon, Spearmint, and Ocotea with stevia extract in a unique blend that supports healthy weight management goals. These ingredients work together to help control hunger, especially when used in conjunction with Slique® Tea or the Slique® Kit. The pleasant citrus combination of Grapefruit, Tangerine, and Lemon essential oils adds a flavorful and uplifting element to any day with the added support of Spearmint that may help with digestion. Ocotea essential oil adds an irresistible, cinnamon-like aroma to help control hunger, while stevia adds an all-natural sweetener that provides a pleasant taste with no added calories."

DIRECTIONS FOR USE

Shake vigorously before use. Add 2-4 drops to 4-6 oz. of your favorite beverage, Slique® Tea, or water. Use between and during meals regularly throughout the day whenever hunger feelings occur.

Note: Stevia extract in this formula may impede diffuser performance, not recommended to use in a diffuser.

SLIQUE® ESSENCE

SLIQUE® GUM
WEIGHTLOSS

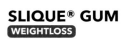

USE BETWEEN MEALS | VEGAN | CONTAINS XYLITOL | CONTAINS SOY | CONTAINS CORN | MINIMUM AGE 12+ | DO NOT FEED TO DOGS

Slique® Gum is not your traditional gum. Take a step back to ancient times when people would chew on gum resins to help clean their teeth and gums and also curb their appetite. The gum tablet starts off as a slight powder and transforms in your mouth to a short-term chewing gum to help keep your cravings at bay. Chew one tablet in the afternoon when your cravings are at their highest. Drink lots of water or have a glass of Slique® Tea to support afternoon cravings as well.

INGREDIENTS
- Isomalt
- Frankincense gum resin (*Boswellia frereana*)
- Gum base
- Sorbitol
- Natural flavors
- Calcium stearate
- Natural green color (Red cabbage juice, Turmeric, Soy protein isolates)
- Stevia (*Stevia rebaudiana*) leaf extract
- Monk fruit
- Xylitol

Fresh Mint Essential Oil Blend
- Peppermint (*Mentha piperita*) oil
- Spearmint (*Mentha spicata*) leaf oil

Allergens - Contains traces of soy. No artificial colors or flavors.

WHAT THE INGREDIENTS DO
- Isomalt - naturally sourced sugar-free sugar replacement made from beet sugar.
- Frankincense gum resin - strengthens teeth and gums and is beneficial to oral health.
- Gum base - proprietary industry formula made from several food-grade raw materials.
- Sorbitol - low calorie fruit-derived sugar.
- Natural flavors - to enhance experience.
- Calcium stearate - calcium combined with vegetable oil used to thicken and stabilize.
- Natural green color - for color.
- Stevia - no calorie natural sweetener.
- Monk fruit - sugar free natural sweetener
- Xylitol - naturally occurring plant-based sugar alcohol (not for dogs).

Slimming Fresh Mint Essential Oil Blend
- Peppermint leaf oil - supports digestive health, stimulates brain function, immune boosting benefits, promotes energy and focus and uplifts emotions.
- Spearmint leaf oil - soothes digestion, promotes energy and is emotionally uplifting.

COMMENTS FROM YOUNG LIVING®
"Ancient travelers throughout the Middle East used raw frankincense resin for its nutritional content and ability to help control hunger. Slique® Gum offers those same benefits in a modern delivery system that helps control food cravings and improve oral health."

DIRECTIONS FOR USE
Chewing 1 gum tablet before or after meals or as desired may help control cravings. CAUTION: Keep away from dogs due to xylitol.

The statements about the supplement and the ingredients have not been evaluated by the Food and Drug Administration. Young Living® products are not intended to diagnose, treat, cure, or prevent any disease.

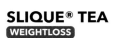

SLIQUE® TEA
WEIGHTLOSS

USE BEFORE 3PM

VEGAN

CONTAINS STEVIA

CONTAINS CAFFEINE

MINIMUM AGE 12+

Slique® Tea - Ocotea Oolong Cacao is a delightful tasting tea served warm or cold. It supports healthy weight loss and emotions by combining natural metabolism supporting Jade oolong and mood enhancing Ecuadorian cacao powder. One tea bag goes a long way! You can use it to make 2-4 total cups of tea. Simply boil 2-4 cups of water, and use one tea bag. For stronger tea, use 1-2 cups of water and for lighter tea use 3-4 cups of water. This tea makes a great sun tea too! Fill a pitcher of filtered water with two Slique® Tea bags in the pitcher. Cover and let sit in the sun for several hours. Refrigerate and serve chilled over ice. Another fun way to use Slique® Tea is with one of Young Living's® shake mixes. Use Slique® Tea chilled as the liquid for any shake mix such as Slique® Shake, Pure Protein™ Complete, or Balance Complete™. Add a few drops of your favorite Vitality™ essential oils and an ounce or two of NingXia Red®. For an added boost, add a NingXia Nitro® tube.

INGREDIENTS
- Jade oolong (*Camellia sinensis*) tea
- Inulin (from chicory root fiber)
- Ocotea (*Ocotea quixos*) leaf
- Cacao powder
- Vanilla (*Vanilla planifolia*) fruit extract
- Sacred Frankincense (*Boswellia sacra*) resin powder
- Stevia (*Stevia rebaudiana*) leaf extract

WHAT THE INGREDIENTS DO
- Jade oolong tea - supports metabolism, heart health, brain function, and sugar levels.
- Inulin - prebiotic to support the gut. Decreases the body's ability to produce some fats.
- Ocotea leaf - helps balance blood sugar levels.
- Cacao powder - enhances mood by increasing endorphin and serotonin levels.
- Vanilla fruit extract - this is not the essential oil. Used as flavoring.
- Sacred Frankincense powder - supports immune function and cell protection.
- Stevia extract - natural sweetener.

COMMENTS FROM YOUNG LIVING®
"Slique® Tea is an exotic drink from Young Living® that has been formulated with natural ingredients to help support individual weight goals. This blend is rich in flavonoids, a dietary compound generally associated with helping maintain certain normal, healthy body functions. It also contains polyphenols, which may be useful as part of a guilt-free weight-management regimen when combined with a healthy diet and physical activity. This unique blend is enhanced with Seed to Seal® Premium Frankincense powder."

DIRECTIONS FOR USE
Bring 8 oz. of water to a rolling boil, let cool for 3 ½ minutes. Place one pouch in a cup, mug, or filter and add water. Steep for at least three minutes. Add your favorite Young Living® Vitality™ essential oils as desired. Use daily before and after workouts, with meals, or any time you need a natural boost. Contains naturally occurring caffeine and tea antioxidants. If you are pregnant, nursing, taking medication, or have a medical condition, consult a health professional prior to use. Not recommended for children.

SLIQUE® TEA

SULFURZYME®
(Capsules & Powder)
MOBILITY • DETOX • LIVER
SKIN • HAIR • NAILS

USE ANYTIME | BEST BETWEEN MEALS | CONTAINS NO OILS | VEGAN | MINIMUM AGE 12+ | ¼-½ DOSAGE IF UNDER 12

Sulfurzyme® is an MSM (organic sulfur) supplement that helps cells to regenerate themselves cleaner and stronger for better mobility, healthier hair, smoother skin, stronger nails. It also helps support a more stable immune system and circulatory system, and supports the liver to cleanse and filter the blood. You get all of these benefits plus more with adding organic natural sulfur amino acids to your diet.

Sulfur is responsible for vital amino acids in our body that support healthy cells, skin, hormones, and enzymes. Sulfur is naturally found in all plant and animal cells. Sulfur amino acids help our body produce glutathione. Glutathione increases energy, improves mental clarity and focus, helps support proper immune function, improves the quality of sleep, supports athletic recovery, slows down the aging process, detoxifies the cells and liver, increases keratin production in skin, hair, and nails, plus more!

Many people claim they have a sulfur allergy. This is incorrect. People cannot be allergic to sulfur as that would be like saying you are allergic to water. Sulfa is commonly mixed up with sulfur and also doctors may refer to "sulfur allergies", but they mean specifically the pharmaceutical called sulfonamide. In an article by William B. Smith and Constance H. Katelaris of the Australian Prescriber entitled "'Sulfur allergy' label is misleading" they state, "Many patients believe that having been labelled 'sulfur allergic' they are also at risk of adverse reactions or allergies from sulfites, sulfates and even elemental sulfur and may attempt to avoid them... Patients who have had allergic reactions to sulfonamide drugs do not need to avoid sulfites, sulfates or sulfur."

Sulfurzyme® powder contains a natural organic form of dietary sulfur. The wolfberries in Sulfurzyme® have a dual action to help allow the MSM to be more bioavailable by allowing it to be more readily assimilated and metabolized by the body. Wolfberries are also an excellent source of prebiotics. Both the powder and the capsules contain prebiotics, but the powder contains even more in the form of fructooligosaccharides.

RECIPES

The NingXia Daily Boost - Try adding ½ tsp. to one full tsp. of Sulfurzyme® powder to 2 oz. of NingXia Red® and one tube of NingXia Nitro® in the morning for 30 days instead of your morning coffee and you'll feel a big difference.

The Red Drink by Dr. Peter Minke - 2 oz. NingXia Red®, ½ tsp. Sulfurzyme®, 16-32 oz. of water, and 3 drops of Lime Vitality™.

NOTE ON ALLERGIES If you are allergic to sulfa, you won't be allergic to sulfur. Your body naturally produces sulfur, so rest assured, using a supplemental form of organic dietary MSM (Methylsulfonylmethane) such as Sulfurzyme®, is a great way to support your overall health.

SULFURZYME® CAPSULES

USE ANYTIME | BEST BETWEEN MEALS | CONTAINS NO OILS | VEGAN | MINIMUM AGE 12+ | ¼-½ DOSAGE IF UNDER 12

INGREDIENTS

Proprietary Sulfurzyme® Blend – 1.8 g
- MSM - Methylsulfonylmethane (an organic form of dietary sulfur)
- Ningxia Wolfberry (Lycium barbarum) fruit (prebiotic)

WHAT THE INGREDIENTS DO
- MSM - replenishes and protects the connection between cells for healthy joint function. Increases glutathione levels, helps speed up post-exercise recovery, improves flexibility, strengthens hair and nails, improves complexion and skin, helps detox the body.
- Ningxia Wolfberry Fruit - prebiotic that supports gut health; a natural polysaccharide that supports the immune system, as well as healthy regeneration of tissues and cells.

Other Ingredients - Hypromellose, Rice Flour, Magnesium stearate, Silica (capsule and substrate).

SULFURZYME® POWDER

USE ANYTIME | BEST BETWEEN MEALS | CONTAINS NO OILS | VEGAN | CONTAINS STEVIA | MINIMUM AGE 12+ | ¼-½ DOSAGE IF UNDER 12

INGREDIENTS

Proprietary Sulfurzyme® Powder Blend – 1.95 g
- MSM - Methylsulfonylmethane (an organic form of dietary sulfur)
- FOS Fructooligosaccharides prebiotic
- Ningxia Wolfberry (*Lycium barbarum*) fruit powder (prebiotic)

Other Ingredients - Stevia (*Stevia rebaudiana*) leaf extract

WHAT THE INGREDIENTS DO
- MSM - replenishes and protects the connection between cells for healthy joint function. Increases glutathione levels, helps speed up post-exercise recovery, improves flexibility, strengthens hair and nails, improves complexion and skin, helps detox the body.
- Ningxia Wolfberry Fruit - prebiotic that supports gut health; a natural polysaccharide that supports the immune system, as well as healthy regeneration of tissues and cells.
- FOS - prebiotic that feeds the good flora in your gut.

Other Ingredients
- Stevia leaf extract - natural sweetener.
- Calcium silicate - anti-caking agent.

COMMENTS FROM YOUNG LIVING®
"Sulfurzyme® combines wolfberry with MSM, a naturally occurring organic form of dietary sulfur needed by our bodies every day to maintain the structure of proteins, protect cells and cell membranes, replenish the connections between cells, and preserve the molecular framework of connective tissue. MSM also supports the immune system, the liver, circulation, and proper intestinal function and works to scavenge free radicals. Wolfberries contain minerals and coenzymes that support the assimilation and metabolism of sulfur. FOS is added to this formula to support normal digestive system health."

DIRECTIONS FOR USE
Capsules: Take 2 capsules two times daily or as needed.
Powder: Mix ½ tsp. with 4-8 oz. of juice or distilled water and take twice daily, one hour before or after meals.

SULFURZYME®

SUPER B™

USE BEFORE BREAKFAST   USE BEFORE 3PM   VEGAN   MINIMUM AGE 12+   ¼-½ DOSAGE IF UNDER 12

Young Living's® Super B™ contains all eight B vitamins - B1, B2, B3, B5, B6, B7, B9, and B12. That is why it is called SUPER B™! B vitamins help keep our cells metabolizing correctly. They have a whole host of benefits. Read below on each B Vitamin and their benefits. Super B™ is infused with Nutmeg essential oil which is known for its energy enhancing qualities.

INGREDIENTS
- B1 (Thiamin HCl) - 25 mg (2083% DV)
- B2 (Riboflavin) - 25 mg (1923% DV)
- B3 (Niacin as Nicotinic acid and Niacinamide) - 35 mg (219% DV)
- B5 (Pantothenic acid as D-calcium pantothenate) - 15 mg (300% DV)
- B6 (Pyridoxine HCl) - 25 mg (1471% DV)
- B7 (Biotin aka Vitamin H) - 150 mcg (500% DV)
- B9 (Folate) - 667 mcg DFE (400 mcg Folic Acid from nature - not synthetic) (167% DV)
- B12 (Methylcobalamin) - 100 mcg (4157% DV)
- Calcium (dicalcium phosphate) - 143 mg (11% DV)
- Magnesium (Magnesium bisglycinate chelate) - 10 mg (2% DV)
- Zinc (Zinc bisglycinate chelate) - 3 mg (27% DV)
- Selenium (Selenium glycinate complex) - 50 mcg (91% DV)
- Manganese (Manganese bisglycinate chelate) - 0.65 mg (28% DV)

Proprietary Super B™ Blend – 30 mg
- PABA (Para amino benzoic acid), Nutmeg (*Myristica fragrans*) seed oil

Other Ingredients
- Cellulose, Stearic acid, Modified Cellulose, Diglycerides, Silicon Dioxide

WHAT THE INGREDIENTS DO
- B1 (Thiamine) - supports a healthy nervous system and helps improve cardiovascular function. It helps to break down fats and proteins. B1 helps convert carbohydrates into glucose to help give energy to the body to perform various functions. It also helps the body withstand stress and maintain a healthy metabolism.
- B2 (Riboflavin) - helps the body break down proteins, fats, and carbohydrates to produce energy. It is a powerful anti-inflammatory that is known to support brain, bone, and eye health. It also supports the liver, blood pressure, and the cardiovascular system. B2 may also support positive moods. It may support the relief of nighttime leg cramps in the elderly as well as healthier pregnancies.
- B3 (Niacin) - is known to help lower cholesterol, increase brain function, support mood swings, help with skin issues, support mental clarity and memory, as well as ease arthritis symptoms. It is important not to take too much Niacin as you can experience what is known as a Niacin flush. Overdosing (250 milligrams or more) on Niacin is uncomfortable but will not harm you. The amount in Super B™ is a good adult amount for daily supplementation.
- B5 (Pantothenic acid) - helps support a healthy metabolism and other bodily functions. It helps convert the food you eat into energy. It works as an anti-inflammatory and supports the immune, nervous, and gastrointestinal systems. B5 is also known to help balance cholesterol levels and reduce stress.
- B6 (Pyridoxine) - supports healthy emotions. It works in the brain to provide healthier cognition. It has been studied to reduce heart disease risk, help aid in hemoglobin production, and support PMS symptoms. It is also used to reduce nausea during pregnancy. B6 supports the digestive tract, heart health, and muscle function.

SUPER B™

WHAT THE INGREDIENTS DO (continued)

- B7 (Biotin or Vitamin H) - helps convert fat, protein, and carbohydrates into energy. This vitamin is important to use if you are pregnant or breastfeeding. It has been touted as a supplement to support healthy hair, skin, and nails.
- B9 (Folate/Natural Folic Acid) - needed for your body to make DNA. Having enough folate may prevent iron deficiency. It helps promote hair, skin and nail health through cell regeneration. Folate is an important supplement for pregnant women to help prevent certain birth defects. It is also noted that folate supports your mood by transforming amino acids from your food into neurotransmitters such as serotonin and dopamine.

  NOTE from YL: "Orgen- FA® is the best source for natural folate we have found in the industry. There is a misconception that folic acid can only be synthetic, but it is simply a term for hydrolyzed (water added to) folates. Orgen-FA® is 100% USDA Certified Organic and it does NOT contain any sort of synthetic folic acid or additives. (It would not be 100% USDA Certified Organic if it did.) It is extracted using hot water and is no different than the folic acid you would get when boiling broccoli. This ingredient is standardized to 5% natural folic acid and the remaining 95% material is naturally occurring co-factors and co-nutrients from organic lemon peel."

- B12 (Methylcobalamin) - plays an important role in helping you make red blood cells. It is known as the "painkilling vitamin". It supports brain health, eye health, skin health, DNA production, cardiovascular support, and converts the food you eat into energy. It also supports improved sleep-wake patterns as well as healthy emotions. There are several forms of B12 and methylcobalamin is the most bioavailable of all forms of B12.
- Calcium - helps prevent bone loss and repairs joints.
- Magnesium - aids in normal function of the cells, nerves, muscles, bones, and heart.
- Zinc - highly absorbable form of zinc. Supports immune function.
- Selenium - is a powerful antioxidant that defends against free radicals in the body.
- Manganese - supports metabolism, blood sugar, and lessens PMS cramps.

Proprietary Super B™ Blend

- PABA - supports skin elasticity and joints; combats hair loss.
- Nutmeg seed oil - supports lymphatic, digestive, and immune health; promotes energy.

Other Ingredients

- Cellulose, Stearic acid, Modified Cellulose, Diglycerides, Silicon Dioxide - tablet base.

SUPER B™

COMMENTS FROM YOUNG LIVING®

"Super B™ is a comprehensive vitamin complex containing all eight essential, energy-boosting B vitamins (B1, B2, B3, B5, B6, B7, B9, and B12). Recently reformulated, it now features Orgen-FA®, a natural folate source derived from lemon peels, and methylcobalamin, a more bioavailable source of B12. Combined with Nutmeg essential oil and bioavailable chelated minerals such as magnesium, manganese, selenium, and zinc, Super B™ not only assists in maintaining healthy energy levels, but it also supports mood and cardiovascular and cognitive function. B vitamins are essential to our health and well-being, and each B vitamin performs a unique and separate function in the body. Unfortunately, they must be replenished daily, as they are not stored in the body."

DIRECTIONS FOR USE

Take two tablets daily.

Customer notes: Split the dose by taking one tablet in the morning and one tablet at lunch. Super B™ is water soluble so it is not necessary to take with food. It is not recommended to take in the evening as this may cause insomnia or restlessness. If it upsets your stomach you may take it with a little food or try taking half a tablet.

Note: This supplement will turn your urine bright yellow. This is normal.

The statements about the supplement and the ingredients have not been evaluated by the Food and Drug Administration. Young Living® products are not intended to diagnose, treat, cure, or prevent any disease.

SUPER C™ *(Chewables & Tablets)*

Vitamin C is something we need daily, as our bodies do not produce it on its own. The benefits of vitamin C are varied, but most of us consider it a wonderful way to strengthen our immune system. Vitamin C has also been touted as a way to support the cardiovascular system, help with prenatal care, support healthy eye function, and skin smoothing! Yes, our favorite vitamin C can help you look younger. When you use isolated vitamin C you are only getting a small amount of its intended benefits. Vitamin C works best when it is consumed as the whole fruit. Fruit purchased at the grocery store is depleted of vital nutrients as they were often picked two weeks prior to you receiving them. Vine-ripening is the best form of whole-fruit nutrition, but if you do not live on or near a farm that allows you to pick ripe fruit and eat it the same day, then you are eating vitamin depleted fruit.

Bioflavonoids are a key part of the whole fruit. They help enhance vitamin C action and are known to support blood circulation and help decrease free-radical damage in the body. Because they are so good at placating oxidative stress, they are able to help support inflammatory conditions in the body. Super C™ from Young Living® allows you to get all the benefits of vine-ripened fruit with all the beautiful bioflavonoids without traveling to a farm or becoming an orchard owner of five varieties of citrus. While some of you have access to these, the majority of us do not. There are two Super C™ products from which to choose in the Young Living® supplement line; tablets and chewables. They are a bit different, so take a look at both to determine your needs.

SUPER C™ CHEWABLES

`IMMUNE SUPPORT`

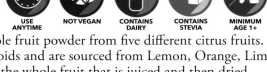

| USE ANYTIME | NOT VEGAN | CONTAINS DAIRY | CONTAINS STEVIA | MINIMUM AGE 1+ |

Super C™ Chewables contain whole fruit powder from five different citrus fruits. These contain powerful bioflavonoids and are sourced from Lemon, Orange, Lime, Tangerine, and Grapefruit. Using the whole fruit that is juiced and then dried to form a powder ensures you get the full botanical synergy of the vitamins. The chewables also contain Acerola fruit extract, Camu camu whole fruit powder, Rose hips fruit powder and Orange peel oil powder. This vitamin C supplement is a powerful way to support your health!

INGREDIENTS
- Calories - 5
- Carbohydrates (Sugars) - 1 g
- Vitamin C (as ascorbic acid) - 150 mg (167% DV)

Proprietary Super C™ Blend – 455 mg
- Acerola (*Malpighia glabra*) fruit extract
- Camu camu (*Myrciaria dubia*) whole fruit powder
- Rose hips (*Rosa canina*) fruit powder

These statements have not been evaluated by the Food and Drug Administration. Young Living® products are not intended to diagnose, treat, cure, or prevent any disease.

INGREDIENTS (continued)

Citrus Bioflavonoids
- Lemon (*Citrus limon*) whole fruit powder
- Orange (*Citrus sinensis*) whole fruit powder
- Lime (*Citrus Aurantifolia*) whole fruit powder
- Tangerine (*Citrus reticulata*) whole fruit powder
- Grapefruit (*Citrus paradisi*) whole fruit powder
- Orange (*Citrus sinesis*) peel oil powder

Other Ingredients - Non-GMO Tapioca dextrose, Sorbitol, Calcium ascorbate, Organic Stevia Blend (Organic Agave Inulin, Stevia [*Stevia rebaudiana*] leaf extract, Natural flavor), Hydroxypropyl cellulose, Stearic acid, Silicon dioxide, Magnesium stearate
Note: Contains milk or milk derivatives.

WHAT THE INGREDIENTS DO

- Ascorbic Acid (Vitamin C) - acts as an antioxidant, protecting cells from free radicals.
- Acerola fruit extract - an antioxidant nutrient, rich in vitamin C.
- Camu camu whole fruit powder - contains powerful antioxidants, including anthocyanins and ellagic acid, is high in vitamin C and helps ease inflammation.
- Rose hips fruit powder - contains antioxidants, protects immune cells from oxidative stress, and encourages white blood cell production.
- Orange peel oil powder - contains limonene, which is a monocyclic, monoterpene that defends against oxidative stress that can negatively affect the immune system.

Citrus Bioflavonoids - support the immune system and enhance the action of vitamin C, promote healthy blood circulation and work to reduce inflammation in the body.
- Orange whole fruit powder - a concentrated source of vitamin C, which doubles as a powerful antioxidant and plays a central role in immune function.
- Lime whole fruit powder - boosts iron absorption, supports blood sugar and cholesterol.
- Tangerine whole fruit powder - contains beneficial compounds with anti-inflammatory properties, aiding in the digestion of fatty foods.
- Grapefruit whole fruit powder - is rich in nutrients, antioxidants and fiber. It provides vitamins A and C, folate (B9), choline, limonins and lycopene.

Other Ingredients
- Non-GMO Tapioca dextrose - simple, easily digested sugar.
- Sorbitol - low calorie fruit-derived sugar.
- Calcium ascorbate - easily digested form of vitamin C.
- Organic Stevia Blend - no-calorie sweetener.
- Hydroxypropyl cellulose - tablet binder.
- Stearic acid - ingredient binder.
- Silicon dioxide - natural anti-caking agent.
- Magnesium stearate - helps lubricate the tablets.

COMMENTS FROM YOUNG LIVING®

"Super C™ combines pure Orange essential oil with a proprietary blend of camu camu, acerola, cherry, and rose hips fruit powder to create a powerful immune-supporting supplement. Together, these premium ingredients deliver desirable polyphenols, carotenoids, and optimal amounts of vitamin C in a convenient chewable tablet."

DIRECTIONS FOR USE

Take 1 chewable tablet three times daily or as needed.

The statements about the supplement and the ingredients have not been evaluated by the Food and Drug Administration. Young Living® products are not intended to diagnose, treat, cure, or prevent any disease.

SUPER C™

SUPER C™ TABLETS

IMMUNE SUPPORT

USE ANYTIME | BEST WITH FOOD | VEGAN | MINIMUM AGE 12+

Super C™ Tablets is a buffered C that differs from the Chewables in that they contain Rutin flower bud powder, Cayenne fruit powder, Orange peel oil, Tangerine rind oil, Grapefruit peel oil, Lemon peel oil, and Lemongrass leaf oil. The tablets do not contain the whole-fruit powders of Orange, Lime, Tangerine, Grapefruit, and Camu camu that are found in the chewables. Instead, it contains the essential oils that allow for better bioavailability of the ingredients and the added benefits of dicalcium phosphate, zinc, manganese, and potassium.

INGREDIENTS

- Calories - 10
- Carbohydrates - 2 g
- Vitamin C (Ascorbic acid) - 1300 mg (1440% DV)
- Calcium (Calcium carbonate and Dicalcium phosphate) - 160 mg (12% DV)
- Zinc (Zinc gluconate) - 1.5 mg (14% DV)
- Manganese (Manganese sulfate) - 2.1 mg (91% DV)

Proprietary Super C™ Blend – 78 mg
- Citrus bioflavonoids, Rutin (*Sophora japonica L*) flower bud powder, Cayenne (*Capsicum annuum*) fruit powder, Orange (*Citrus sinensis*) peel oil, Tangerine (*Citrus reticulata*) rind oil, Grapefruit (*Citrus paradisi*) peel oil, Lemon (*Citrus limon*) peel oil, Lemongrass (*Cymbopogon flexuosus*) leaf oil

Other Ingredients - Cellulose, Stearic acid, Potassium (Potassium chloride), Silicon dioxide, Modified cellulose, Magnesium stearate

WHAT THE INGREDIENTS DO

- Ascorbic Acid (Vitamin C) - acts as an antioxidant, protecting cells from free radicals.
- Calcium - supports bone health, muscle contractions, and weight maintenance.
- Zinc - promotes a healthy immune system. Aids in healing of wounds.
- Manganese - supports nutrient absorption and bone health.

Proprietary Super C™ Blend
- Citrus bioflavonoids - help maximize the benefits of vitamin C.
- Rutin flower bud powder - antioxidant; supports circulation and blood vessels.
- Cayenne fruit powder - supports circulation, metabolism, and digestion.
- Orange peel oil - supports immune system, improves blood flow, and anti-inflammatory.
- Tangerine rind oil - supports immune system.
- Grapefruit peel oil - supports fat burning and sugar cravings.
- Lemon peel oil - cleanses toxins from body and stimulates lymphatic drain.
- Lemongrass leaf oil - supports immune and circulatory systems.

Other Ingredients - Cellulose, Stearic acid, Potassium (Potassium chloride), Silicon dioxide, Modified cellulose, Magnesium stearate - tablet substrate

COMMENTS FROM YOUNG LIVING®

"Super C™ not only contains 1440% of the recommended dietary intake of vitamin C per serving, but it is also fortified with rutin, citrus bioflavonoids, and minerals to balance electrolytes and enhance the effectiveness and absorption of vitamin C. The essential oils that are added may also increase bioflavonoid activity."

DIRECTIONS FOR USE

For reinforcing immune strength, take 2 tablets daily. For maintenance, take 1 tablet daily. Best if taken with meals for those with sensitive stomachs.

SUPER C™ TABLETS

SUPER CAL™ PLUS
BONE AND IMMUNE HEALTH

BEST WITH FOOD · VEGAN · CONTAINS CORN · MINIMUM AGE 12+ · ½ DOSAGE IF UNDER 12

Start your morning off with supporting those bones! Eat a little something with these because it needs some fat to get into your system. Even just a handful of nuts is good. This is not your mother's calcium supplement. Oh no! It is far better and so much more bioavailable. You will absolutely love Super Cal™ Plus. It should be part of your daily regimen because the calcium is sourced from bioavailable red algae.

INGREDIENTS
- Vitamin D (D3 as cholecalciferol) - 10 mcg (50% DV)
- Vitamin K (K2 as menquinone-7) - 30 mcg (25% DV)
- Calcium (from Red Algae) - 260 mg (20% DV)
- Magnesium (as magnesium citrate) - 119 mg (30% DV)

Super Cal™ Plus Dual Action Blend – 1134 mg
- Marine minerals, Fermented polysaccharide complex, L-lysine, L-arginine, Winged treebine (*Cissus quadrangularis*) root extract PE 2.5%, Hops (*Humulus lupulus*) flower extract PE 4 -1, Tea (*Camellia sinensis*) leaf extract

Super Cal™ Plus Essential Oil Blend – 5.5 mg
- Idaho Blue Spruce (*Picea pungens*) wood/branch/leaf oil, Black Spruce (*Picea mariana*) wood/branches/needle oil, Copaiba (oleoresin) (*Copaifera officinalis*) wood oil, Vetiver (*Vetiveria zizanoides*) root oil, Peppermint (*Mentha piperita*) aerial parts oil.

Other Ingredients - Stearic acid, Non-GMO cornstarch, Hypromellose

WHAT THE INGREDIENTS DO
- Vitamin D - supports healthy bones and helps support immune function.
- Vitamin K - helps to push calcium into the bones.
- Calcium - helps prevent bone loss.
- Magnesium - supports the immune system, nerves, heart, eyes, brain, and muscles.

Super Cal™ Plus Dual Action Blend
- Marine minerals - support tissues and bones; help maintain fluid and pH balance.

Fermented Polysaccharide Complex
- L-lysine - converts fatty acids into energy; supports absorption of calcium; supports stress.
- L-arginine - stimulates the release of hormones and insulin, promotes increased blood flow.
- Winged treebine root extract - supports blood and heart health.
- Hops flower extract - helps to maintain a healthy weight by fighting oxidative stress.
- Tea leaf extract - supports blood, skin, liver, and brain health.

Super Cal™ Plus Essential Oil Blend
- Idaho Blue Spruce oil - contains high amounts of alpha-pinene and limonene for bone health.
- Black Spruce oil - alpha-pinene, camphene, and beta-pinene for bone and muscle health.
- Copaiba oil - supports inflammatory response in muscles and joints.
- Vetiver oil - supports joints and skin.
- Peppermint oil - supports bones, muscles, joints, and ligaments.

Other Ingredients - Stearic acid, Non-GMO cornstarch, Hypromellose - capsule base.

COMMENTS FROM YOUNG LIVING®
"Using a marine mineral blend derived from red algae that's harvested off the coast of Iceland, Super Cal™ Plus harnesses the power of naturally derived ingredients to bring you the vital minerals found in the most complete bone-support supplement. This unique seaweed absorbs calcium, magnesium, and other trace minerals from ocean water, bringing them together to support overall bone health, including bone-density support."

DIRECTIONS FOR USE
Take 2 capsules daily with food. It is best to split the dose in two, twice daily.

The statements about the supplement and the ingredients have not been evaluated by the Food and Drug Administration. Young Living® products are not intended to diagnose, treat, cure, or prevent any disease.

SUPER CAL™ PLUS

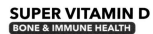

SUPER VITAMIN D
BONE & IMMUNE HEALTH

BEST WITH FOOD

VEGAN

MINIMUM AGE 12+

¼-½ DOSAGE IF UNDER 12

We should get most of our vitamin D from sun exposure. When you expose your skin to the sun, your body is able to create its own vitamin D. Sunscreens and locations with low sun exposure can leave many people vitamin D deficient. According to a Journal of Pharmacology & Pharmacotherapeutics study on vitamin D, almost 50% of the worldwide population is vitamin D deficient. They consider it a pandemic called "hypovitaminosis D" and is mainly the outcome of reduced outdoor lifestyle and activities as well as air pollution that has caused a decline in sunlight exposure.

Another reason people may not be getting enough natural vitamin D is that many people do not understand how to expose their skin properly, without getting burned. To get good sun exposure for optimal vitamin D production, simply expose the lower back, or an area that does not commonly see the sun, for 5-10 minutes per day. Arms and facial skin have built up more pigment on most people, which causes UVB to have a much lower absorption rate.

Vitamin D is vital to support the regulation of calcium and phosphate in the body to support healthy bones, muscles, and teeth. Vitamin D is also important to help boost cellular energy, enhance skin growth and repair, support healthy immune and cardiovascular systems, as well as even help you lose weight and potentially combat symptoms of depression. A 2017 review article of literature on vitamin D was published in the Neuropsychiatry Volume 7, Issue 5 journal that found that there was a great enough relationship between vitamin D deficiency and depression that they recommended getting your vitamin D levels tested if you are experiencing depression.

Most vitamin D supplements on the market today are D3 (cholecalciferol) from lanolin. Lanolin is extracted from sheep wool and is often contaminated with pesticides or other toxins found in the chemicals sheep are often dipped in or sprayed with. Young Living's® Super Vitamin D is naturally sourced from sustainable D3 from lichen which is a plant-like growth native to North America, Scandinavia, and Asia. Lichen is a slow growing combination of algae, fungi, and cyanobacteria that looks like a crusty leaf that grows on rocks, walls, and trees. It is a cross between an algae and a fungus. It absorbs D from the sun as a means to protect itself.

A common question regarding Super Vitamin D is, "Why is there no Vitamin K, Magnesium, or Calcium in this supplement?" Many D supplements combine these for specific bone health. Young Living® wanted to provide a clean Vitamin D. This allows people who are taking other vitamins to make sure their regimen works specifically for their needs. If you need bone support, you can easily combine Super Vitamin D with K, Magnesium, and Calcium, by using CardioGize™ (for K2) and Super Cal™ Plus (for K2, Calcium, and Magnesium).

SUPER VITAMIN D

INGREDIENTS
- Serving Size 2 Tablets (640 mg)
- Vitamin D - 50 mcg / 2,000 IU (250% DV) (1,000 IU per tablet)

Super Vitamin D Blend – 54 mg
- Organic Lemon Balm (*Melissa officinalis*) extract
- Vitamin D3 Lichen extract
- Melissa (*Melissa officinalis*) plant oil
- Lime (*Citrus aurantifolia*) peel oil

Other Ingredients
- Mannitol, Sodium starch glycolate, Natural mixed berry flavor, Citric acid, Hydroxypropyl cellulose, Stevia (*Stevia rebaudiana*) leaf extract, Magnesium stearate

WHAT THE INGREDIENTS DO
Super Vitamin D Blend – 54 mg
- Organic Lemon Balm (*Melissa officinalis*) extract - used to support emotional and mental health. It is also an excellent flavoring.
- Vitamin D3 (cholecalciferol) Lichen extract - a naturally sourced D3 from of sustainable vegan lichen that is more easily absorbed. Supports respiratory and immune system health. Helps to balance calcium for bone growth and healthy muscles.
- Melissa (*Melissa officinalis*) plant oil - known to help reduce stress and regulate hormones through mood balance. It may increase GABA by blocking GABA antagonists. Melissa contains a polyphenol called rosmarinic acid which has a positive effect on cognition and mood balance. It also allows for more bioavailability of other ingredients.
- Lime (*Citrus aurantifolia*) peel oil - adds flavor and bioavailability to the vitamin D. It helps improve fatty liver and helps to decrease the production of bile in the liver when used with D3.

Other Ingredients
- Mannitol - type of sugar alcohol as a sweetener.
- Sodium starch glycolate - natural base; not from gluten.
- Vitamin D3 lichen extract - D3 that is more easily absorbed.
- Natural mixed berry flavor - sourced from nature.
- Citric acid - naturally sourced from citrus fruit and an excellent antioxidant.
- Hydroxypropyl cellulose - naturally derived tablet binder.
- Stevia (*Stevia rebaudiana*) leaf extract - natural sweetener.
- Magnesium stearate - a natural "flow agent" that helps the consistency of the ingredients.

COMMENTS FROM YOUNG LIVING®
"Who doesn't need a super boost of sunshine? With our proprietary formula and delivery system, Young Living's® plant-based Super Vitamin D is highly absorbable, vegan friendly, and completely synthetic free. Dissolvable in a delicious mixed berry-flavored tablet, Super Vitamin D is a super source of vitamin D that helps support bone growth and healthy muscle. Vitamin D plays a key function in respiratory health, and through its innate and adaptive defense mechanisms, it supports the body's respiratory immune system.* This dissolvable tablet is made with lemon balm extract and vitamin D to support mood and hormone regulation."

DIRECTIONS FOR USE
Take 2 tablets daily with food.
Place in mouth and allow to dissolve for 5-10 seconds, then chew for optimal results.
Best taken with a little fat to enhance absorption.
Contains no gluten, soy, dairy, egg, fish, shellfish, or nut-containing ingredients.

The statements about the supplement and the ingredients have not been evaluated by the Food and Drug Administration. Young Living® products are not intended to diagnose, treat, cure, or prevent any disease.

SUPER VITAMIN D

THYROMIN™

HORMONES • NATURAL HRT

USE JUST BEFORE BED

NOT VEGAN

CONTAINS PORK

CONTAINS BEEF GELATIN

MINIMUM AGE 19+

Thyromin™ is a glandular supplement containing bovine (cow) thyroid powder, porcine (pig) pituitary powder, and porcine (pig) adrenal powder. These work well for those with poor functioning thyroids because the extracts contain active hormones. Thyromin™ is an excellent alternative for those who wish to support their thyroid and adrenals in a more natural way. Many medical doctors are now seeing the greater benefits to prescribing bovine and porcine glandular supplements over the traditional synthetic counterparts. Many older research claims online have a negative view simply because there was not enough data. As more and more people are seeing major benefits from glandular supplementation, the newer articles are changing to reflect a more positive view. As you research this on your own, it is recommended that you check the date of the article and only look at more recent studies and reviews.

INGREDIENTS
- Vitamin E as mixed tocopherols - 10 mg (67%)
- Iodine from whole plant Kelp and potassium iodide - 547 mcg (356%)

Thyromin™ Blend – 439.7 mg
- Parsley leaf powder
- Bovine thyroid powder (cow)
- Pituitary powder from porcine (pig)
- Adrenal powder from porcine (pig)
- L-tyrosine
- L-cystine
- L-cysteine HCL
- Essential oils - Peppermint, Spearmint, Myrtle, Myrrh

Other Ingredients - Gelatin, Magnesium carbonate, Potassium citrate, Magnesium stearate.

WHAT THE INGREDIENTS DO
- Vitamin E - high antioxidant property.
- Iodine - needed to make thyroid hormone.
- Parsley leaf powder - improves digestion, and helps promote menstrual flow.
- Bovine thyroid powder - helps to replace missing or lacking thyroid hormones.
- Pituitary powder from porcine - helps to replace missing or lacking pituitary hormones.
- Adrenal powder from porcine - helps to replace missing or lacking adrenal hormones.
- L-tyrosine - an amino acid that helps improve mental performance, alertness, and memory.
- L-cystine - an amino acid that is the basic building block of glutathione, for longevity, liver detoxification, and cognitive health. Helps fight oxidative stress.
- L-cysteine HCL - supports anti-aging properties in cells; supports the immune system.
- Essential oils - Peppermint, Spearmint, Myrtle, Myrrh - makes ingredients bioavailable.

Other Ingredients - Gelatin, Magnesium carbonate, Potassium citrate, Magnesium stearate - capsule base and substrate.

COMMENTS FROM YOUNG LIVING®
"Thyromin™ is a special blend of porcine glandular extracts, herbs, amino acids, minerals, and Seed to Seal® Premium essential oils in a perfectly balanced formula that maximizes nutritional support for healthy thyroid function. The thyroid gland regulates body metabolism, energy, and body temperature."

DIRECTIONS FOR USE
Take 1 capsule. (Best before bed on an empty stomach.)

The statements about the supplement and the ingredients have not been evaluated by the Food and Drug Administration. Young Living® products are not intended to diagnose, treat, cure, or prevent any disease.

THYROMIN™

YL VITALITY DROPS

ELECTROLYTES

USE ANYTIME   VEGAN   CONTAINS STEVIA   MINIMUM AGE 6+

If you are not a fan of drinking plain water, need the benefits of natural electrolytes, or simply want great tasting water, then the YL Vitality Drops are for you! They come in two delicious flavors. The Grapefruit Bergamot has a more fruity flavor, while the Lavender Lemonade is a more mature tasting lemonade.

INGREDIENTS

- Calories - 0
- Sodium - 5 mg (0% DV)
- Potassium - 7 mg (0% DV)
- Electrolyte blend, Water, Citric acid, Malic acid, Stevia (Stevia rebaudiana) leaf extract, Quillaja extract, Xanthan gum

Grapefruit Bergamot Flavor
- Bergamot (*Citrus bergamia*) peel oil
- Grapefruit (*Citrus paradisi*) rind oil

Lavender Lemon Flavor
- Lavender (*Lavandula angustifolia*) oil
- Lemon (*Citrus limon*) peel oil

WHAT THE INGREDIENTS DO

- Water - base ingredient for the drops.
- Citric acid - naturally sourced from citrus fruit and an excellent antioxidant.
- Malic acid - a component of most fruits; promotes energy production, increases endurance, and helps prevent muscle fatigue while exercising; natural preservative.
- Stevia (*Stevia rebaudiana*) leaf extract - natural no-calorie sweetener.
- Electrolyte blend - supports the pH and function of your body fluids, cells, and organs. Extracted from the Great Salt Lake: sodium (retains fluids), chloride (balances blood volume and pressure), magnesium (helps regulate muscle function), calcium (supports nerves, blood, bones, teeth, and muscles), and potassium (regulates fluids, nerve signals, and muscle contractions).
- Quillaja extract - a naturally derived emulsifier for consistency.
- Xanthan gum - a naturally derived stabilizer and thickener.

Grapefruit Bergamot Flavor
- Bergamot - flavor enhancer with calming effects.
- Grapefruit - flavor enhancer with flushing effects.

Lavender Lemon Flavor
- Lavender - flavor enhancer with calming effects.
- Lemon - flavor enhancer with detox and flushing effects.

COMMENTS FROM YOUNG LIVING®

"Water never tasted so good! YL Vitality Drops lets you hydrate naturally without sugar or artificial colors with the delicious flavors of both Grapefruit Bergamot and Lavender Lemonade that take your water or favorite beverage to the next level. Formulated with naturally occurring electrolytes from the Great Salt Lake and all-natural flavors, including Vitality™ essential oils, a few drops of YL Vitality Drops will keep you hydrated and feeling great!"

DIRECTIONS FOR USE

Add a small squirt of YL Vitality Drops to 8 ounces of cold water. If desired, add more drops according to taste preference. Do not drink directly from the bottle.

The statements about the supplement and the ingredients have not been evaluated by the Food and Drug Administration. Young Living® products are not intended to diagnose, treat, cure, or prevent any disease.

YL VITALITY DROPS

NOTE ON LABELING REGULATIONS

The ingredients on the physical label is always correct as to the ingredients, however, the supplement "daily value" percentages may be different because they are constantly changing as new data from studies become available. Young Living® reformulates supplements on an ongoing basis due to their desire to provide the best ingredients possible. If you have an older product, the newer one may have changed. Additionally, the Young Living® website is not always updated as fast as the labels are, so please refer to the product label in your hand.

ABBREVIATION KEY

- DV = Daily Value
- IU = International Units
- mg = milligrams
- mcg = micrograms
- ml = milliliters
- RAE = Retinol Activity Equivalents
- DFE = Dietary Folate Equivalents

UNITS CONVERSIONS

- 1,000 IU = 25 mcg
- 1,000 mcg = 1 mg
- 1,000 mg = 1 ml
- 1 ml = 20 drops
- 50 mg = 1 drop

USAGE

USE ANYTIME | USE BEFORE BREAKFAST | USE JUST BEFORE BED | USE 1 HOUR BEFORE MEAL | USE BEFORE 3PM | USE 1-4 HRS AFTER DINNER | BEST WITH FOOD | WITHOUT FOOD | BEST BEFORE A WORKOUT | KEEP REFRIGERATED

ANIMAL INGREDIENTS

CONTAINS DAIRY | CONTAINS PORK | CONTAINS BEEF | CONTAINS BEEF GELATIN | CONTAINS EGG | CONTAINS FISH | CONTAINS BEE PRODUCTS | CONTAINS SHELLFISH

POTENTIAL ALLERGENS

CONTAINS STEVIA | CONTAINS XYLITOL | CONTAINS SOY | CONTAINS BARLEY | CONTAINS CORN | CONTAINS NUTS | CONTAINS COCONUT

AGE MINIMUMS & DOSAGE ALTERNATIVES

MINIMUM AGE 1+ | MINIMUM AGE 2+ | MINIMUM AGE 4+ | MINIMUM AGE 6+ | MINIMUM AGE 12+ | MINIMUM AGE 14+ | MINIMUM AGE 18+ | MINIMUM AGE 21+ | ½ DOSAGE IF UNDER 12 | 2X ADULT DOSAGE

OTHER CAUTIONS AND CONSIDERATIONS

DON'T USE WITH BLOOD THINNERS | CAUTION IF PREGNANT | DO NOT FEED TO DOGS | WOMEN SPECIFIC | MEN SPECIFIC | VEGAN | NOT VEGAN | CONTAINS CAFFEINE

INGREDIENTS

SECTION FOUR
the ingredients

VITAMINS

A (Beta-carotene) Fat Soluble
- Balance Complete™ (25% DV)
- IlluminEyes™ 1300 mcg (144% DV)
- KidScents® MightyVites™ 180 mcg (20% DV)
- Master Formula™ 675 mcg RAE (4500 IU) (75% DV) - Micronized Nutrient Capsule

A (Retinyl acetate)
- Slique® Shake (8% DV)

B1 (Thiamin HCl) Water Soluble
- Balance Complete™ (25% DV)
- KidScents® MightyVites™ 0.8 mg (70% DV)
- Master Formula™ 11 mg (917% DV) - Micronized Nutrient Capsule
- Pure Protein™ Complete 0.75 mg (63% DV)
- Slique® Shake (20% DV)
- Super B™ 25 mg (2083% DV)

B2 (Riboflavin) Water Soluble
- Balance Complete™ (25% DV)
- Essentialzymes-4™ 8.3 mg (638% DV)
- KidScents® MightyVites™ 0.9 mg (70% DV)
- Master Formula™ 10 mg (769% DV) - Micronized Nutrient Capsule
- Pure Protein™ Complete 0.85 mg (65% DV)
- Slique® Shake (25% DV)
- Super B™ 25 mg (1923% DV)

B3 (Niacin/Niacinamide) Water Soluble
- Balance Complete™ (30% DV)
- KidScents® MightyVites™ 9 mg (60% DV)
- Master Formula™ 17 mg (106% DV) - Micronized Nutrient Capsule
- NingXia Zyng® 10 mg (60% DV)
- Pure Protein™ Complete 10 mg (63% DV)
- Slique® Shake (30% DV)
- Super B™ 35 mg (219% DV)

B5 (Pantothenic acid as D-calcium pantothenate) Water Soluble
- Balance Complete™ (25% DV)
- KidScents® MightyVites™ 1.8 mg (35% DV)
- Master Formula™ 19 mg (380% DV) - Micronized Nutrient Capsule
- Mineral Essence™ ionic trace amounts
- NingXia Zyng® 5 mg (100% DV)
- Pure Protein™ Complete 5 mg (100% DV)
- Slique® Shake (10% DV)
- Super B™ 15 mg (300% DV)

B6 (Pyridoxine HCl) Water Soluble
- Balance Complete™ (25% DV)
- EndoGize™ 25 mg (1470% DV)
- KidScents® MightyVites™ 2.2 mg (130% DV)
- Master Formula™ 11 mg (647% DV) - Micronized Nutrient Capsule
- Mineral Essence™ ionic trace amounts
- NingXia Nitro® (50% DV)
- NingXia Zyng® 1.5 mg (90% DV)
- PowerGize™ 12 mg (691% DV)
- Pure Protein™ Complete 1 mg (59% DV)
- Slique® Shake (20% DV)
- Super B™ 25 mg (1471% DV)

B7 (Biotin or Vitamin H) Water Soluble
- Balance Complete™ (30% DV)
- KidScents® MightyVites™ 40 mcg (130% DV)
- Master Formula™ 300 mcg (1000% DV) - Micronized Nutrient Capsule
- Pure Protein™ Complete 150 mcg (500% DV)
- Slique® Shake (8% DV)
- Super B™ 150 mcg (500% DV)

B9 (Folate) Water Soluble
- Balance Complete™ (30% DV)
- CardoGize™ 165 mcg DFE (40% DV)
- KidScents® MightyVites™ 153 mcg DFE - 90 mcg folic acid (38% DV)
- Master Formula™ 583.3 mcg DFE (146% DV) - Micronized Nutrient Capsule
- Slique® Shake (15% DV)
- Super B™ 667 mcg DFE (400 mcg Folic Acid from nature - not synthetic) (167% DV)

B12 (Methylcobalamin) Water Soluble
- KidScents® MightyVites™ 3.2 mcg (130% DV)
- Master Formula™ 12 mcg (500% DV) - Micronized Nutrient Capsule
- Pure Protein™ Complete 3 mcg (125% DV)
- Slique® Shake (6% DV)
- Super B™ 100 mcg (4157% DV)

C (from food sources) Water Soluble
- IlluminEyes™ 10mg (11% DV)
- KidScents® MightyVites™ 27 mg (30% DV)
- Slique® Bars Tropical Berry (15% DV)

INGREDIENTS

C (Ascorbic Acid) Water Soluble
- Balance Complete™ (25% DV)
- Slique® Shake (20% DV)
- Super C™ Chewables 150 mg (167% DV)
- Super C™ Tablet 1,300 mg (1440% DV)

C (Calcium Ascorbate) Water Soluble
- Master Formula™ 61 mg (68% DV) - Phyto-Caplet
- MegaCal™ 8.2 mg (9% DV)

Coenzyme Q10 (ubiquinone) Fat Soluble
- CardioGize™
- MindWise™ 31.8 mg
- OmegaGize3® 40 mg

D3 (Cholecalciferol) Fat Soluble
- Balance Complete™ (25% DV)
- KidScents® MightyVites™ 5 mcg (25% DV)
- Master Formula™ 10 mcg (400 IU) (50% DV) - Liquid Vitamin Capsule
- MindWise™ 20 mcg (100% DV)
- OmegaGize3® 24 mcg (120 % DV)
- Super Cal™ Plus 10 mcg (50% DV)
- Super Vitamin D 50 mcg or 2,000 iu (250% DV)

E (d-alpha tocopherol acetate) Fat Soluble
- AminoWise® 10.8 mg (72% DV)
- Balance Complete™ (15% DV)
- CBD by Nature's Ultra - Joint & Muscle Balm
- IlluminEyes™ 10 mg (67% DV)
- KidScents® MightyVites™ 30 mg (200% DV)
- Master Formula™ 33.5 mg (223% DV) - Liquid Vitamin Capsule
- NingXia Zyng® 2 mg (15% DV)
- Thyromin™ 10 mg (67% DV)

K2 Fat Soluble
- CardioGize™ 100 mcg (83% DV)
- Master Formula™ 50 mcg (42% DV) - Liquid Vitamin Capsule
- Super Cal™ Plus 30 mcg (25% DV)

INGREDIENTS

MINERALS

Boron
- Mineral Essence™ ionic trace amounts

Boron Citrate
- Master Formula™ - Micronized Nutrient Capsule

Calcium
- ICP™ 14 mg (2% DV)
- MegaCal™ 206 mg (16% DV)
- NingXia Red® 40 mg (4% DV)
- Pure Protein™ Complete 135 mg (10% DV)
- Slique® Bars Tropical Berry (2% DV)
- Slique® Shake (2% DV)
- Super Cal™ Plus 260 mg (26% DV)

Calcium (Red Algae)
- Super Cal™ Plus 260 mg (26% DV)

Calcium ascorbate
- MegaCal™
- Super C™ Chewables

Calcium carbonate
- AlkaLime®
- ICP™ 14mg/serving
- ImmuPro™ 84 mg (6% DV)
- KidScents® MightyZyme™ 50mg
- Life 9® 63.9 mg (4% DV)
- Master Formula™ 200 mg (5% DV) - Phyto-Caplet
- MegaCal™
- Sulfurzyme® Powder 8 g (<1% DV)
- Super C™ Tablet 160 mg (12% DV)

Calcium citrate
- AminoWise® 67 mg (5% DV)

Calcium (dicalcium phosphate)
- AlkaLime®
- Essentialzyme™ 70 mg (6% DV)
- JuvaTone® 344 mg (35% DV)
- Super B™ 143 mg (11% DV)
- Super C™ Tablet 160 mg (12% DV)

Calcium fructoborate
- AgilEase™

Calcium glycerophosphate
- MegaCal™

Calcium lactate pentahydrate
- MegaCal™

Calcium silicate
- AminoWise®

Calcium Stearate
- Slique® Gum

Calcium Sulfate
- AlkaLime®

Calcium (tricalcium phosphate)
- Balance Complete™ 40%

Chloride
- Mineral Essence™ 1,000 mg (45% DV)

Chromium
- Balance Complete™ (30% DV)
- Master Formula™ 120 mcg (343% DV) - Micronized Nutrient Capsule

Copper (Copper bisglycinate chelate)
- ImmuPro™ 0.16 mg (18% DV)

Copper (Copper citrate)
- JuvaTone® 1.6 mg (80% DV)

Copper (Copper gluconate)
- Slique® Shake (25% DV)
- MegaCal™

Copper (Copper glycinate chelate)
- Master Formula™ 350 mcg (39% DV) - Micronized Nutrient Capsule

Hyaluronic acid (Sodium hyaluronate)
- AgilEase™

Iodine
- Balance Complete™ (25% DV)
- NingXia Nitro® 75 µg (50% DV)
- Slique® Shake (6% DV)

Iodine from Kelp
- Master Formula™ - Micronized Nutrient Capsule
- MulitGreens™
- Thyromin™ 547 mcg (365% DV)

Iron
- Balance Complete™ (2% DV)
- FemiGen™ 0.8 mg (4% DV)
- ICP™ 1mg (2% DV)
- JuvaPower® 1.7 mg (10% DV)
- Master Formula™ 10 mg (56% DV) - Micronized Nutrient Capsule
- Mineral Essence™ ionic trace amounts
- MultiGreens™ 0.8 mg (4% DV)
- NingXia Red® 0.4 mg (2% DV)
- Pure Protein™ Complete 7 mg (41% DV)
- Slique® Bars Tropical Bar (4% DV)
- Slique® Shake (30% DV)

Lithium
- Mineral Essence™ ionic trace amounts

Magnesium
- Balance Complete™ (35% DV)
- KidScents® MightyVites™ 4.5 mg (2% DV)
- KidScents® Unwind™ 42mg (10% DV)
- Master Formula™ 60 mg (14% DV) - Micronized Nutrient Capsule
- MegaCal™ 191 mg (46% DV)
- Mineral Essence™ 350 mg (80% DV)
- Slique® Shake (20% DV)
- Super B™ 10 mg (2% DV)

Magnesium (magnesium bisglycinate)
- PowerGize™ 20 mg (5% DV)
- Super B™ 10 mg (2% DV)

Magnesium carbonate
- FemiGen™ 5 mg (2% DV)
- MegaCal™
- Thyromin™

Magnesium citrate
- AminoWise®
- MegaCal™
- Super Cal™ 119 mg (30% DV)
- KidScents® Unwind™ 42mg (10% DV)

Magnesium oxide
- Balance Complete™
- Slique® Shake

Magnesium phosphate
- AlkaLime®

Magnesium stearate (natural flow agent)
- BLM™
- Detoxzyme®
- Essentialzymes-4™
- ImmuPro™
- JuvaTone®
- KidScents® MightyVites™
- KidScents® MightyZyme™
- KidScents® Unwind™
- Master Formula™ - Micronized Nutrient Capsule
- Olive Essentials™
- Sulfurzyme® Capsules
- Super C™ Chewables
- Thyromin™

Magnesium sulfate
- MegaCal™ 320 mcg (14% DV)

Manganese
- Master Formula™ 2 mg (87% DV) - Micronized Nutrient Capsule
- Slique® Shake (150% DV)
- Super B™ 0.65 mg (28% DV)

Manganese citrate
- BLM™

Manganese sulfate
- Super C™ Tablet 2.1 mg (91% DV)
- Mega Cal™ 320 mcg (15% DV)

Methylsulfonylmethane (MSM or sulfur)
- BLM™
- Sulfurzyme® Capsules
- Sulfurzyme® Powder

Molybdenum
- Balance Complete™ (20% DV)
- Master Formula™ 75 mcg (167% DV) - Micronized Nutrient Capsule
- Slique® Shake (60% DV)

Phosphorus
- Balance Complete™ (25% DV)
- Slique® Shake (25% DV)

Potassium
- Balance Complete™ 330 mg (9% DV)
- NingXia Red® 414 mg (9% DV)
- Pure Protein™ Complete 1375.4 mg (8% DV)
- Super C™ Tablet 20 mg (<1% DV)
- YL Vitality Drops 7 mg

Potassium bicarbonate
- AlkaLime®

Potassium chloride
- AlkaLime®
- Master Formula™ 50mg (<2% DV) - Phyto-Caplet
- Super C™ Tablet 20 mg (<1% DV)

Potassium citrate
- AminoWise® 50 mg (1% DV)
- Thyromin™

Potassium iodide
- Slique® Shake

Potassium phosphate
- AlkaLime®

Potassium sulfate
- AlkaLime®

Salt
- Mineral Essence™

Selenium (selenomethionine)
- Balance Complete™ (30% DV)

Selenium (Sodium selenite - inorganic)
- Slique® Shake (50% DV)

Selenium (from yeast)
- CardioGize™ 100 mcg (182% DV)

Selenium (from organic food)
- KidScents® MightyVites™ 8 mcg (15% DV)
- Mineral Essence™ ionic trace amounts

Selenium (selenium amino acid complex)
- Master Formula™ 75 mcg (136% DV) - Micronized Nutrient Capsule

Selenium (selenium glycinate chelate / complex)
- ImmuPro™ 68 mcg (124% DV)
- Super B™ 50 mcg (91% DV)

Silica (natural substrate for anti-caking)
- Allerzyme™
- AminoWise®
- CardioGize™
- CortiStop®
- Detoxzyme®
- Digest & Cleanse®
- KidScents® MightyVites™
- KidScents® MightyZyme™
- Life 9®
- Longevity™
- MultiGreens™
- Prostate Health™
- Sulfurzyme® Capsules

Silicon
- ComforTone®
- Mineral Essence™ ionic trace amounts

Silicon dioxide
- BLM™
- ComforTone®
- Essentialzymes-4™
- ImmuPro™
- JuvaTone®
- Master Formula™ - Micronized Nutrient Capsule
- Master Formula™ - Phyto-Caplet
- OmegaGize3®
- PowerGize™
- Slique® CitriSlim™
- Super C™ Chewables

Sodium
- Balance Complete™ 115 mg (5% DV)
- Essentialzymes-4™ 10 mg (<1% DV)
- JuvaPower® 25 mg (1% DV)
- JuvaTone® 16mg (<1% DV)
- Mineral Essence™ 10 mg / serving
- MultiGreens™ 8mg (<1% DV)
- NingXia Red® 35 mg (2% DV)
- Pure Protein™ Complete 200 mg (9% DV)
- Slique® Bars Tropical Berry 70 mg (3% DV)
- Slique® Shake (17% DV)
- YL Vitality Drops 5 mg

Sodium bicarbonate
- AlkaLime®

Sodium chloride
- Pure Protein™ Complete

Sodium citrate
- AminoWise®
- Slique® Shake

Sodium hyaluronate (Hyaluronic acid)
- AgilEase™

Sodium phosphate
- AlkaLime®

Sodium selenite
- Slique® Shake

Sodium sulfate
- AlkaLime®

Sulfur
- BLM™ (as MSM)
- Mineral Essence™ ionic trace amounts
- Sulfurzyme® Capsules (as MSM)
- Sulfurzyme® Powder (as MSM)

Thallium
- Mineral Essence™ ionic trace amounts

Zinc (from organic food blend)
- KidScents® MightyVites™ 1.1 mg (10% DV)

Zinc (Zinc aspartate)
- EndoGize™ 2 mg (20% DV)

Zinc (Zinc bisglycinate chelate)
- ImmuPro™ 5 mg (45% DV)
- Super B™ 3 mg (27% DV)

Zinc (Zinc gluconate)
- AminoWise® 2.1 mg (19% DV)
- MegaCal™ 320 mcg (3% DV)
- Slique® Shake 2 mg (20% DV)
- Super C™ Tablet 1.5 mg (14% DV)

Zinc (Zinc glycinate chelate)
- Master Formula™ 15 mg (136% DV) - Micronized Nutrient Capsule
- PowerGize™ 5 mg (45% DV)

Zinc (Zinc picolinate)
- Pure Protein™ Complete 15 mg (136% DV)

Zinc oxide
- Balance Complete™

INGREDIENTS

DIGESTIVE ENZYMES

Alpha-galactosidase
Breaks down polysaccharides, beans, and vegetables.
- Allerzyme™
- Detoxzyme®

Amylase
Breaks down starches, breads, and pasta.
- Allerzyme™
- Balance Complete™
- Detoxzyme®
- EndoGize™
- Essentialzymes-4™
- KidScents® MightyZyme™
- Pure Protein™ Complete
- Slique® CitriSlim™

Betaine HCL (Betaine hydrochloride)
Aids digestion, helps absorb nutrients.
- Essentialzyme™
- FemiGen™

Bromelain
Breaks down meat, dairy, eggs, and grains.
- Allerzyme™
- Balance Complete™
- Detoxzyme®
- Essentialzyme™
- Essentialzymes-4™
- KidScents® MightyZyme™
- Pure Protein™ Complete

Cellulase
Breaks down man-made and plant fibers.
- Allerzyme™
- Detoxzyme®
- EndoGize™
- Essentialzymes-4™
- KidScents® MightyZyme™
- Pure Protein™ Complete
- Slique® CitriSlim™

Diastase (barley malt)
Breaks down grain sugars and starches.
- Allerzyme™

Glucoamylase
Breaks down starchy foods and cereals.
- Detoxzyme®
- EndoGize™

Invertase
Breaks down table sugar.
- Allerzyme™
- Detoxzyme®

Lactase
Breaks down lactose (dairy sugars).
- Allerzyme™
- Balance Complete™
- Detoxzyme®
- Pure Protein™ Complete

Lipase
Breaks down dietary fats and oils.
- Allerzyme™
- Balance Complete™
- Detoxzyme®
- Essentialzymes-4™
- ICP™
- KidScents® MightyZyme™
- Pure Protein™ Complete
- Slique® CitriSlim™

Pancreatin (from pig pancreatic glands)
Helps produce other enzymes. For those with a poorly performing pancreas.
- Essentialzyme™
- Essentialzymes-4™

Pancrelipase (from pig pancreatic glands)
For those with a poorly performing pancreas.
- Essentialzyme™

Papain
Digestive aid.
- Balance Complete™
- Essentialzyme™
- Essentialzymes-4™
- Pure Protein™ Complete

Peptidase
Finishes breaking down proteases.
Helps support immune system.
- Allerzyme™
- Essentialzymes-4™
- ICP™
- KidScents® MightyZyme™

Phytase
Helps with bone health and minerals.
- Allerzyme™
- Detoxzyme®
- Essentialzymes-4™
- ICP™
- KidScents® MightyZyme™

INGREDIENTS

Protease 3.0
Higher acid to break down animal protein.
- Essentialzymes-4™
- ICP™
- KidScents® MightyZyme™

Protease 4.5
Lower acidic content.
- Detoxzyme®
- Essentialzymes-4™
- ICP™
- KidScents® MightyZyme™

Protease 6.0
Carries away toxins in the blood. Least acidic.
- Allerzyme™
- EndoGize™
- Essentialzymes-4™
- ICP™
- KidScents® MightyZyme™
- Pure Protein™ Complete
- Slique® CitriSlim™

Trypsin
Breaks down proteins.
- Essentialzyme™

AMINO ACIDS

Amino Acids (general)
- AminoWise®
- Mineral Essence™
- NingXia Red®

Acetyl-L-Carnitine (ALCAR)
- MindWise™

B-alanine
- AminoWise®

Branched-chain amino acids
- AminoWise®

L-alpha glycerylphosphorylcholine (GPC)
- MindWise™

L-a-phosphatidylserine
- CortiStop®

L-a-phosphatidylcholine
- CortiStop®

L-arginine
- AminoWise®
- EndoGize™
- MultiGreens™
- Super Cal™ Plus

L-carnitine
- FemiGen™

L-citrulline
- AminoWise®

L-cysteine
- MultiGreens™

L-cysteine HCL (hydrochloride)
- FemiGen™
- JuvaTone®
- Thyromin™

L-cystine
- FemiGen™
- Thyromin™

L-glutamine
- AminoWise®
- Pure Protein™ Complete

L-isoleucine
- Pure Protein™ Complete

L-leucine
- Pure Protein™ Complete

L-lysine
- Pure Protein™ Complete
- Super Cal™ Plus

L-methionine
- Pure Protein™ Complete

L-phenylalanine
- FemiGen™

L-taurine
- AminoWise®
- JuvaPower®

L-theanine
- KidScents® Unwind™

L-tyrosine
- MultiGreens™
- Thyromin™

L-valine
- Pure Protein™ Complete

INGREDIENTS

PREBIOTICS

Prebiotic from Inulin (chicory root)
- Slique® Tea

Prebiotics (Wolfberry fiber)
- Master Formula™ -
  Micronized Nutrient Capsule
- MightyPro™
- NingXia Red®
- Sulfurzyme® Powder
- Sulfurzyme® Capsules

**Prebiotics
(Fructooligosaccharides FOS)**
- AminoWise®
- KidScents® MightyPro™
- Master Formula™ -
  Phyto-Caplet
- Sulfurzyme® Powder

PROBIOTICS

Probiotics
- Life 9®
- MightyPro™
- Pure Protein™ Complete

Lactobacillus acidophilus
- Pure Protein™ Complete

Probiotics in Life 9®
1. *Lactobacillus acidophilus*
2. *Lactobacillus plantarum*
3. *Lactobacillus rhamnosus*
4. *Lactobacillus salivarius*
5. *Streptococcus thermophilus*
6. *Bifidobacterium breve*
7. *Bifidobacterium bifidum*
8. *Bifidobacterium longum*
9. *Bifidobacterium lactis*

Probiotics in MightyPro™
1. *Lactobacillus acidophilus*
2. *Lactobacillus plantarum*
3. *Lactobacillus rhamnosus GG AF*
4. *Streptococcus thermophilus*
5. *Lactobacillus rhamnosus 6594*
6. *Lactobacillus paracasei*
7. *Bifidobacterium infantis BI-26*

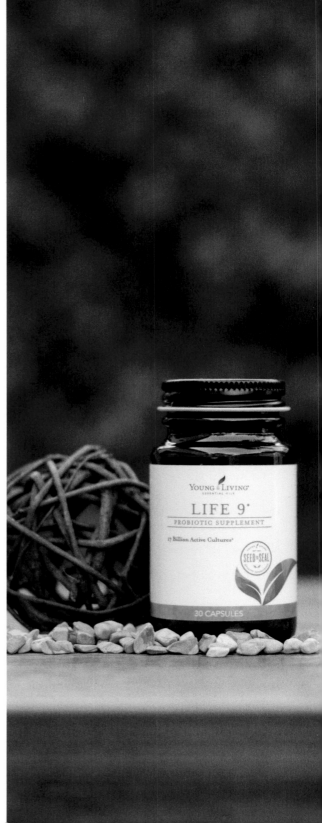

INGREDIENTS

NUTRIENTS, HERBS, & OTHER INGREDIENTS

5-HTP (*Griffonia simplicifolia* seed extract)
- KidScents® Unwind™

Acai Puree
- MindWise™

Acerola Cherry Powder
- Super C™ Chewables

Acerola Fruit Extract (Malpighiaglabra)
- IlluminEyes™
- Master Formula™ - Phyto-Caplet
- Super C™ Chewables

Acerola Juice Concentrate
- NingXia Nitro®

Adrenal Powder
- Thyromin™

Alfalfa Grass Juice Powder
- Slique® Shake

Alfalfa Leaf Powder
- Essentialzyme™
- KidScents® MightZyme™

Alfalfa Leaf/Stem Extract
- MultiGreens™

Alfalfa Sprout Powder
- Essentialzyme™
- JuvaTone®

Almonds
- Slique® Bars

Aloe Vera Leaf Extract
- Balance Complete™
- ICP™
- JuvaPower®

American Ginseng Root
- FemiGen™

Amla Fruit Extract
- KidScents® MightyVites™

Anise Fruit Oil
- ParaFree™

Anise Seed
- JuvaPower®

Annatto
- KidScents® MightyVites™

Apple Fruit Skin Extract
(*Malus domestica*)
- Master Formula™ - Phyto-Caplet

Apple Juice Powder
- KidScents® MightyZyme™

Apple Pectin
- ComforTone®

Apricot Kernel Oil
- CBD - Calm Roller

Arabinogalactan
- ImmuPro™

Argan Oil
- CBD - Calm Roller

Arnica Flower (Arnica montana)
- CBD - Joint & Muscle Balm

Aronia Juice Concentrate
- NingXia Red®

Ashwagandha Root Powder
- EndoGize™
- PowerGize™

Astragalus Root Powder
- CardioGize™

Atlantic Kelp
- Master Formula™ -
  Micronized Nutrient Capsule

Avocado Oil
- CBD - Calm Roller

Barberry Bark
- ComforTone®

Barley Grass (Hordeum vulgare)
- Allerzyme™
- Balance Complete™
- Master Formula™ -
  Micronized Nutrient Capsule

Barley Grass Juice Concentrate
(*Hordeum vulgare*)
- MultiGreens™

Barley Grass Leaf Powder
(*Hordeum vulgare*)
- KidScents® MightyVites™

Barley Sprouted Seed
- JuvaPower®

Baru Nuts
- Slique® Bars

Basil Leaf Concentrate
(Ocimum basilicum)
- Master Formula™ - Phyto-Caplet

Bee Pollen
- Essentialzymes-4™
- MultiGreens™

Bee Propolis
- JuvaTone®

Beeswax *(Cera alba)*
- CBD - Joint & Muscle Balm

Beet Root Juice Powder
- JuvaPower®
- JuvaTone®
- KidScents® MightyVites™

Bentonite
- ComforTone®

Berberine
- JuvaTone®
- Rehemogen™

Bilberry Fruit Extract
- Master Formula™ - Phyto-Caplet

Bilberry Juice Concentrate
- NingXia Nitro®

Bing Cherries
- Slique® Bars

Bitter Orange Unripened Fruit Extract
(Citrus aurantium)
- Slique® CitriSlim™

Black Carrot Extract
- Slique® Shake

Black Cohosh Root Extract
- CortiStop®
- FemiGen™

Black Currant Fruit Extract
- Master Formula™ - Phyto-Caplet

Black Currant Juice Concentrate
- NingXia Nitro®

Blackberry Fruit Concentrate
- Master Formula™ - Phyto-Caplet

Blackberry Juice Concentrate
- NingXia Zyng®

Black Pepper Fruit Extract
- EndoGize™

Blueberry Fruit Concentrate
- Master Formula™ - Phyto-Caplet

Blueberry Juice Concentrate
- NingXia Nitro®
- NingXia Red®

Bovine (cow)
- ComforTone® (Bovine gelatin)
- CortiStop® (Bovine gelatin)
- EndoGize™ (Bovine gelatin)
- Essentialzymes-4™ (Bovine gelatin)
- FemiGen™ (Bovine gelatin)
- MultiGreens™ (Bovine gelatin)
- PD 80/20™ (Bovine gelatin)
- Slique® CitriSlim™ (Bovine gelatin)
- Thyromin™ (Bovine thyroid powder)

Broccoli Floret/Stalk Powder
- JuvaPower®
- KidScents® MightyVites™

Broccoli Floret/Stem Concentrate
- Master Formula™ - Phyto-Caplet

Broccoli Seed Concentrate
- Master Formula™ - Phyto-Caplet

Brown Rice Bran
- Balance Complete™

Brussels Sprout Head Concentrate
- Master Formula™ - Phyto-Caplet

Buckthorn Bark
- Rehemogen™

Burdock Root
- ComforTone®
- Rehemogen™

Cabbage Palm Fruit Concentrate
- Master Formula™ - Phyto-Caplet

Cacao Nibs
- Slique® Bars

Cacao Powder (Ecuadorian)
- Slique® Tea

INGREDIENTS

Cactus Cladode Powder
- CardioGize™

Caffeine (Natural)
- NingXia Nitro® (green tea extract)
- NingXia Zyng® (white tea extract)
- Slique® CitriSlim™ (Guarana fruit)
- Slique® Shake (Guarana fruit)
- Slique® Tea (Jade Oolong Tea and Ecuadorian cacao powder)
- Master Formula™ (Green tea)

Camellia Seed Oil
- CBD - Calm Roller

Camellia Sinensis Leaf Extract
(Jade oolong green tea)
- CBD - Joint & Muscle Balm
- Master Formula™ - Phyto-Caplet
- Slique® Tea

Camu Camu Whole Fruit Concentrate
- Master Formula™ - Phyto-Caplet

Camu Camu Whole Fruit Powder
- Super C™ Chewables

Cane Sugar (evaporated)
- NingXia Zyng® 8 gm
- Pure Protein™ Complete

Cannabidiol (CBD) by Nature's Ultra
- CBD - Cinnamon Dropper (500 mg or 1000 mg per 30 ml)
- CBD - Citrus Dropper (500 mg or 1000 mg per 30 ml)
- CBD - Mint Dropper (500 mg or 1000 mg per 30 ml)
- CBD - Pet Dropper (500 mg or 1000 mg per 30 ml)
- CBD - Calm Roller (300 mg or 600 mg per 10 ml)
- CBD - Joint & Muscle Balm (300 mg or 600 mg per 50 g)

Caprylic/Capric Glycerides
- Slique® CitriSlim™

Caraway Fruit Oil
- Digest & Cleanse®

Carbonated Water
- NingXia Zyng®

Cardamom Seed Powder
- CardioGize™

Carrageenan
- SleepEssence™

Carrot Root Concentrate
- Master Formula™ - Phyto-Caplet

Carrot Root Powder
- Essentialzyme™
- KidScents® MightyZyme™

Cascara Sagrada Bark
- ComforTone®
- Rehemogen™

Cassia Branch/Stem Concentrate
- Master Formula™ - Phyto-Caplet

Cassia Dried Bark Powder
- Slique® CitriSlim™

Cat's Claw Bark Powder
- CardioGize™

Cayenne Fruit
- ComforTone®
- Super C™ Tablet

Cellulose
- ICP™
- JuvaTone®

Cellulose Film-Coating
- JuvaTone®

Cherry Juice Concentrate
- NingXia Nitro®
- NingXia Red®

Chia Seeds
- Slique® Bars

Chicory Root
- Balance Complete™
- Slique® Bars

Chocolate Oil
- NingXia Nitro®

Chokeberry Fruit Concentrate
- Master Formula™ - Phyto-Caplet

Choline (as choline bitartrate)
- JuvaTone®
- Master Formula™ - Phyto-Caplet
- MultiGreens™
- NingXia Nitro®

INGREDIENTS

Chromium Amino Nicotinate
- Balance Complete™
- Slique® Shake (10% DV)

Cinnamon Bark
- Balance Complete™

Citric Acid
- AlkaLime®
- AminoWise®
- KidScents® MightyPro™
- MegaCal™
- MindWise™
- NingXia Zyng®

Citrus Bioflavonoids
(whole fruit powder)
- Master Formula™ - Micronized Nutrient Capsule
- Super C™ Chewables
- Super C™ Tablet

Citrus Flavonoids
(from Tangerine peel)
- KidScents® MightyVites™

Clove Bud
- K & B™

Cocoa Powder
- Pure Protein™ Complete

Coconut
- Slique® Bars

Coconut Fruit Oil
- CBD Droppers
- Digest & Cleanse®
- Inner Defense®
- Longevity™
- SleepEssence™

Coconut Nectar
- NingXia Nitro®

Coenzyme Q10 (ubiquinone) Fat Soluble
- CardioGize™
- MindWise™ 31.8 mg
- OmegaGize3® 40 mg

Coffea Arabica Fruit Extract
- Master Formula™ - Phyto-Caplet

Collards Leaf Concentrate
(Brassica oleracea acehala)
- Master Formula™ - Phyto-Caplet

Corn
- AgilEase™
- AlkaLime®
- Allerzyme™
- Slique® Gum
- Slique® Shake
- Super Cal™ Plus
- SleepEssence™

Cow (see Bovine)

Cramp Bark
- FemiGen™

Cucumber Fruit Powder
- JuvaPower®

Cumin Seed Oil
- ParaFree™

Cumin Seed Powder
- Detoxzyme®
- Essentialzyme™

Curcuminoids Complex Rhizome Extract (Turmeric)
- AgilEase™

D-Ribose
- NingXia Nitro®

DHA (Docosahexaenoic acid)
- OmegaGize3® 310 mg

DHEA (derived from wild yam)
- CortiStop®
- EndoGize™
- PD 80/20™ 100 mg

Damiana Leaf
- FemiGen™

Dandelion Root Extract
- K & B™
- JuvaTone®

Dates
- Slique® Bars

Desert Hyacinth Root Powder
- PowerGize™

Dextrates
- KidScents® MightyZyme™

Dextrose
- ImmuPro™

Dietary Fiber
- Balance Complete™ 4 g (14%)
- ICP™ 2 g
- JuvaPower® 2 g
- Pure Protein™ Complete 2 g
- Slique® Shake - 5 g (20% DV)

Dill Seed
- JuvaPower®

Di-methylglycine HCL
- FemiGen™

Distilled Water (see also Water)
- Rehemogen™

Dong Quai Root Powder
- CardioGize™
- FemiGen™

Echinacea Root
- ComforTone®
- JuvaTone®

Eleuthero Root
- MultiGreens™

EPA (Eicosapentaenoic acid)
- OmegaGize3® 135mg

Epimedium Aerial Parts
- EndoGize™
- FemiGen™

Epimedium Leaf Powder
- PowerGize™

Erythritol
- KidScents® MightyPro™
- KidScents® Unwind™

Ethanol Alcohol
- K & B™
- Rehemogen™

European Elder Fruit Concentrate
- Master Formula™ - Phyto-Caplet

Evening Primrose Oil
- CBD by Nature's Ultra - Calm Roller

Fennel Fruit
- K & B™

Fennel Seed
- ComforTone®
- ICP™
- JuvaPower®

Fenugreek Seed Extract
- PowerGize™

Fermented Polysaccharide Complex
- Super Cal™ Plus

Fiber
- Balance Complete™ 4 g (14%)
- ICP™ 2 g
- JuvaPower® 2 g
- Pure Protein™ Complete 2 g
- Slique® Shake - 5 g (20% DV)

Fish (Basa)
- OmegaGize3®

Fish (Tilapia, Carp)
- Inner Defense®
- ParaFree™

Fish Gelatin
- Inner Defense®
- OmegaGize3®
- ParaFree™

Flax Seed Powder
- ICP™
- JuvaPower®

Fractionated Coconut Oil
- Digest & Cleanse®
- Longevity™

Frankincense Resin
(Boswellia frereana)
- Slique® Gum

Frankincense resin powder
(Boswellia sacra)
- AgilEase™
- Slique® Tea

Fructooligosaccharides (FOS)
- AminoWise®
- KidScents® MightyPro™
- Master Formula™ - Phyto-Caplet
- Sulfurzyme® Powder

INGREDIENTS

Fructose
- Balance Complete™
- KidScents® MightyVites™

Garlic Bulb Extract
- CardioGize™
- ComforTone®

Garlic Clove Concentrate
- Master Formula™ - Phyto-Caplet

Gelatin from Cow or Pork
- BLM™ (Pork)
- ComforTone® (Cow)
- CortiStop® (Cow)
- EndoGize™ (Cow)
- Essentialzymes-4™ (Cow)
- FemiGen™ (Cow)
- MultiGreens™ (Cow)
- PD 80/20™ (Cow)
- Prostate Health™ (Pork)
- Slique® CitriSlim™ (Cow - liquid cap)
- Thyromin™ (Cow)

Geranium Aerial Parts
- K & B™

German Chamomile Flower Extract
- K & B™
- ComforTone®

Ginger Root
- ComforTone®
- JuvaPower®

Glucosamine Sulfate
- AgilEase™ (from non-GMO corn)
- BLM™ (from shellfish - crab and shrimp)

Glycerin
- Inner Defense®
- MindWise™
- ParaFree™
- SleepEssence™

Goldenberries
- Slique® Bars

Grape Extracts (Red & White)
- Slique® Shake

Grape Seed Extract
- NingXia Red®

Grapefruit Extract
- Slique® Shake

Grapefruit Whole Fruit Extract
- Slique® CitriSlim™

Grapefruit Whole Fruit Powder
- Master Formula™ - Micronized Nutrient Capsule

Green Tea Extract
- CBD - Joint & Muscle Balm
- Master Formula™ - Phyto-Caplet
- NingXia Nitro®
- Slique® Shake
- Slique® Tea

Guar Gum (organic)
- Master Formula™ - Phyto-Caplet

Guar Gum Seed Powder
- Balance Complete™
- ICP™

Guarana Seed Extract
- Slique® Shake

Guarana Whole Fruit Extract
(Paulinia cupana)
- Slique® CitriSlim™

Guava Fruit Extract
- KidScents® MightyVites™

Gumbase
- Slique® Gum

HPMC Targeted Release Capsule
(Hydroxypropylmethylcellulose)
Derived from vegetable cellulose
- Life 9®

Hawthorn Berry Powder
- CardioGize™

Hemp Seed Oil
- CBD - Calm Roller

Holy Basil Aerial Parts Extract
- KidScents® MightyVites™

Honey
- Mineral Essence™
- Slique® Bars

Hops Flower Extract
- Super Cal™ Plus

INGREDIENTS

Hydroxypropyl Cellulose
- ImmuPro™
- Super C™ Chewables

Hydroxytyrosol
- Olive Essentials™

Hypromellose (veggie capsule)
- Allerzyme™
- CardioGize™
- Detoxzyme®
- Digest & Cleanse®
- Essentialzymes-4™
- Longevity™
- Master Formula™ - Liquid Vitamin
- Master Formula™ - Micronized Nutrient Capsule
- Olive Essentials™
- PowerGize™
- Slique® CitriSlim™
- Sulfurzyme® Capsules

Inositol
- JuvaTone®
- Master Formula™ - Micronized Nutrient Capsule

Isomalt (from beet sugar)
- Slique® Gum

Isomalto-oligosaccharide
- Slique® Shake

Jade Oolong Tea *(Camellia sinensis)*
- Slique® Tea

Japanese Sophora Flower Extract
- Master Formula™ - Phyto-Caplet

Jojoba Seed Oil *(Simmondsia chinensis)*
- CBD - Joint & Muscle Balm

Juniper Berry Extract
- K & B™

Juniper Branch/Leaf/Fruit
- K & B™

Kelp Whole Thallus
- MultiGreens™

Kiwi Juice Concentrate
- NingXia Nitro®

Konjac
- Balance Complete™

Korean Ginseng Extract
- NingXia Nitro®

Lecithin
- Balance Complete™
- EndoGize™
- SleepEssence™

Lemon Fruit Powder (whole fruit)
- AlkaLime®
- Master Formula™ - Micronized Nutrient Capsule

Licorice Root Extract
- FemiGen™
- Rehemogen™

Lime Fruit Powder
- AminoWise®
- Master Formula™ - Micronized Nutrient Capsule

Longjack Root Extract
- EndoGize™
- PowerGize™

Luo Han Guo Fruit Extract
- MindWise™
- Pure Protein™ Complete
- Balance Complete™

Lutein (from marigold flower)
- IlluminEyes™

Lycopene
- Master Formula™ - Micronized Nutrient Capsule

MCT (Medium-chain triglycerides)
- Balance Complete™
- Longevity™
- MindWise™
- Slique® Shake

Maitake Mushroom Mycelia Powder
- ImmuPro™

Malic Acid
- KidScents® MightyVites™
- MegaCal™
- MindWise™
- NingXia Red®
- Slique® Shake

INGREDIENTS

Maltodextrin
- ImmuPro™
- Master Formula™ - Phyto-Caplet

Mangosteen Fruit Concentrate
- Master Formula™ - Phyto-Caplet

Marigold Flower Extract
- IlluminEyes™

Marine Minerals
- Super Cal™ Plus

Melatonin
- ImmuPro™ 4.2 mg
- SleepEssence™ 3.2 mg

Menthol
- CBD - Joint & Muscle Balm

Microcrystalline Cellulose
- KidScents® MightyZyme™
- Life 9®
- Master Formula™ - Micronized Nutrient Capsule
- Master Formula™ - Phyto-Caplet
- Olive Essentials™

Mixed Carotenoids
- Balance Complete™
- OmegaGize3®

Mixed Tocopherols
- Balance Complete™
- Longevity™

Modified Cornstarch
- SleepEssence™

Mojave Yucca Root
- ICP™

Motherwort Herb Powder
- CardioGize™

Muira Puama Bark
- EndoGize™
- FemiGen™
- PowerGize™

Mulberry Leaf Extract
- NingXia Nitro®

Mushroom Mycelia Powder
- ImmuPro™

Natural Flavors
- AminoWise®
- Balance Complete™
- KidScents® MightyVites™
- MindWise™
- NingXia Nitro®
- NingXia Zyng®
- Pure Protein™ Complete
- Slique® Gum
- Slique® Shake

Natural Fruit Punch Flavor
- KidScents® MightPro™

Natural Mixed Berry Flavor
- KidScents® MightyZyme™

Natural Sweetener
- KidScents® MightyVites™
- Slique® Gum

Neem Oil
- CBD - Calm Roller

Neohesperidin Derivative
- Balance Complete™

Ningxia Wolfberry Fruit Powder
- AminoWise®
- KidScents® MightyPro™
- Master Formula™ - Micronized Nutrient Capsule
- Sulfurzyme® Capsules
- Sulfurzyme® Powder

Ningxia Wolfberry Puree
- NingXia Red®

Nonfat Dry Milk
- Balance Complete™

Non-GMO Cornstarch
- Super Cal™ Plus

Non-GMO Tapioca Dextrose
- Slique® Shake
- Super C™ Chewables

Oat Bran Powder
- ICP™
- JuvaPower®

Ocotea Leaf (Ocotea quixos)
- Slique® Tea

Ocotea Leaf Powder
- Slique® CitriSlim™

Olive Fruit Oil
- ParaFree™

Olive Leaf Extract *(olea europaea)*
- Master Formula™ - Micronized Nutrient Capsule

Omega-3 Fatty Acids
- OmegaGize3® (from fish oil) 445mg

Onion Bulb Extract
- Master Formula™ - Phyto-Caplet

Orange Fruit Juice Powder
- KidScents® MightyVites™

Orange Whole Fruit Extract
- Slique® CitriSlim™

Orange Whole Fruit Powder
- Master Formula™ - Micronized Nutrient Capsule

Oregano Leaf Concentrate
- Master Formula™ - Phyto-Caplet

Oregon Grape Root
- JuvaTone®
- Rehemogen™

Organic Coconut Palm Sugar
- Slique® Shake

Organic Ground Nutmeg
- Pure Protein™ Complete (Vanilla Spice)

Organic Pumpkin Seed Protein
- Slique® Shake

Organic Quinoa Powder
- Slique® Shake

Orgen-Kid® Amala Fruit Extract
- KidScents® MightyVites™

Orgen-Kid® Annatto Seed Extract
- KidScents® MightyVites™

Orgen-Kid® Curry Leaf Extract
(Murraya koenigii)
- KidScents® MightyVites™

Orgen-Kid® Guava Fruit Extract
- KidScents® MightyVites™

Orgen-Kid® Holy Basil Aerial Parts Extract
- KidScents® MightyVites™

Orgen-Kid® Lemon Peel Extract
- KidScents® MightyVites™

Orgen-Kid® Sesbania Leaf Extract
(Sesbania grandiflora)
- KidScents® MightyVites™

PABA
- Master Formula™ - Micronized Nutrient Capsule
- Super B™

Palm Olein
- Master Formula™ - Phyto-Caplet

Parsley Leaf Extract
- JuvaTone®
- K & B™
- Thyromin™

Pea Protein Isolate
- Slique® Shake

Peach Bark
- Rehemogen™

Pear Juice Concentrate
- NingXia Zyng®

Pectin
- NingXia Red®
- NingXia Nitro®

Peppermint Leaf
- JuvaPower®

Phosphatidylcholine
- EndoGize™

Piperine Whole Fruit Extract
- AgilEase™

Pituitary Powder
- Thyromin™

Plantain Leaf
- Allerzyme™

Plum Juice Concentrate
- NingXia Red®

Poke Root
- Rehemogen™

Polyphenols Extract
- AminoWise®

INGREDIENTS

Pomegranate Fruit Extract
- MindWise™

Pomegranate Juice Concentrate
- MindWise™
- NingXia Red®

Porcine/Pork
- BLM™ (porcine gelatin)
- Essentialzyme™ (pancreas from pig)
- Prostate Health™ (porcine gelatin)
- Thyromin™ (pig gland powders)

Potato Skin Extract
- Slique® Bars

Pregnenolone
- CortiStop®
- PD 80/20™ 400 mg

Prickly Ash Bark
- Rehemogen™

Proprietary V-Fiber Blend
- Balance Complete™

Psyllium Seed
- ComforTone®
- ICP™
- JuvaPower®

Pterostilbene
- Slique® CitriSlim™

Pumpkin Seed Oil
- Prostate Health™

Purified Water (see also Water)
- OmegaGize3®
- NingXia Nitro®

Quinoa Crisps
- Slique® Bars

Raspberry Fruit Concentrate
- Master Formula™ - Phyto-Caplet

Raspberry Fruit Powder
- ImmuPro™

Raspberry Juice Concentrate
- NingXia Nitro®

Red Cabbage Juice
- Slique® Gum

Red Clover Blossom
- Rehemogen™

Reishi Whole Mushroom Powder
- ImmuPro™

Retinyl Palmitate
- NingXia Zyng®

Rhododendron Leaf Extract
- MindWise™

Rice Bran (natural filler for volume control)
- Detoxzyme®
- ICP™
- JuvaPower®

Rice Bran Oil
- OmegaGize3®

Rice Flour
- BLM™
- CortiStop®
- Essentialzymes-4™
- PD 80/20™
- PowerGize™
- Slique® CitriSlim™
- Sulfurzyme® Capsules

Roman Chamomile Aerial Parts
- K & B™

Rose Hips Fruit Powder
- Super C™ Chewables

Rosehip Seed Oil
- CBD - Calm Roller

Royal Jelly
- K & B™
- Rehemogen™
- Mineral Essence™

Rutin Flower Bud Powder
- Super C™ Tablet

Sacha Inchi Seed oil (*Plukenetia volubilis*)
- MindWise™

Safflower (*Carthamus tinctorius*)
- CBD - Joint & Muscle Balm

Sage Aerial Parts
- K & B™

INGREDIENTS

Sarsaparilla Root
- Rehemogen™

Saw Palmetto Fruit Extract
- Prostate Health™

Sea Salt
- Slique® Bars

Sesame Seed Oil
- ParaFree™

Shea Butter *(Butyrospermum parkii)*
- CBD - Joint & Muscle Balm

Shellfish (crab and shrimp)
- BLM™

Slippery Elm Bark
- JuvaPower®

Sorbitol
- KidScents® MightyZyme™
- SleepEssence™
- Slique® Gum
- Super C™ Chewables

Soy
- CortiStop®
- EndoGize™
- Essentialzyme™
- Slique® Gum

Spinach Leaf Concentrate
- Master Formula™ - Phyto-Caplet

Spinach Leaf Powder
- JuvaPower®

Spirulina
- MultiGreens™

Spirulina Algae
- Master Formula™ - Micronized Nutrient Capsule

Squalane
- CBD - Joint & Muscle Balm

Squaw Vine Aerial Parts
- FemiGen™

Stearic Acid
- Super Cal™ Plus
- KidScents® MightyZyme™
- Super C™ Chewables
- Master Formula™ - Phyto-Caplet

Stevia Leaf Extract *(Stevia rebaudiana)*
- AlkaLime®
- AminoWise®
- CBD Droppers
- ImmuPro™
- KidScents® MightyVites™
- KidScents® MightyZyme™
- KidScents® Unwind™
- MegaCal™
- NingXia Red®
- NingXia Zyng®
- Pure Protein™ Complete
- Slique® Essence Oil
- Slique® Shake
- Slique® Tea
- Sulfurzyme® Powder
- Super C™ Chewables

Stillingia Root
- Rehemogen™

Strawberry Fruit Juice Powder
- ImmuPro™
- KidScents® MightyVites™
- Slique® Shake

Sugar (from fruit juice)
- NingXia Red® 5 g
- NingXia Nitro® 4 g

Sunflower Lecithin (non-GMO)
- Master Formula™ - Liquid Vitamin
- Master Formula™ - Phyto-Caplet
- MindWise™

Sweet Almond Oil
- CBD - Calm Roller

Sweet Cherry Fruit Concentrate
- Master Formula™ - Phyto-Caplet

Tangerine Whole Fruit Powder
- Master Formula™ - Micronized Nutrient Capsule

Tapioca Maltodextrin
- AminoWise®

Tapioca Starch
- AminoWise®

Tartaric Acid
- AlkaLime®
- NingXia Red®

INGREDIENTS

Tea Leaf Extract
- Super Cal™ Plus

Thyme Leaf Powder
- Essentialzyme™

Thyroid Powder (from cow)
- Thyromin™

Tomato Fruit Concentrate
- Master Formula™ - Phyto-Caplet

Tomato Fruit Flakes
- JuvaPower®

Tribulus Fruit Extract
- EndoGize™
- PowerGize™

Turmeric Rhizome Extract
- AgilEase™

Turmeric Root Concentrate
- Master Formula™

Turmeric Root Powder
- MindWise™
- Slique® Gum (for color)

Type II Collagen
- AgilEase™
- BLM™

Uva-ursi Leaf Extract
- K & B™

Vanilla Extract
- NingXia Red®
- Slique® Tea

Water
- Allerzyme™
- CardioGize™
- ComforTone®
- Detoxzyme®
- Digest & Cleanse®
- Inner Defense®
- K & B™
- Longevity™
- MindWise™
- Olive Essentials™
- ParaFree™
- Prostate Health™
- SleepEssence™

Whey Protein Concentrate
- Balance Complete™

White Tea Leaf Extract
- NingXia Zyng® - 35 mg

Wild Yam Root (see also DHEA)
- FemiGen™

Winged Treebine Root Extract
- Super Cal™ Plus

Wolfberries *(Lycium barbarum)*
- Slique® Bars

Wolfberry Fruit Polysaccharide
- ImmuPro™

Wolfberry Fruit Powder
(Lycium barbarum)
- AminoWise®
- IlluminEyes™
- KidScents® MightyPro™
- KidScents® MightyVites™
- Master Formula™ - Micronized Nutrient Capsule
- Slique® Shake
- Sulfurzyme® Capsules
- Sulfurzyme® Powder

Wolfberry Puree
- NingXia Red®
- NingXia Zyng®

Wolfberry Seed Oil
- NingXia Nitro®

Xanthan Gum
- Balance Complete™
- NingXia Nitro®
- Pure Protein™ Complete
- Slique® Shake

Xylitol
- Balance Complete™
- KidScents® MightyPro™
- KidScents® Unwind™
- MegaCal™
- Slique® Gum

Yerba Mate Oil
- NingXia Nitro®

Zeaxanthin (from marigold flower)
- IlluminEyes™

ESSENTIAL OILS

Angelica root oil
(Angelica archangelica)
- CardioGize™

Anise fruit oil
(Pimpinella anisum)
- Allerzyme™
- Essentialzymes-4™
- MindWise™

Anise seed oil
(Pimpinella anisum)
- ComforTone®
- Detoxzyme®
- Digest & Cleanse®
- Essentialzyme™
- ICP™
- JuvaPower®

Black Pepper oil
(Piper nigrum)
- NingXia Nitro®

Blue Tansy flowering top oil
(Tanacetum annuum)
- JuvaTone®

Camphor bark oil
(Cinnamomum camphora)
- CBD - Joint & Muscle Balm

Canadian Fleabane flowering top oil
(Conyza canadensis)
- CortiStop®
- EndoGize™

Caraway fruit oil
(Carum Carvi)
- Digest & Cleanse®

Cardamom seed oil
(Elettaria cardamomum)
- CardioGize™
- Master Formula™ - Liquid Vitamin

Cassia branch/leaf oil
(Cinnamomum aromaticum)
- EndoGize™
- Slique® CitriSlim™

Cinnamon bark oil
(Cinnamomum verum)
- Inner Defense®
- Slique® Bars

Cinnamon bark oil
(Cinnamomum zeylanicum)
- CardioGize™
- CBD - Cinnamon Dropper

Clary Sage flowering top oil
(Salvia sclarea)
- CortiStop®
- EndoGize™
- FemiGen™

Clove flower bud oil
(Syzygium aromaticum)
- AgilEase™
- BLM™
- Essentialzyme™
- Inner Defense®
- Longevity™
- Master Formula™ - Liquid Vitamin
- OmegaGize3®

Clove leaf oil
(Eugenia caryophyllus)
- CBD - Joint & Muscle Balm

Copaiba wood oil
(Copaifera officinalis)
- AgilEase™
- Super Cal™ Plus

Cumin seed oil
(Cuminum cyminum)
- Detoxzyme®

Cypress leaf/nut/stem oil
(Cupressus sempervirens)
- CardioGize™

Eucalyptus Globulus leaf oil
(Eucalyptus globulus)
- CBD - Calm Roller

Eucalyptus Radiata leaf oil
(Eucalyptus radiata)
- Inner Defense®

Fennel seed oil
(Foeniculum vulgare)
- Allerzyme™
- CortiStop®
- Detoxzyme®
- Digest & Cleanse®
- Essentialzyme™
- Essentialzymes-4™
- FemiGen™
- ICP™
- JuvaPower®
- Master Formula™ - Liquid Vitamin
- MindWise™
- Prostate Health™
- Slique® CitriSlim™

Frankincense gum/resin oil
(Boswellia carterii)
- CBD - Calm Roller
- CortiStop®
- Longevity™

Geranium aerial parts oil
(Pelargonium graveolens)
- JuvaTone®
- Prostate Health™

INGREDIENTS

German Chamomile flower oil
(Matricaria recuita)
- ComforTone®
- OmegaGize3®
- JuvaTone®

Ginger root oil
(Zingiber officinale)
- Allerzyme™
- ComforTone®
- Digest & Cleanse®
- EndoGize™
- Essentialzymes-4™
- ICP™
- Master Formula™ - Liquid Vitamin Capsule

Grapefruit rind oil
(Citrus paradisi)
- CBD - Citrus Dropper
- Slique® Essence Oil
- Slique® Shake

Helichrysum flower oil
(Helichrysum italicum)
- CardioGize™
- CBD - Joint & Muscle Balm

Idaho Balsam Fir branch/leaf oil
(Abies balsamea)
- Slique® CitriSlim™

Idaho Blue Spruce
(Picea pungens)
- Super Cal™ Plus

Juniper leaf oil
(Juniperus osteosperma)
- Allerzyme™
- K & B™

Lavender oil
(Lavandula angustifolia)
- CardioGize™
- CBD - Calm Roller
- KidScents® Unwind™
- Prostate Health™
- SleepEssence™

Lemon Myrtle leaf oil
(Backhousia citriodora)
- Slique® CitriSlim™

Lemon peel oil
(Citrus limon aka Citrus medica limonum)
- AlkaLime®
- AminoWise®
- CBD - Joint & Muscle Balm
- Digest & Cleanse®
- Inner Defense®
- JuvaTone®
- NingXia Red®
- MegaCal™
- MindWise™

Lemon peel oil continued
- MultiGreens™
- Slique® Essence Oil
- Slique® Shake

Lemongrass leaf oil
(Cymbopogon flexuosus)
- Allerzyme®
- Essentialzymes-4™
- ICP™
- Inner Defense®
- MultiGreens™
- Slique® CitriSlim™

Lime peel oil
(Citrus aurantifolia)
- AlkaLime®
- AminoWise®
- MegaCal™
- MindWise™
- Super Vitamin D

Melissa leaf/flower oil
(Melissa officinalis)
- MultiGreens™
- Super Vitamin D

Myrrh gum/resin oil
(Commiphora Myrrha)
- EndoGize™

Myrtle leaf oil
(Myrtus communis)
- JuvaTone®
- Prostate Health™

Northern Lights Black Spruce™ tree oil
(Picea mariana)
- AgilEase™
- Super Cal™ Plus

Nutmeg oil
(Myristica fragrans)
- NingXia Nitro®

Ocotea leaf oil
(Ocotea quixos)
- ComforTone®
- Slique® CitriSlim™
- Slique® Essence Oil
- Slique® Shake

Orange peel oil
(Citrus aurantium dulcis)
- CBD - Calm Roller

Orange peel oil
(Citrus sinensis)
- Balance Complete™
- CBD - Citrus Dropper
- ImmuPro™
- Longevity™
- NingXia Red®
- Slique® Bars

INGREDIENTS

Oregano leaf/stem oil
(Origanum vulgare)
- Inner Defense®

Parsley leaf oil
(Petroselinum crispun)
- Olive Essentials™

Patchouli flower oil
(Pogostemon cablin)
- Allerzyme™

Peppermint leaf oil
(Mentha piperita)
- Allerzyme™
- CBD - Joint & Muscle Balm
- CBD - Mint Dropper
- ComforTone®
- CortiStop®
- Digest & Cleanse®
- Essentialzyme™
- KidScents® MightyZyme™
- MindWise™
- NingXia Nitro®
- Prostate Health™
- Slique® Gum

Pomegranate seed oil
(Punica granatum)
- Slique® CitriSlim™

Roman Chamomile flower oil
(Chamaemelum nobile)
- KidScents® Unwind™

Rosemary leaf oil
(Rosmarinus officinalis)
- CardioGize™
- ComforTone®
- Essentialzymes-4™
- ICP™
- Inner Defense®
- JuvaTone®
- MultiGreens™
- Olive Essentials™

Rue flower oil
(Ruta graveolens)
- SleepEssence™

Sage leaf oil
(Salvia officinalis)
- FemiGen™

Spearmint leaf oil
(Mentha spicata)
- CBD - Mint Dropper
- OmegaGize3®
- NingXia Nitro®
- Slique® CitriSlim™
- Slique® Essence Oil
- Slique® Gum
- Slique® Shake

Tangerine rind oil
(Citrus reticulata)
- ComforTone®
- NingXia Red®
- Slique® Essence Oil
- SleepEssence™
- Slique® Shake

Tarragon leaf oil
(Artemisia dracunculus)
- Allerzyme™
- ComforTone®
- Essentialzyme™
- Essentialzymes-4™
- ICP™

Tea Tree leaf oil
(Melaleuca alternifolia)
- CBD - Joint & Muscle Balm

Turmeric root oil
(Curcuma longa)
- Master Formula™ - Liquid Vitamin

Thyme leaf oil
(Thymus vulgaris)
- Inner Defense®
- Longevity™

Valerian root oil
(Velariana officianalis)
- SleepEssence™

Vanilla Oil
(Vanilla planifolia)
- NingXia Nitro®
- Slique® Bars

Vetiver root oil
(Vetiveriz zizanoides)
- CBD - Calm Roller
- SleepEssence™
- Super Cal™ Plus

Wintergreen leaf oil
(Gaultheria procumbens)
- AgilEase™
- CBD -Joint & Muscle Balm

Wormwood oil
(Gaultheria artemisia absinthium)
- CBD - Joint & Muscle Balm

Ylang Ylang flower oil
(Cananga odorata)
- CBD - Calm Roller
- FemiGen™

Yuzu peel oil
(Citrus junos)
- NingXia Red®

INGREDIENTS

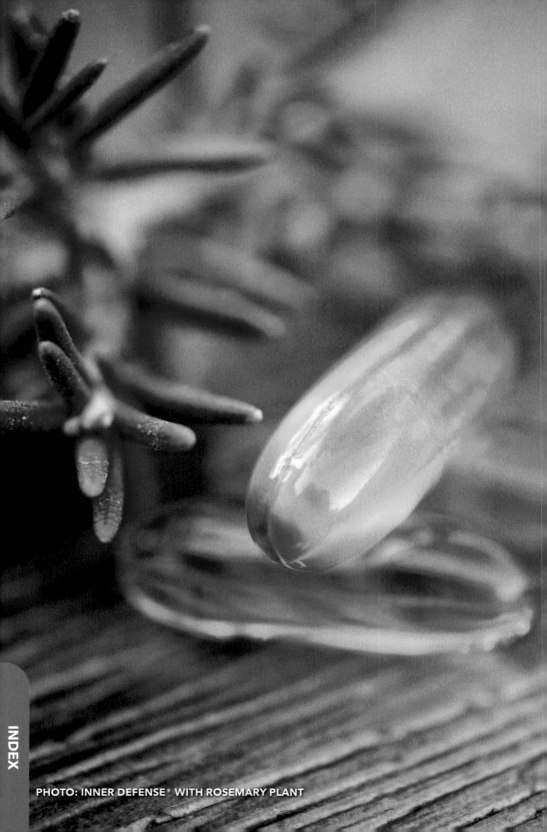

PHOTO: INNER DEFENSE® WITH ROSEMARY PLANT

SECTION FIVE
the index

Page numbers in colored text are the main content for that subject.

INDEX

B

C

INDEX

INDEX

INDEX

INDEX

INDEX

INDEX

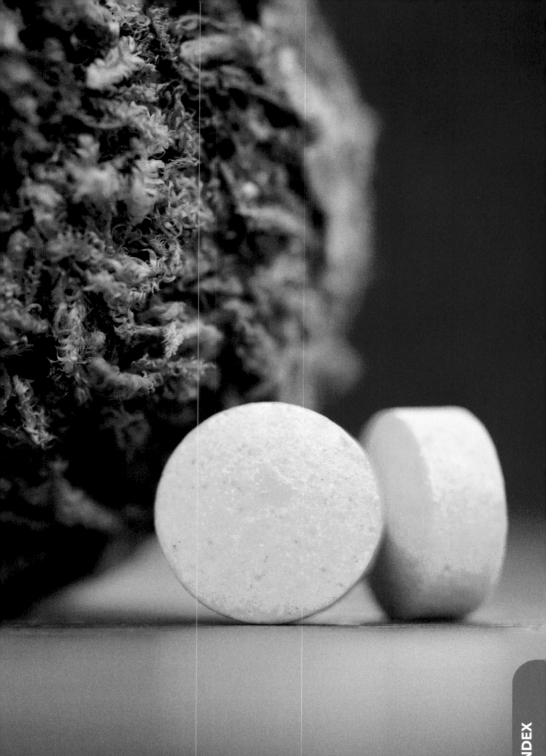

SUPPLEMENT SCHEDULE

PERSONAL PROTOCOL

√	TIME	SUPPLEMENT	DOSE

SUPPLEMENT SCHEDULE

√	TIME	SUPPLEMENT	DOSE

PERSONAL PROTOCOL

SUPPLEMENT SCHEDULE

PERSONAL PROTOCOL

√	TIME	SUPPLEMENT	DOSE

SUPPLEMENT SCHEDULE

√	TIME	SUPPLEMENT	DOSE

PERSONAL PROTOCOL

SUPPLEMENT SCHEDULE

PERSONAL PROTOCOL

√	TIME	SUPPLEMENT	DOSE

ADDITIONAL RESOURCES

For free bonus items visit **www.31oils.com/freebonus**

ONLINE RESOURCES
www.31oils.com (books and learning tools)
www.VitalityEDU.com/jen (Jen's Story)
www.facebook.com/groups/TheHumanBody
www.facebook.com/JenOSullivanAuthor
www.JensTips.com (YouTube)
@JenAuthor on Instagram
Mobile App: "THE EO BAR"

BOOKS AVAILABLE BY JEN
For bulk purchasing of any of her books please go to www.31oils.com

WELLNESS (ESSENTIAL OILS)
Covers the Essential Oil PSK. Available at www.31oils.com/wellness

PURPOSE (THIEVES® LINE)
Covers the Thieves® line. Available at www.31oils.com/purpose

ABUNDANCE (NINGXIA RED® & SUPPLEMENTS)
NingXia Red® and supplements. Available at www.31oils.com/abundance

VITALITY: THE YOUNG LIVING® LIFESTYLE
All about the Young Living® lifestyle and products.
Available on Amazon and at www.31oils.com/vitality

THE RECIPE BOOK WITH JEN O'SULLIVAN
Over 250 recipes for essential oil enthusiasts. Recipes that work!
Available on Amazon and at www.31oils.com/recipe

THE ESSENTIAL OIL TRUTH: THE FACTS WITHOUT THE HYPE
48 micro lessons to help you understand the world of oils.
Available on Amazon and at www.31oils.com/truth

FRENCH AROMATHERAPY: ESSENTIAL OIL RECIPES & USAGE GUIDE
The user guide for the French method with over 300 recipes.
Available on Amazon and at www.31oils.com/french

ESSENTIAL OIL MAKE & TAKES:
Over 70 DIY Projects and Recipes for the Perfect Class
Available on Amazon and at www.31oils.com/make-takes

LIVE WELL: FOR WELLNESS, PURPOSE, AND ABUNDANCE
PSK mini is Available on Amazon and at www.31oils.com/live-well

THE OIL GUIDE
The best resource for those just starting out. www.31oils.com/oilguide

ESSENTIALLY DRIVEN: THE BUSINESS HANDBOOK
The quick guide to starting your business the right way.
Available on Amazon and at www.31oils.com/essentially-driven

ABOUT THE AUTHOR, JEN O'SULLIVAN

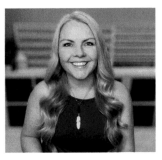

Jen O'Sullivan believes that getting to the root of the problem is vital to full health and restoration and utilizes a whole-body system approach of care with her students and customers. She has been with Young Living since 2007, and absolutely adores helping people on their path to wellness. She is known for her up-front and to-the-point education style. Jen has studied health and nutrition since 2007 and has the ability to take complicated information and share it in a way that makes it easy to understand. Jen is certified in French Medicinal Aromatherapy through the School for Aromatic Studies and has been a professional educator since 1999, at both the collegiate and high school levels. She is lovingly known as "The oil lady to the oil ladies" and is the author of eight Amazon best-sellers. She has developed one of the largest and most comprehensive essential oil education and recipe usage apps on the market today called "The EO Bar". Her online education group of over a quarter of a million oil enthusiasts called "The Human Body and Essential Oils" (www.Facebook.com/groups/TheHumanBody) is her main group where she teaches proper usage and safety with essential oils. She also has a full on-line educational school called Vitality EDU (www.VitalityEDU.com) where she offers certification courses as well as free and tuition based education. Jen lives in Southern California with her husband and high school sweetheart Tim and their son Jacob, and fur-baby, Dash the min pin.

Get over $2,000 in free bonus items!
www.31oils.com/freebonus

Be blessed!